T0180156

Measuring Spinal Cord Injury

Giovanni Galeoto
Anna Berardi • Marco Tofani
Maria Auxiliadora Marquez
Editors

Measuring Spinal Cord Injury

A Practical Guide of Outcome Measures

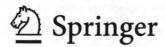 Springer

Editors
Giovanni Galeoto
Department of Human Neurosciences
Sapienza University of Rome
Rome
Italy

Anna Berardi
Department of Human Neurosciences
Sapienza University of Rome
Rome
Italy

Marco Tofani
Department of Neurorehabilitation and
Robotics
Bambino Gesù Paediatric Hospital
Rome
Italy

Maria Auxiliadora Marquez
Universidad Fernando Pessoa-Canarias
Las Palmas
Spain

ISBN 978-3-030-68384-9   ISBN 978-3-030-68382-5   (eBook)
https://doi.org/10.1007/978-3-030-68382-5

This Springer imprint is published by the registered company Springer Nature Switzerland AG
The registered company address is: Gewerbestrasse 11, 6330 Cham, Switzerland

Contents

Introduction on Measuring Spinal Cord Injury

Giorgio Scivoletto, Giovanni Galeoto,
Marco Tofani, Anna Berardi,
and Maria Auxiliadora Marquez

1 Introduction

Every year, around the world, between 250,000 and 500,000 people suffer a spinal cord injury (SCI). There is no reliable estimate of global prevalence, but the estimated annual global incidence is 40–80 cases per million. Traffic accidents were typically the most common cause of SCI, followed by falls in the elderly population [1]. Substantial variation in mortality and longevity within the SCI population, compared to the general population, and between World Health Organization regions and country income level was found. People with an SCI are two to five times more likely to die prematurely than people without an SCI, with worse survival rates in low- and middle-income countries [2].

Living with an SCI requires strategies to face a wide range of health-related problems. Apart from the paralysis, problems in various body functions, such as the bladder, bowel and sexual function, autonomic function, and pain, will be of concern. Functional problems can lead to limitations in activities and participation restrictions typically related to mobility, self-care activities, difficulties in regaining work, maintaining social relationships, participating in leisure activities, and being active members of the community [3, 4]. Participation restrictions are highly dependent on environmental factors, such as mobility equipment and transportation [5]. After an SCI, long-term functional outcomes result in a combination of acute neurological recovery and medical intervention, rehabilitation, and social participation [6]. Establishing the value of medical interventions from multiple parties' perspective is essential to the availability and adoption of therapies [7]. This study was conducted by a research group comprised of medical doctors and health professionals from the "Sapienza" University of Rome and from "Rehabilitation & Outcome Measure Assessment" (R.O.M.A.) association. R.O.M.A. association in the last few years has dealt with several studies and validated Italy's outcome measures for the spinal cord injury population [8–21].

The research group aims to develop a systematic review to identify all the evaluation tools developed and validated to measure different aspects of SCI. This study aims to provide clini-

G. Scivoletto
Foundation Santa Lucia, Rome, Italy

G. Galeoto · A. Berardi
Department of Human Neurosciences, Sapienza University of Rome, Rome, Italy

M. Tofani (✉)
Department of Neurorehabilitation and Robotics, Bambino Gesù Paediatric Hospital, Rome, Italy
e-mail: marco.tofani@uniroma1.it

M. Auxiliadora Marquez
Universidad Fernando Pessoa-Canarias, Las Palmas, Spain

© The Author(s), under exclusive license to Springer Nature Switzerland AG 2021
G. Galeoto et al. (eds.), *Measuring Spinal Cord Injury*,
https://doi.org/10.1007/978-3-030-68382-5_1

cians and researchers information regarding the existing outcome measures to assess people with SCI based on reviewing, analyzing, comparing, and critically appraising the available outcome measures and their distribution in the international literature.

2 Spinal Cord and International Classification of Functioning Disability and Health

The International Classification of Functioning, Disability, and Health (ICF) [22] provides a comprehensive and universally accepted framework to classify and describe functioning, disability, and health. According to the ICF framework, the problems associated with a disease may involve *body functions and body structures* and the *activities and participation* in life situations. Health status and disability are modified by contextual factors such as environmental and personal factors [22]. According to ICF, many people living with SCI face different body function problems and structure domains according to lesion levels and according to early post-acute or long-term settings. These differences also appear in the activity and participation domains. New efforts to understand differences within people living with SCI, according to the ICF framework, were made.

Table 1 describes the ICF core set for acute SCI [23]. The formal consensus process integrating evidence from preparatory studies and expert knowledge at the ICF Core Set conference for SCI led to the definition of a Comprehensive ICF Core Set for SCI in the early post-acute context for multidisciplinary assessment and clinical studies.

A formal consensus process integrating evidence and expert opinion based on the ICF framework and classification led to the definition of ICF core sets for SCI in the long-term context. The brief ICF core set includes 33 second-level categories that were selected out of the second-level categories of the comprehensive ICF core set, using a two-step ranking procedure and a final cutoff decision. Table 2 describes the ICF

Table 1 ICF core set for acute SCI adapted and modified from Kirchberger et al. [23]

Body functions	b730	Muscle power functions
	b620	Urination functions
	b525	Defecation functions
	b280	Sensation of pain
	b440	Respiration functions
	b735	Muscle tone functions
	b152	Emotional functions
	b810	Protective functions of the skin
Body structures	s120	Spinal cord and related structures
	s430	Structure of respiratory system
	s610	Structure of urinary system
Activities and participation	d420	Transferring oneself
	d410	Changing basic body position
	d445	Hand and arm use
	d530	Toileting
	d550	Eating
	d450	Walking
	d510	Washing oneself
	d540	Dressing
	d560	Drinking
Environmental factors	e310	Immediate family
	e355	Health professionals

core set for people living with SCI in a long-term context [24].

Tables 1 and 2 just described well represent the needs of people living with an SCI during the early phase or the life-span perspective. Researchers, clinicians, and students should approach the ICF framework for clinical practice, research, and health reporting.

3 Outcome Measures

An outcome measure is a tool used to investigate a different aspect of patients' status. An outcome measure can provide baseline data and/or provide information on patient change during recovery and/or rehabilitation. According to the ICF framework, different outcome measures could investigate body function and structure, activity and

Table 2 ICF core set for people living with SCI in a long-term context adapted and modified from Cieza et al. [24]

Body functions	b730	Muscle power functions
	b620	Urination functions
	b280	Sensation of pain
	b525	Defecation functions
	b640	Sexual functions
	b810	Protective functions of the skin
	b735	Muscle tone functions
	b710	Mobility of joint functions
	b152	Emotional functions
Body structures	s120	Spinal cord and related structures
	s610	Structure of urinary system
	s810	Structure of areas of skin
	s430	Structure of respiratory system
Activities and participation	d530	Toileting
	d420	Transferring oneself
	d230	Carrying out daily routine
	d465	Moving around using equipment
	d410	Changing basic body position
	d445	Hand and arm use
	d470	Using transportation
	d455	Moving around
	d520	Caring for body parts
	d550	Eating
	d240	Handling stress and other psychological demands
Environmental factors	e310	Immediate family
	e120	Products and technology for personal indoor and outdoor mobility and transportation
	e115	Products and technology for personal use in daily living
	e150	Design, construction, and building products and technology of buildings for public use
	e155	Design, construction, and building products and technology of buildings for private use
	e110	Products or substances for personal consumption
	e355	Health professionals
	e340	Personal care providers and personal assistants
	e580	Health services, systems, and policies

participation, environmental and personal factors. Some of the assessment tools commonly used in clinical practice can also link to the ICF domains. Regardless of the area investigated, the outcome measures have a different structure and basic concept. For a comprehensive overview, the main categories of outcome measures are presented:

3.1 Patient-Reported Outcome Measure (PROM)

Self-report measures are typically captured in the form of a questionnaire. The questionnaires are scored by applying a predetermined point system to the patient's responses. Although self-report measures seem subjective, PROM objectifies a patient's perception. PROM can be pencil-based or in electronic format. When examining equivalence between paper and electronic versions, formats are usually judged by authors to be equivalent [25].

3.2 Clinician-Reported Outcomes (ClinRo)

The use of a ClinRO assessment requires specialized professional training to evaluate the patient's health status. Conducted and reported by a trained health care professional, the ClinRO assessment reflects the evaluation of a patient's reported condition. A ClinRO assessment that is an appropriate outcome assessment in one context of use may or may not be adequate in a different context. ClinRO assessments are commonly used in end points that form the basis for reviewing and approving medical interventions [26].

3.3 Observer-Reported Outcomes (ObsRo)

An ObsRO is a measurement based on an observation by someone other than the patient or a health professional. In general, ObsRO is reported by a parent, caregiver, or someone who observes the patient in daily life and is particularly useful for patients who cannot report for themselves (e.g., infants or individuals who are cognitively impaired) [27].

3.4 Performance-Based Outcome Measure (PbOM)

Performance-based measures involve presenting examinees with functional tasks in a standardized format. The clinician does not apply judgment to quantifying the performance but is administering and monitoring the performance of the PbOM. A performance-based measure entails having the patient prepare a meal using a lab/hospital-based mock kitchen. For instance, rather than merely asking a patient or a collateral informant about the patient's cooking skills and safety (limited by their insight, candor, and objectivity), or going to the patient's home and watching them prepare a meal (while potentially valuable and informative, can be impractical), the patient's performance of a defined task is quantified in a specified way, and it does not rely on judgment to determine the rating [28].

4 International Project for Measuring SCI

"Good science and good clinical practice depend upon sound information, which in turn relies on sound measurement. Measurement enables health care professionals and researchers to describe, predict and evaluate in order to provide benchmarks and summarize change related to the condition and care of individuals with spinal cord injury." This is the incipit to the Spinal Cord Injury Rehabilitation (SCIRE) collaboration (https://scireproject.com/). SCIRE outcome measures provide information on the psychometric properties and the clinical use of 104 measures, giving the reader the necessary confidence to move their clinical practice and research forward on a more rigorous basis. The project started to analyze and search different outcome measures in studies involving the SCI population investigating

psychometric properties, namely reliability, validity, and responsiveness. SCIRE's efforts provided in these years the development of the spinal cord injury outcome measures toolkit: a standardized set of outcome measures for use in the SCI practice consisting of 33 outcome measures that have been psychometrically validated for the SCI population. The outcome measures are grouped into different categories: assistive technology, community integration, lower limb and walking, mental health, neurological impairment and autonomic dysfunction, pain, quality of life and health status, self-care and daily living, skin health, spasticity, upper limb and wheeled mobility.

Another concrete effort to spread evidence-based practice using validated outcome measures is the Rehabilitation Measures Database (www.sralab.org/rehabilitation-measures). The database is organized for a specific health condition and can be filtered according to specific categories (e.g., assessment type, area of assessment, costs). There is a specific section for the SCI population; however, for each category, the database reports the purpose of the scale, time, and administration, psychometric properties, population, references.

In conclusion, the international landscape is engaging in promoting using valid outcome measures that can lead to better quality of care, reduced health care costs, and promote a continuous evaluation of the effectiveness of health interventions. Health care workers are called to improve their work and credentials continually. The adaptation of valid outcome measures is an ethical and moral issue and a duty enshrined in their individual professional profiles. The present manual aims to propose a critical and systematic analysis of the validated outcome measures for the SCI population at international levels. We hope that less experienced readers will be inspired to approach their work with seriousness and determination. Instead, we trust that more experienced readers will enthusiastically grasp our effort to systematize the outcome measures available to the population with SCI. Our hope is to create an international synergy to improve the care process and the quality of people's lives.

References

1. Singh A, Tetreault L, Kalsi-Ryan S, Nouri A, Fehlings MG. Global prevalence and incidence of traumatic spinal cord injury. Clin Epidemiol. 2014. https://doi.org/10.2147/CLEP.S68889.

2. Chamberlain JD, Meier S, Mader L, Von Groote PM, Brinkhof MWG. Mortality and longevity after a spinal cord injury: systematic review and meta-analysis. Neuroepidemiology 2015. https://doi.org/10.1159/000382079

3. Gerhart KA, Bergstrom E, Charlifue SW, Menter RR, Whiteneck GG. Long-term spinal cord injury: functional changes over time. Arch Phys Med Rehabil. 1993. https://doi.org/10.1016/0003-9993(93)90057-H.

4. Lidal IB, Huynh TK, Biering-Sørensen F. Return to work following spinal cord injury: a review. Disabil Rehabil. 2007. https://doi.org/10.1080/09638280701320839.

5. Whiteneck G, Meade MA, Dijkers M, Tate DG, Bushnik T, Forchheimer MB. Environmental factors and their role in participation and life satisfaction after spinal cord injury. Arch Phys Med Rehabil. 2004. https://doi.org/10.1016/j.apmr.2004.04.024.

6. McKinley W, Meade MA, Kirshblum S, Barnard B. Outcomes of early surgical management versus late or no surgical intervention after acute spinal cord injury. Arch Phys Med Rehabil. 2004. https://doi.org/10.1016/j.apmr.2004.04.032.

7. Walton MK, Powers JH, Hobart J, et al. Clinical outcome assessments: conceptual foundation-report of the ISPOR clinical outcomes assessment-emerging good practices for outcomes research task force. Value Heal. 2015. https://doi.org/10.1016/j.jval.2015.08.006.

8. Castelnuovo G, Giusti EM, Manzoni GM, et al. What is the role of the placebo effect for pain relief in neurorehabilitation? Clinical implications from the Italian consensus conference on pain in neurorehabilitation. Front Neurol. 2018. https://doi.org/10.3389/fneur.2018.00310.

9. Marquez MA, De Santis R, Ammendola V, et al. Cross-cultural adaptation and validation of the "spinal cord injury-falls concern scale" in the Italian population. Spinal Cord. 2018;56(7):712–8. https://doi.org/10.1038/s41393-018-0070-6.

10. Berardi A, De Santis R, Tofani M, et al. The Wheelchair Use Confidence Scale: Italian translation, adaptation, and validation of the short form. Disabil Rehabil Assist Technol. 2018;13(4) https://doi.org/10.1080/17483107.2017.1357053.

11. Anna B, Giovanni G, Marco T, et al. The validity of rastersterography as a technological tool for the objectification of postural assessment in the clinical and educational fields: pilot study. In: Advances in intelligent systems and computing; 2020. https://doi.org/10.1007/978-3-030-23884-1_8.

12. Panuccio F, Berardi A, Marquez MA, et al. Development of the pregnancy and motherhood evaluation questionnaire (PMEQ) for evaluating and measuring the impact of physical disability on pregnancy and the management of motherhood: a pilot study. Disabil Rehabil. 2020:1–7. https://doi.org/10.1080/09638288.2020.1802520.

13. Amedoro A, Berardi A, Conte A, et al. The effect of aquatic physical therapy on patients with multiple sclerosis: a systematic review and meta-analysis. In: Mult Scler Relat Disord; 2020. https://doi.org/10.1016/j.msard.2020.102022.

14. Dattoli S, Colucci M, Soave MG, et al. Evaluation of pelvis postural systems in spinal cord injury patients: outcome research. J Spinal Cord Med. 2018;43:185–92.

15. Berardi A, Galeoto G, Guarino D, et al. Construct validity, test-retest reliability, and the ability to detect change of the Canadian occupational performance measure in a spinal cord injury population. Spinal Cord Ser Cases. 2019. https://doi.org/10.1038/s41394-019-0196-6.

16. Ponti A, Berardi A, Galeoto G, Marchegiani L, Spandonaro C, Marquez MA. Quality of life, concern of falling and satisfaction of the sit-ski aid in sit-skiers with spinal cord injury: observational study. Spinal Cord Ser Cases. 2020. https://doi.org/10.1038/s41394-020-0257-x.

17. Panuccio F, Galeoto G, Marquez MA, et al. General sleep disturbance scale (GSDS-IT) in people with spinal cord injury: a psychometric study. Spinal Cord. 2020. https://doi.org/10.1038/s41393-020-0500-0.

18. Monti M, Marquez MA, Berardi A, Tofani M, Valente D, Galeoto G. The multiple sclerosis intimacy and sexuality questionnaire (MSISQ-15): validation of the Italian version for individuals with spinal cord injury. Spinal Cord. 2020. https://doi.org/10.1038/s41393-020-0469-8.

19. Galeoto G, Colucci M, Guarino D, et al. Exploring validity, reliability, and factor analysis of the Quebec user evaluation of satisfaction with assistive technology in an Italian population: a cross-sectional study. Occup Ther Heal Care. 2018. https://doi.org/10.1080/07380577.2018.1522682.

20. Colucci M, Tofani M, Trioschi D, Guarino D, Berardi A, Galeoto G. Reliability and validity of the Italian version of Quebec user evaluation of satisfaction with assistive technology 2.0 (QUEST-IT 2.0) with users of mobility assistive device. Disabil Rehabil Assist Technol. 2019. https://doi.org/10.1080/17483107.2019.1668975.

21. Berardi A, Galeoto G, Lucibello L, Panuccio F, Valente D, Tofani M. Athletes with disability' satisfaction with sport wheelchairs: an Italian cross sectional study. Disabil Rehabil Assist Technol. 2020. https://doi.org/10.1080/17483107.2020.1800114.

22. World Health Organization. The ICF: an overview. Geneva: WHO; 2001.

23. Kirchberger I, Cieza A, Biering-Sørensen F, et al. ICF Core sets for individuals with spinal cord injury in the early post-acute context. Spinal Cord. 2010. https://doi.org/10.1038/sc.2009.128.
24. Cieza A, Kirchberger I, Biering-Sørensen F, et al. ICF Core sets for individuals with spinal cord injury in the long-term context. Spinal Cord. 2010. https://doi.org/10.1038/sc.2009.183.
25. Campbell N, Ali F, Finlay AY, Salek SS. Equivalence of electronic and paper-based patient-reported outcome measures. Qual Life Res. 2015. https://doi.org/10.1007/s11136-015-0937-3.
26. Powers JH, Patrick DL, Walton MK, et al. Clinician-reported outcome assessments of treatment benefit: report of the ISPOR clinical outcome assessment emerging good practices task force. Value Heal. 2017. https://doi.org/10.1016/j.jval.2016.11.005.
27. Benjamin K, Vernon MK, Patrick DL, Perfetto E, Nestler-Parr S, Burke L. Patient-reported outcome and observer-reported outcome assessment in rare disease clinical trials: an ISPOR COA emerging good practices task force report. Value Heal. 2017. https://doi.org/10.1016/j.jval.2017.05.015.
28. Moore DJ, Palmer BW, Patterson TL, Jeste DV. A review of performance-based measures of functional living skills. J Psychiatr Res. 2007. https://doi.org/10.1016/j.jpsychires.2005.10.008.

Psychometric Properties of Assessment Tools

Marco Monticone, Giovanni Galeoto, Anna Berardi, and Marco Tofani

1   Introduction

Clinicians and researchers are encouraged to proficiently analyze the psychometric properties of assessment tools essential for evaluating patients with medical problems [1]. Advances in diagnosis and care are possible when appropriate assessment tools are made available to decision makers. They know the measure used is adequate for its purpose, how it compares with similar measures, and how to interpret findings [2]. For every patient or population group, several instruments can be used to evaluate clinical conditions or health status. However, many instruments have been poorly or incompletely validated over time, thus limiting their use for specific diseases or among populations and countries [3]. Assessment is common in the medical sciences and varies from questions asked during history-taking to physical evaluations, imaging techniques, laboratory tests, or self-reported questionnaires.

Irrespective of the tool clinicians and researchers may wish to select, a correct way of assessment aims to replace an empirical approach with a scientific methodology, therefore increasing the effectiveness of everyday practice [4].

This study was conducted by a research group comprised of medical doctors and health professionals from the "Sapienza" University of Rome and "Rehabilitation & Outcome Measure Assessment" (R.O.M.A.) association. R.O.M.A. association in the last few years has dealt with several studies and validated outcome measures in Italy for the spinal cord injury (SCI) population [5–18].

This chapter serves as a synthetic guide to present the core psychometric properties of measurement instruments in the medical field. The method of assessments, strengths, and criticisms for each psychometric property is directly based on current literature in the field. Terminology and definitions based on recent consensus-based standards for the selection of health measurement instruments (also known as COSMIN) are reported throughout the chapter [19].

2   Reliability

This method is defined as "the degree to which the measurement is free from measurement error" [19], and when repeated measurements are conducted, it is worthy of investigation. Reliability

M. Monticone
Physical Medicine and Rehabilitation, Department of Medical Sciences and Public Health, University of Cagliari, Cagliari, Italy

G. Galeoto (✉) · A. Berardi
Department of Human Neurosciences, Sapienza University of Rome, Rome, Italy
e-mail: giovanni.galeoto@uniroma1.it

M. Tofani
Department of Neurorehabilitation and Robotics, Bambino Gesù Paediatric Hospital, Rome, Italy

© The Author(s), under exclusive license to Springer Nature Switzerland AG 2021
G. Galeoto et al. (eds.), *Measuring Spinal Cord Injury*,
https://doi.org/10.1007/978-3-030-68382-5_2

varies depending on issues that include the instrument under investigation, the evaluators, and the patients under study. These possibilities led to different types of reliability: (1) test–retest reliability, when measurements are repeated over time; (2) inter-rater reliability, when they are conducted by different evaluators but on the same occasion; (3) intra-rater reliability, when they are conducted by the same evaluator but on different occasions, and (4) internal consistency, when different sets of items from the same tool are employed [1, 19].

When test–retest, inter, and intra-rater reliability are addressed, readers should know they state the way evaluations can be distinguished from each other despite the presence of measurement error. Statistics to calculate test–retest, inter, and intra-rater reliability vary according to variables adopted. When continuous variables are studied, the adoption of intraclass correlation coefficients, which consist of a ratio of variances, is recommended [20]. The coefficient values vary from 0 (i.e., the error variance is considered negligible compared to patient variance) to 1 (i.e., the error variance is very large regarding patient variance as may happen when homogenous samples are encountered). A coefficient value of 0.70 is considered acceptable, and values of 0.80 and 0.90 as good and very good [21]. When categorical variables are studied, literature advises the use of Cohen's kappa, which adjusts for the agreement expected by chance, calculated by assuming independence of measurements as obtained by multiplications of the marginals. Estimates vary from −1 to 1: figures equal to 1 state there is a perfect agreement; figures of 0 mean there is no agreement, which can be expected by chance; figures near to −1 are usually caused by reversed scaling by one of the two raters. Cohen's kappa may be influenced by sample differences, marginals distribution, number of classes, and between-raters' systematic differences [22].

Measurement error constitutes a related but different concept from reliability and corresponds to the difference between an amount that can be measured and its true value [23]. It can be calculated in three ways. First, the standard error of measurement corresponds to the standard devia-

tion around a single measurement. It is a measure of how far apart the findings of repeated measures are. Clinicians and researchers easily interpret it as it is reported in the reference unit of the tool under study [24]. It is calculated by the following formula:

$$SEM = SD\sqrt{1 - ICC_{2,1}}$$

where ICC corresponds to test–retest reliability of the reference population as assessed by intraclass coefficient correlation statistics.

Second, the limits of agreement represent a graphical method to compare two measurements where differences between the two techniques are plotted against the averages of the two techniques. Relating the limits of agreement to the tool range may give an impression of the magnitude of the measurement error. By definition, 95% of the differences between repeated measurements fall between the limits of agreement [1, 24]. Third, by the coefficient of variation, which relates the standard deviation of repeated measurements to the mean value, with higher percentage figures representing higher heterogeneity [1, 24].

Internal consistency is defined as "the degree of interrelatedness among the items" and represents the level to which items belonging to an assessment tool assess the same construct [19]. There are three parameters for calculating internal consistency: Cronbach's alpha, inter-item correlations, and item-total correlations. The first determines how closely related a set of items are as a group, with values greater than 0.7 and 0.8 showing acceptable and good internal consistency, respectively. The second indicates whether an item is part of the assessment tool, with values higher than 0.7 suggesting items evaluating the same construct. The third gives an indication of whether the items discriminate patients on the construct under investigation, with figures below 0.3 suggesting a low contribution to distinctions [25].

Sample size. A minimum number of 50 patients are required in order to calculate reliability by avoiding the risk of bias due to insufficient populations [26].

3 Validity

Validity is defined as "the degree to which an instrument truly measures the construct it purports to measure" [1, 19]. An adequate definition of the construct (i.e., an explanatory variable to be measured which is not directly observable) is imperative. The construct itself has to be part of the conceptual model within a theoretical and clinical framework. There are three different types of validity: content validity, criterion validity, and construct validity.

3.1 Content Validity

This has been defined as "the degree to which the content of a measurement instrument is an adequate reflection of the construct to be measured" [19]. It has been recommended as the starting point of each validation process [3]. With special reference to multi-item measures, content validity aims to investigate their relevance and comprehensiveness about the construct under study. The first issue evaluates if all items refer to relevant aspects of the construct to be measured, whether they are all relevant for the population being studied, and if they are really relevant for the object of the tool usage. The second issue investigates if the construct chosen is entirely covered by the items. Content validity can be qualitatively evaluated by an independent panel of independent experts to avoid the risk of bias. A full description of the outcome measure, including procedures of administration, has to be warranted [27].

An additional aspect of the content validity is represented by face validity, which has been defined as "the degree to which a measurement instrument looks, indeed, as though it is an adequate reflection of the instrument to be measured."[19] It stands for an overall view of the tool and it is related to a subjective assessment. This property is still undervalued because no standards as to how it should be evaluated are clearly recommended.

3.2 Criterion Validity

It has been defined as "the degree to which the scores of a measurement instrument are an adequate reflection of a gold standard (i.e., diagnostic test that is regarded as definitive in determining whether an individual has a disease process)" [19]. Criterion validity can be subdivided into two main sides: (1) concurrent validity and (2) predictive validity. When assessing the first side, clinicians and researchers take into account, and at the same time, the score deriving from the gold standard they have chosen and that from the measurement under investigation. When the second side is addressed, clinicians and researchers aim to know whether the outcome measure under study forecasts the gold standard. The hypothesis is that the outcome measure should perform as efficiently as the gold standard for both sides. Moreover, an appropriate target population should be individuated. The level of agreement of the gold standard and the instrument under study should be stated as early as possible, and the scores should be obtained independently. Statistics to apply depends again on the variables included: criterion validity is expressed through sensitivity and specificity estimates whether the gold standard and the instrument under study show dichotomous outcomes; receiver operating characteristics curves are advised if the tool relies upon an ordinal or a continuous scale; correlation coefficients are adopted if a continuous gold standard variable is represented [1]. Sample size: a minimum number of 50 patients are required [26].

3.3 Construct Validity

It has been defined as "the degree to which the scores of a measurement instrument are consistent with hypotheses, e.g., with regard to internal relationships, relationships with scores of other instruments or differences between relevant groups" [19]. In other terms, evaluating this property, clinicians and researchers state a measurement tool that validly assesses the construct under investigation. There are three subtypes of construct validity: (1) structural validity, (2) hypothesis testing, and (3) cross-cultural validity.

The first subtype is defined as "the degree to which the scores of a measurement instrument are an adequate reflection of the dimensionality of the construct to be measured" [19]. Overall structural validity can be assessed by factorial analyses that mainly include exploratory factor analysis (EFA) and confirmatory factor analysis (CFA). EFA is chosen when there are no clear ideas on the factorial characteristics (i.e., number and types of dimensions) composing a multi-item instrument. An initial analysis is initially performed using Cattel's scree test to determine the line plot of extracted factors with eigenvalues greater than 1 selected. Furthermore, orthogonal (also known as Varimax) rotation of the item is habitually applied, leading to defining a component matrix made of all the items under study. Those with loadings on dimensions greater than 0.50 are included in the factor. The expected explained variance by this factor analysis should be more than 50% to be considered acceptable [28]. CFA is implemented when, based on previous researches and findings, predefined hypotheses on dimensions are available. Each item needs to be specified to load onto its subscale, as originally described. Model fit is assessed using the ratio between the χ^2-test and degrees of freedom (i.e., χ^2/d.f.), the comparative fit index, the normed fit index, and the root-mean square error of approximation and its 90% confidence intervals [29]. The following thresholds are considered to represent a good fit: χ^2/d.f. < 3, comparative fit index $\geq$ 0.90, normed fit index $\geq$ 0.90 and root-mean square error of approximation $\leq$0.08 [30]. Sample size: from 4 to 10 patients per item with a minimum of 100 patients are required [26].

The second subtype of construct validity occurs when hypotheses are formulated a priori on the relationships of scores on the instrument under investigation with scores deriving from other measures evaluating related or dissimilar constructs. One idea suggests formulating a series of hypotheses between the tool under study and related measures, describing the expected direction (i.e., positive or negative) and magnitude (i.e., small, moderate, large) of the above relationships. It is important to evaluate if the findings are consistent with the preformulated hypotheses by counting how many are established and how many refuted (usually they are expressed in percentage), and discuss the findings [31]. Sample size: a minimum of 50 patients are recommended are preferred [26].

The third subtype (i.e., cross-cultural validity) is defined as "the degree to which the performance of the items on a translated or culturally adapted tool is an adequate reflection of the performance of items in the original version of the instrument" [19]. This issue is important after the translation of a questionnaire. There may be differences in cultural aspects; some items may be irrelevant in other cultures, causing the risk of lowering the subsequent psychometric assessment [32, 33]. The first step is represented by the *forward translation*, where items are translated to retain the tool's original concepts. Two professional translations conduct two independent translations and ensure the language is compatible with a reading age of 14 years. Discrepancies are resolved through reconciliation which ends when a common adaptation is agreed. The second step is defined as *backward translation*. Two bilingual translators independently back-translate the initial translation; the researchers review these translations and ensure the adapted version essentially reflects the same item content as the original version. The third step is the *evaluation of the pre-final version by an expert committee*, where the translations are submitted to a bilingual committee of clinicians and methodologists who explore items semantic, idiomatic, and conceptual equivalence and answers to identify any discrepancies or mistakes. This third step ends when a pre-final version is agreed upon. A fourth step is represented by the *on-field test of the pre-final version*, where the pre-final version is tested to assess the comprehensibility and cognitive equivalence of the translation; this is pursued by cognitive interviews performed by trained psychologists (and eventually by health carers) who administer the instrument to selected subjects. At conclusion, the expert committee reviews the results, identifying any modification to improve the adapted form further. Finally, the step consisting of the *evaluation of the process by the developers*, where the shared version of the questionnaire is sent to the developers to receive further suggestions and final approval. All of the above steps rely on qualitative assessment. However, the new tool actually performs as the original version in different populations can be tested through factor analysis methods (especially CFA) or logistic regression analysis techniques [1].

4   Responsiveness

This psychometric property has been defined as "the ability of an instrument to detect change over time in the construct to be measured" [19], as it is important to know if the clinical status of patients has changed over time. When a tool shows to be responsive to change if patients change on the construct of interest, their scores on the measurement tool assess this construct change accordingly. Responsiveness is crucial with longitudinal studies and when evaluation scopes are pursued.

There are two ways of assessing responsiveness: almost similar to what above describes validity but based on a criterion that uses a construct approach. When a gold standard for change is available, a criterion approach is recommended to assess the degree in the scores of the tool under study is an adequate reflection of changes in scores of the gold standard. An appropriate target population should be individuated. The level of agreement between changes of the gold standard and the instrument under study should be defined. The scores should be obtained independently and over the same time period. Coefficients correlations are used when the gold standard is a continuous (i.e., change in score) variable and receiver operating characteristics (ROC) curves when it is a dichotomous (i.e., change vs. no change) variable. The area under the ROC curve is considered to measure an instrument's ability to distinguish between patients who are considered improved (or deteriorated) from those who are not considered improved (or deteriorated) in relation to the gold standard. An area under the curve of at least 0.70 is considered an appropriate responsive measure [34]. Hypothesis testing is useful to test the responsiveness of a measure when no gold standard is available. The hypotheses test correlations between changes in scores of the tool under study and changes in scores on other measures with satisfactory responsiveness. Relative correlations (i.e., comparisons between comparisons) can also be considered. The hypotheses should include the expected direction and magnitude between the change scores [34–36]. Previous studies should help formulate hypotheses.

4.1   Inappropriate Measures of Responsiveness

A series of methods to evaluate responsiveness, such as effect size, Guyatt's approach, the standardized response means, and the paired *t*-test, have been suggested and widely used over time. Effect size calculates on a whole sample by dividing the pre- and posttest scores by the pretest standard deviation (SD). As for Guyatt's approach, the change computed on the whole sample gets divided by the pretest SD calculated only for those subjects whose status remains unchanged. The standardized response mean (also known as the responsiveness treatment coefficient or efficacy index) is the ratio between individual change and the SD of that change. As for all of the measures, estimates of 0.20, 0.50, and 0.80 represent small, moderate, and large changes. However, evidence concludes they are inadequate measures of responsiveness as they express the magnitude of the change scores and not the validity of those changes. The paired *t*-test measures the change scores' statistical significance and not, again, the validity of the change scores [35, 36].

5 Interpretability

Interpretability has been defined as "the degree to which one can assign qualitative meaning, that is clinical or commonly understood connotations, to an instrument's qualitative scores or change in scores" [19]. It is crucial for every measurement instrument and a powerful information for clinicians and researchers as it refers to what the scores on an instrument mean. The minimum detectable change and the minimal important change get reported when addressing the meaning of change scores.

5.1 Minimum Detectable Change

It is the change beyond measurement error. In other words, it corresponds to a change that falls outside the limits of agreement as calculated by the Bland and Altman method [37] and can be estimated by the following formula:

$$MDC = SEM * z \text{ value} * \sqrt{2}$$

where SEM is the standard error of measurement, and z value corresponds to 1.96 or 1.64 when 95% or 90% confidence levels are chosen, respectively.

If a subject achieves a change score greater than the threshold estimated as per the MDC, it is possible to state (with % confidence) this change is real and not due to measurement error. A smaller change in score should be attributed to measurement error [24].

5.2 Minimal Important Change (MIC)

It is defined as "the smallest change in score in the construct to be measured which patients perceive as important" [19]. When outcomes based on patients' perspectives are considered, the MIC should consider their perspective, while when different instruments are used the clinician's point of view is of importance [38, 39]. MIC is estimated by anchor-based or distribution-based methods.

Anchor-based methods. They utilize an external criterion, or anchor, to determine clinically important improvements or to worsen. A globally perceived effect for patients' or clinicians' use and evaluated by the question: "Overall, how much did the treatment you received help your current problem?" or "Overall, how much did the treatment you delivered help your patient's current problem?"; then the perceived effect is determined using a Likert-type scale characterized by improvement levels (e.g., "it helped a lot" and "it helped"), no change level (e.g., "it did not help") and worsening levels (e.g., it made things worse; it made things much worse) [40]. A first method based on the use of an anchor is the mean change method, where the minimal important change corresponds to the mean change in score on the measurement instrument in the subcategory of patents who are minimally importantly changed. A second method is based on the receiver operating characteristics curves: subjects are dichotomized into two groups based on the global perceived effect scores (e.g., improved vs. nonimproved; improved vs. worsened); sensitivity (i.e., the probability that the measure correctly classifies subjects who demonstrate change when an external criterion of clinical change is used) and specificity (i.e., the probability that the measure correctly classifies subjects who do not demonstrate change when the external criterion is used) of each value of change in the measure are calculated and used to plot the curve. Sensitivity values and false-positive rates (1-specificity) are then plotted at the y and x-axis on the curve. Using the Youden index, an optimal cutoff point (i.e., the minimal important change figure) is computed and taken as the MIC, which indicates the change score associated with the least misclassification [34–36].

Anchor-based methods represent powerful methods to calculate the minimal important change as they explicitly define and incorporate the concept of minimal importance; however, they limit by not considering the variability of tool scores within the sample.

5.3 Distribution-Based Approaches

They are based on the distributional features of the population under study and explicit the observed change in the outcome measure to some form of variation to get a standardized metric. Several methods have been proposed over time, such as the effect size and the standard error of measurement; they should be used with caution because they do not directly indicate the importance of the observed change [34–36].

Two issues are crucial before addressing interpretability: (1) scores distribution and (2) floor and ceiling effects. The first delineate if the sample is distributed over the whole range of the scale, whether the study sample has high or low scores, or patients are clustered at points on the scale. The second is again important as patients at both ends of a measurement tool cannot show any further improvements or worsen [1].

6 Additional Properties [41, 42]

6.1 Floor and Ceiling Effects

These terms describe how subjects have scored at or near the possible lower or upper limit, preventing from measuring variance above a certain level. They are recognized when more than 15% of patients achieve the lowest (i.e., floor) or the highest (i.e., ceiling) possible score.

6.2 Precision

It represents the instrument's exactness, which is based on the number and accuracy of distinctions made. This issue is raised concerning response categories and numerical values, and for the relationship between the range of difficulty of the items and the distribution of what is being measured. Advanced statistical methods (e.g., the Rasch analysis) or simpler techniques such as ordering the items based on their mean scores may provide a system for examining an instrument's interval characteristics.

6.3 Acceptability

It describes how easy the measure is for respondents to complete. Patients are investigated about the response rate (i.e., missing values) and the time to complete the tool.

6.4 Feasibility

It constitutes how easily the instrument can be administered and processed, including the extent of effort, burden, and disruption to staff and clinical care arising from the use. It also requires gathering information on professional expertise to apply or interpret the instrument and an instruction manual (including its clarity).

7 Conclusions

Researchers are encouraged to ensure outcome measures are psychometrically sound, and they are administered thoughtfully and analyzed correctly. All measures should meet the classical requirements of reliability, validity, and responsiveness. Conducting an appropriate evaluation is a difficult task: evaluating outcome measures should be carefully oriented, using well-chosen judgment criteria defined in terms of precise objective and referring to international standards. The importance of appropriate assessment is clearly demonstrated by the growing number of studies devoted to identifying the best criteria for choosing and applying. Development and refinements of measurement tools are recommended over time as part of an ongoing process. More robust validation is possible when a measurement instrument that has shown an acceptable degree of validity in one situation is also validated in another context, disease, or population. More evidence is recommended to test and enlarge psychometric properties. Despite encouraging results and ongoing processes as described above, improving the quality of assessment still constitutes an important challenge for most medical fields. Better assessment will undoubtedly lead to better planning of care, better communication among health professionals, better evaluations of treatment efficacy, better clinical research, and better knowledge about patients' needs and expectations.

References

1. de Vet HCW, Terwee CB, Mokkink LB, Knol DL. Measurement in medicine. Cambridge: Cambridge University Press; 2011. https://doi.org/10.1017/CBO9780511996214.
2. Clinton-McHarg T, Yoong SL, Tzelepis F, et al. Psychometric properties of implementation measures for public health and community settings and mapping of constructs against the consolidated framework for implementation research: a systematic review. Implement Sci. 2016. https://doi.org/10.1186/s13012-016-0512-5.
3. O'Connor A, McGarr O, Cantillon P, McCurtin A, Clifford A. Clinical performance assessment tools in physiotherapy practice education: a systematic review. Physiother (United Kingdom). 2018. https://doi.org/10.1016/j.physio.2017.01.005.
4. Walters SJ, Stern C, Robertson-Malt S. The measurement of collaboration within healthcare settings: a systematic review of measurement properties of instruments. JBI Database Syst Rev Implement Reports. 2016. https://doi.org/10.11124/JBISRIR-2016-2159.
5. Castelnuovo G, Giusti EM, Manzoni GM, et al. What is the role of the placebo effect for pain relief in neurorehabilitation? Clinical implications from the Italian consensus conference on pain in neurorehabilitation. Front Neurol. 2018. https://doi.org/10.3389/fneur.2018.00310.
6. Marquez MA, De Santis R, Ammendola V, et al. Cross-cultural adaptation and validation of the "spinal cord injury-falls concern scale" in the Italian population. Spinal Cord. 2018;56(7):712–8. https://doi.org/10.1038/s41393-018-0070-6.
7. Berardi A, De Santis R, Tofani M, et al. The Wheelchair Use Confidence Scale: Italian translation, adaptation, and validation of the short form. Disabil Rehabil Assist Technol. 2018;13(4) https://doi.org/10.1080/17483107.2017.1357053.
8. Anna B, Giovanni G, Marco T, et al. The validity of rasterstereography as a technological tool for the objectification of postural assessment in the clinical and educational fields: pilot study. In: Advances in Intelligent Systems and Computing; 2020. https://doi.org/10.1007/978-3-030-23884-1_8.
9. Panuccio F, Berardi A, Marquez MA, et al. Development of the pregnancy and motherhood evaluation questionnaire (PMEQ) for evaluating and measuring the impact of physical disability on pregnancy and the management of motherhood: a pilot study. Disabil Rehabil. August 2020:1–7. https://doi.org/10.1080/09638288.2020.1802520.
10. Amedoro A, Berardi A, Conte A, et al. The effect of aquatic physical therapy on patients with multiple sclerosis: a systematic review and meta-analysis. Mult Scler Relat Disord. 2020. https://doi.org/10.1016/j.msard.2020.102022
11. Dattoli S, Colucci M, Soave MG, et al. Evaluation of pelvis postural systems in spinal cord injury patients: outcome research. J Spinal Cord Med. 2018;43:185–92.
12. Berardi A, Galeoto G, Guarino D, et al. Construct validity, test-retest reliability, and the ability to detect change of the Canadian occupational performance measure in a spinal cord injury population. Spinal Cord Ser Cases. 2019. https://doi.org/10.1038/s41394-019-0196-6.
13. Ponti A, Berardi A, Galeoto G, Marchegiani L, Spandonaro C, Marquez MA. Quality of life, concern of falling and satisfaction of the sit-ski aid in sit-skiers with spinal cord injury: observational study. Spinal Cord Ser Cases. 2020. https://doi.org/10.1038/s41394-020-0257-x.
14. Panuccio F, Galeoto G, Marquez MA, et al. General sleep disturbance scale (GSDS-IT) in people with spinal cord injury: a psychometric study. Spinal Cord. 2020. https://doi.org/10.1038/s41393-020-0500-0.
15. Monti M, Marquez MA, Berardi A, Tofani M, Valente D, Galeoto G. The multiple sclerosis intimacy and sexuality questionnaire (MSISQ-15): validation of the Italian version for individuals with spinal cord injury. Spinal Cord. 2020. https://doi.org/10.1038/s41393-020-0469-8.
16. Galeoto G, Colucci M, Guarino D, et al. Exploring validity, reliability, and factor analysis of the Quebec user evaluation of satisfaction with assistive Technology in an Italian Population: a cross-sectional study. Occup Ther Heal Care. 2018. https://doi.org/10.1080/07380577.2018.1522682.
17. Colucci M, Tofani M, Trioschi D, Guarino D, Berardi A, Galeoto G. Reliability and validity of the Italian version of Quebec user evaluation of satisfaction with assistive technology 2.0 (QUEST-IT 2.0) with users of mobility assistive device. Disabil Rehabil Assist Technol. 2019. https://doi.org/10.1080/17483107.2019.1668975.
18. Berardi A, Galeoto G, Lucibello L, Panuccio F, Valente D, Tofani M. Athletes with disability' satisfaction with sport wheelchairs: an Italian cross sectional study. Disabil Rehabil Assist Technol. 2020. https://doi.org/10.1080/17483107.2020.1800114.
19. Mokkink LB, Terwee CB, Patrick DL, et al. The COSMIN study reached international consensus on taxonomy, terminology, and definitions of measurement properties for health-related patient-reported outcomes. J Clin Epidemiol. 2010. https://doi.org/10.1016/j.jclinepi.2010.02.006.
20. McGraw KO, Wong SP. Forming inferences about some Intraclass correlation coefficients. Psychol Methods. 1996. https://doi.org/10.1037/1082-989X.1.1.30.

21. Nunnally JC. Psychometric theory. 1979. https://doi.org/10.1109/PROC.1975.9792

22. Cohen J. A coefficient of agreement for nominal scales. Educ Psychol Meas. 1960. https://doi.org/10.1177/001316446002000104.

23. Streiner DL, Norman GR. A Practical guide to their development and use: health measurement scales. 2008. https://doi.org/10.1093/acprof:oso/9780199231881.001.0001.

24. Portney A, Washington RD. Review of: foundations of clinical research applications to practice (3rd edition). J Allied Health. 2010;8:3.

25. Bland JM, Altman DG. Statistics notes: Cronbach's alpha. BMJ. 1997. https://doi.org/10.1136/bmj.314.7080.572.

26. Kline P. Handbook of psychological testing. London: Routledge; 2013. https://doi.org/10.4324/9781315812274.

27. Chiarotto A, Ostelo RW, Boers M, Terwee CB. A systematic review highlights the need to investigate the content validity of patient-reported outcome measures for physical functioning in patients with low back pain. J Clin Epidemiol. 2018. https://doi.org/10.1016/j.jclinepi.2017.11.005.

28. Child D. The essentials of factor analysis (2nd ed.). Cassell Educational; 1990.

29. Browne MW, Cudeck R. Alternative ways of assessing model fit. Sociol Methods Res. 1992. https://doi.org/10.1177/0049124192021002005.

30. Hu LT, Bentler PM. Cutoff criteria for fit indexes in covariance structure analysis: conventional criteria versus new alternatives. Struct Equ Model. 1999. https://doi.org/10.1080/10705519909540118.

31. Smith GT. On construct validity: issues of method and measurement. Psychol Assess. 2005. https://doi.org/10.1037/1040-3590.17.4.396.

32. Beaton DE, Bombardier C, Guillemin F, Ferraz MB. Guidelines for the process of cross-cultural adaptation of self-report measures. Spine (Phila Pa 1976) 2000. https://doi.org/10.1097/00007632-200012150-00014.

33. Wild D, Grove A, Martin M, et al. Principles of good practice for the translation and cultural adaptation process for patient-reported outcomes (PRO) measures: report of the ISPOR task force for translation and cultural adaptation. Value Heal. 2005. https://doi.org/10.1111/j.1524-4733.2005.04054.x.

34. Zweig MH, Campbell G. Receiver-operating characteristic (ROC) plots: a fundamental evaluation tool in clinical medicine. Clin Chem. 1993. https://doi.org/10.1093/clinchem/39.4.561.

35. Revicki D, Hays RD, Cella D, Sloan J. Recommended methods for determining responsiveness and minimally important differences for patient-reported outcomes. J Clin Epidemiol. 2008. https://doi.org/10.1016/j.jclinepi.2007.03.012.

36. Husted JA, Cook RJ, Farewell VT, Gladman DD. Methods for assessing responsiveness. A critical review and recommendations. J Clin Epidemiol. 2000. https://doi.org/10.1016/S0895-4356(99)00206-1.

37. Bland JM, Altman DG. Measuring agreement in method comparison studies. Stat Methods Med Res. 1999. https://doi.org/10.1191/096228099673819272.

38. Cook CE. Clinimetrics corner: the minimal clinically important change score (MCID): a necessary Pretense. J Man Manip Ther. 2008. https://doi.org/10.1179/jmt.2008.16.4.82e.

39. Engel L, Beaton DE, Touma Z. Minimal clinically important difference. A review of outcome measure score interpretation. Rheum Dis Clin North Am. 2018. https://doi.org/10.1016/j.rdc.2018.01.011.

40. Kamper SJ, Maher CG, Mackay G. Global rating of change scales: a review of strengths and weaknesses and considerations for design. J Man Manip Ther. 2009. https://doi.org/10.1179/jmt.2009.17.3.163.

41. Terwee CB, Bot SDM, de Boer MR, et al. Quality criteria were proposed for measurement properties of health status questionnaires. J Clin Epidemiol. 2007. https://doi.org/10.1016/j.jclinepi.2006.03.012.

42. Barat M, Franchignoni F. Assessment in physical medicine and rehabilitation. Pavia: Maugeri Foundation Books; 2004.

Methodological Approach to Identifying Outcome Measures in Spinal Cord Injury

Giovanni Galeoto, Marco Tofani, Giulia Grieco, Marina D'Angelo, and Anna Berardi

1   Introduction

Measuring health status and health interventions is fundamental to guarantee the quality of services and good health for all. The biomedical model of health had focused well-being assessment and related interventions on strictly biomedical parameters in the past. The biopsychosocial model's emergence has instead overturned this paradigm, defining health as a set of biological, psychological, and environmental contingencies. The *International Classification of Functioning, Disability, and Health (ICF)*—approved by the World Health Assembly in 2001 [1]—describes a universal framework of functioning, and health examining different components: body functions and structures, activities and participation, and contextual factors. The increasing recognition of the patient perspective and, more specifically, functioning and health has led to an impressive effort in research to develop concepts and instruments to measure them [2].

G. Galeoto · A. Berardi (✉)
Department of Human Neurosciences,
Sapienza University of Rome, Rome, Italy
e-mail: anna.berardi@uniroma1.it

M. Tofani
Department of Neurorehabilitation and Robotics,
Bambino Gesù Paediatric Hospital, Rome, Italy

G. Grieco · M. D'Angelo
R.O.M.A. Rehabilitation Outcome Measures
Assessment, Non-Profit Organization, Rome, Italy

Comparing selected instruments may provide clinicians and researchers with new insights when selecting health-status measures for clinical studies [3]. High-quality clinical care requires people to provide information regarding how they feel, their symptoms, the possibility of restoring community living, and achieving a satisfying life quality. Keeping in mind the great varieties of areas to consider, how can clinicians choose the more appropriate outcome measures? In the specific context of the SCI population, different efforts are made: the ICF framework was investigated [4, 5], using the Delphi method with occupational therapists [6], physical therapists [7], and customers [8].

Furthermore, many authors tried to investigate the appropriateness of outcome measures for newly acquired SPI population [9] or for measuring function or mobility [10]. Studies suggested a good general methodology, but with a limited sample. Furthermore, for the development of clinical practice guidelines including recommendations for assessments in initial SCI rehabilitation, the psychometric properties of outcome measures and their clinical relevance need to be considered [9, 11]. Unfortunately, in everyday clinical activities, this is a widespread practice. In many countries, the lack of interest and funding opportunities in validating outcome measures may also lead to a worse quality of care and poor adherence/compliance of healthcare plans. The COSMIN (*COnsensus-based Standards for the selection of*

G. Galeoto et al. (eds.), *Measuring Spinal Cord Injury*,
https://doi.org/10.1007/978-3-030-68382-5_3

health Measurement INstruments) initiative aims to improve the selection of outcome measurement instruments in research and clinical practice by developing tools for selecting the most suitable instrument for the situation at issue. Recently, a comprehensive methodological guideline for systematic reviews of the *Patient-Reported Outcome Measures* (PROM) was developed by the COSMIN initiative [12]. In addition, the COSMIN checklist was adapted for assessing the risk of bias in studies on measurement properties in systematic reviews of PROMs [13]. A Delphi study was also performed to develop standards and criteria for assessing the content validity of PROMs [14]. The COSMIN is an international initiative consisting of a multidisciplinary team of researchers with expertise in epidemiology, psychometrics, and qualitative research. Their expertise is in health care and in performing systematic reviews of outcome measurement instruments in the development and evaluation of outcome measurement instruments. Therefore, the purpose of the present chapter is to illustrate COSMIN-based methodology used to identify outcome measures in the SCI population throughout a systematic review. The authors present assessment tools for various clinical uses in the health sciences, following validity, reliability, and responsiveness parameters. It is essential to develop clinical practice and research that practical and appropriate measures become universally accepted; this would allow comparisons and meta-analysis of high-quality randomized controlled trials of people with this increasingly common injury. This research hopes to emphasize the need for consensus among researchers as to which tools must be studied in-depth or adapted to other national contexts, or which measurement instruments should be standardized to develop universal norms and standards for people with SCI.

2   Materials and Methods

A research group comprised of medical doctors and health professionals from the "Sapienza" University of Rome and the "Rehabilitation &

Outcome Measure Assessment" (R.O.M.A.) association conducted this study. The R.O.M.A. association in the last few years has dealt with several studies and validation of many outcome measures in Italy for the spinal cord injury (SCI) population [15–28].

This chapter focuses on the methodological approach to identifying outcome measures in the SCI population and guides the methodology of further chapters of the book. Systematic reviews and meta-analyses are essential tools for conducting accurate and reliable summary of the evidence. The present investigation follows *the Preferred Reporting Items for Systematic reviews and Meta-Analyses (PRISMA)* guidelines [29]. PRISMA is an evidence-based minimum set of items for reporting in systematic reviews and meta-analyses. PRISMA focuses on reporting of reviews randomized trials but can also be used as a basis for reporting systematic reviews of other types of research, particularly evaluations of interventions.

The COSMIN methodology for systematic reviews of Patient-Reported Outcome Measures [12] was used. In assessing the quality of a PROM, we distinguish three domains, i.e., reliability, validity, and responsiveness. Each domain contains one or more measurement properties, i.e., quality aspects of measurement instruments. The domain reliability contains three measurement properties: internal consistency, reliability, and measurement error. The domain validity also contains three measurement properties: content validity (including face validity), structural validity, hypotheses testing for construct validity, cross-cultural validity, and criterion validity. The domain responsiveness contains only one measurement property, which is also called responsiveness [12].

2.1   Protocol Registration

The present systematic review was registered to *PROSPERO* database. The protocol was accepted in August 2020 (code CRD42020199454), it is available at www.crd.york.ac.uk/prospero/display_record.php?RecordID=199454. PROSPERO is an international database of prospectively registered systematic reviews in health and social care, welfare, public health, education, crime, justice, and international development, where there is a health-related outcome.

2.2   Literature Search

A comprehensive search strategy was performed using different databases, namely MEDLINE, SCOPUS, CINAHL, and WEB OF SCIENCES. As recommended by Cochrane methodology [30], the search strategy was performed from inception until May 2020. Searches were carried out in July 2020 and updated in October 2020, using the following search terms: "spinal cord injury or sci or paraplegic or quadriplegic" AND "scale or test or questionnaire or assessment or measure or inventory or instrument" AND "validated tool or validated instrument or validated questionnaire or validated survey."

The search strategy was adjusted for each database with regard to filters or limits.

2.3   Inclusion Criteria and Data Extraction

As mentioned before, the purpose of the present systematic review was to critical appraise, compare, and summarize the quality of measurement properties of available outcome measures for people living with SCI. Therefore, general inclusion criteria were defined following the extended PICO format:
- Patient: at least three people living with SCI
- Intervention: assessment of all relevant aspects of body function and structure, psychosocial domain, environment, health, and clinical aspects
- Comparison: no comparator
- Outcome: clinometric properties, country-based validations, recommendation for clinical uses
- Study design: cross-sectional study, validation/psychometric study

Additionally, no language restriction has been imposed. Systematic reviews, observational studies,

and clinical trials were excluded. Articles got excluded if either the study did not investigate one or more psychometric properties, or if the outcome measure was used to investigate clinical outcomes, instrument test (such as dynamometers), or item banks. Cross-sectional studies, as well as validation studies involving people with different health conditions, also were excluded. Four rehabilitation professionals (GG, BA, TM, PF) firstly screened one database each, by reading title and abstract. Then, the same reviewers were divided into two groups. To guarantee an independent and unconditional review process, each group evaluated the full texts primarily selected by the others. In case no agreement was achieved between the two primary reviewers, a third and fourth reviewer made decision on articles' inclusion. This process led to select articles to include in the systematic review. Articles' information was then categorized by authors, year of publication, title, study design, sample size, psychometric properties. In the end, articles were categorized based on domains and area of intervention. For more information, please see Results section.

3   Results

The study selection process is shown in Fig. 1.

A total of 6256 records were identified and screened through the initial search strategy. After removing duplicates, 3333 papers were screened. Of these, 476 were included in this systematic review. Results show 298 assessment tools that evaluate people with SCI. Articles were organized according to the year of publication, author(s), title, language, outcome measures, and psychometric properties; and further divided according to the area of competence. In the next chapters, readers can choose the area of interest and/or analyze the most appropriate outcome measures by following the macro-areas below:
- Walking and balance (Table 1)
- Activity of daily living (Table 2)
- Assistive devices management (Table 3)
- Caregiving (Table 4)
- Neurological status (Table 5)
- Nursing and clinical evaluation (Table 6)

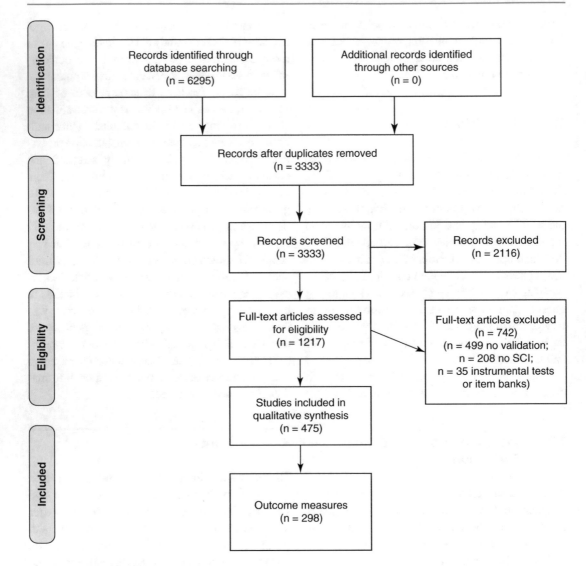

Fig. 1 Flow chart of the included study

- Pediatrics (Table 7)
- Psychological evaluation (Table 8)
- Quality of life (Table 9)
- Upper limb function (Table 10)
- Urological aspects (Table 11)

4 Conclusion

This chapter describes the methodological approach to identifying outcome measures for the SCI population. The systematic review found a total of 476 relevant research papers. The 11 categories into which the different outcome measures have been divided will be fundamental to identifying valid and reliable tools. This work can potentially be a starting point for having internationally comparable data and producing clinical studies with robust evidence. The aim is to maximize the quality of care and improve the quality of life of people living with SCI.

Table 1 Scale, test, or questionnaire measuring walking and balance in people with spinal cord injury

Name of the scale, test, or Questionnaire (acronym)
10-Meter Walking Test (10MWT)
6-Min Push Test (6MPT)
6-Minute Walking Test (6MWT)
Activity-Based Balance Level Evaluation (ABLE) Scale
Activity-Specific Balance Confidence Scale (ABC SCALE)
Alternating Reach Test
Berg Balance Scale (BBS)
Bilateral Reach (BR)
Community Balance and Mobility Scale (CB&M)
Coordinated Stability
Five Times Sit-To-Stand Test (FTSST)
Function In Sitting Test (FIST)
Function Reach (FR)
Limits of Stability (LOS)
Locomotor Stages in Spinal Cord Injury (LOSSCI)
Maximal Balance Range
Mini-Best
Modified Function In Sitting Test (FIST-SCI)
Motor Assessment Scale (MAS)
Neuromuscular Recovery Scale (NRS)
Reach Area (RA)
Seated Reach Distance
Sequential Weight Shifting (SWS)
Sitting Balance Measure (SBM)
Sitting Balance Score (SBS)
Spinal Cord Injury Functional Ambulation Inventory (SCI-FAI)
Spinal Cord Injury Functional Ambulation Profile (SCI-FAP)
Standing And Walking Assessment Tool (SWAT)
Standing Balance Assessment For Spinal Cord Injury (SBASCI)
Test-Table-Test (TTT)
Thoracic–Lumbar Control Scale
Timed Up and Go Test (TUGT)
Trunk Control Scale
Trunk Impairment Classification System (TIC)
T-Shirt Test
Upper Body Sway
Walking Index for Spinal Cord Injury (WISCI)
Walking Index for Spinal Cord Injury II (WISCI II)

Table 2 Scale, test, or questionnaire measuring activities of daily living in people with spinal cord injury

Name of the scale, test, or questionnaire (acronym)
Access to Information Anche Technology (AIT)
Attention to Clothing and Impact of its Restrictive Factors (ACIRF)
Barriers to Physical Activity Questionnaire for People With Mobility Impairments (BPAQ-MI)
Canadian Occupational Performance Measure
Clinical Outcome Variables Scale (COVS)
Craig Handicap Assessment and Reporting Technique (CHART)
Craig Handicap Assessment and Reporting Technique (CHART) Short Form
Craig Hospital Inventory of Environmental Factors (CHIEF)
Exercise Self-Efficacy Scale (ESES)
Frenchay Activities Index (FAI)
Functional Assessment Measure (FAM)
Functional Independence Measure—Five Additional Mobility and Locomotor Items (FIM-5-AML)
Functional Independence Measure—Self Report (FIM-SR)
Functional Independence Measure (FIM)
Ghent Participation Scale (GPS)
Housing Enabler Instrument (HEI)
ICF Measure of Participation and Activities Questionnaire (IMPACT-S)
ICF Core Sets for SCI
Impact on Participation and Autonomy Questionnaire (IPA)
International Spinal Cord Injury Activities and Participation (SCIA&P) Basic Data Set
International Spinal Cord Injury Community Survey (InSCI)
Keele Assessment of Participation (KAP)
Leisure Time Physical Activity Questionnaire for People With Spinal Cord Injury (LTPA)
Level of Rehabilitation Scale-III (LORS-III)
Life Habits Assessment (Life-H 3.1)
Moorong Self-Efficacy Scale (MSES)
New Measure of Participation PAR-PRO
Nottwil Environmental Factors Inventory (NWFI)—Short Version
Occupational Performance History Interview (OPHI)
Participation Measure–Post-Acute Care (PM-PAC)

(continued)

Table 2 (continued)

Name of the scale, test, or questionnaire (acronym)
Participation Objective and Participation Subjective (POPS)
Physical Activity Instrument—SCI (PAI-SCI)
Physical Activity Recall Assessment for People With Spinal Cord Injury (PARA-SCI)
Physical Activity Scale for Individuals With Physical Disabilities (PASIPD)
Quadriplegia Index of Function (QIF)
Reintegration to Normal Living (RNL)
Risk Inventory for Persons With Spinal Cord Injury (RIPSCI)
Spinal Cord Independence Measure I (SCIM-I)
Spinal Cord Independence Measure II (SCIM-II)
Spinal Cord Independence Measure III (SCIM-III)
Spinal Cord Independence Measure- Self Report (SCIM-SR)
Spinal Cord Injury Functional Index (SCI-FI Short Forms)
Spinal Cord Injury Functional Index (SCI-FI)
Spinal Cord Index of Function (SIF)
Sunnaas ADL Index
The Physical Activity Recall Assessment for People With Spinal Cord Injury (PARA-SCI)
Transfer Assessment Instrument (TAI)
World Health Organization Disability Assessment Scale (WHODAS II)

Table 3 Scale, test, or questionnaire measuring assistive devices management in people with spinal cord injury

Name of the scale, test, or questionnaire (acronym)
Adapted Manual Wheelchair Circuit (AMWC)
Assistive Technology Predisposition Assessment (ATD PA)
Assistive Technology Predisposition Assessment (ATD PA) Device From
Electronic Mobile Shower Commode Assessment Tool (Emast) 1.0
Functional Tasks for Persons Who Self-Propel A Manual Wheelchair
Manual Wheelchair Propulsion Tests (MWPT)
Manual Wheelchair Slalom Test (MWST)
Obstacle Course Assessment of Wheelchair User Performance (OCAWUP)
Quebec User Evaluation With Assistive Technology (Version 2.0) (QUEST 2.0)
Queensland Evaluation of Wheelchair Skills (QEWS)
Self-Efficacy in Wheeled Mobility (SEWM)
Test of Wheeled Mobility (TOWM)
Treadmill-Based Wheelchair Propulsion Test (WPTTreadmill)

Table 3 (continued)

Name of the scale, test, or questionnaire (acronym)
Wheelchair Circuit
Wheelchair Components Questionnaire for Condition (WCQC)
Wheelchair Maintenance Training Questionnaire (WMT-Q)
Wheelchair Outcome Measure (Whom)
Wheelchair Propulsion Test (WPT)
Wheelchair Skills Test (WST)
Wheelchair Use Confidence Scale (Wheelcon)
Wheelchair User's Shoulder Pain Index (WUSPI)
Wheelie Test

Table 4 Scale, test, or questionnaire measuring caregiving in people with spinal cord injury

Name of the scale, test, or questionnaire (acronym)
Caregiver Burden Index (CBI)
Caregiver Burden Scale (CBS)
Family Needs Questionnaire (FNQ)
Zarit Caregiver Burden Interview Short Form (ZBI)

Table 5 Scale, test, or questionnaire measuring neurological status in people with spinal cord injury

Name of the scale, test, or questionnaire (acronym)
American Spinal Cord Injury Association (ASIA)
Ashworth Scale (AS)
Cervical Spine Injury Recovery Prediction Scale (CSIRPS)
Knee-Up Test
Modified Ashworth Scale (MAS)
Modified Modified Ashworth Scale (MMAS)
Modified Tardieu Scale (MTS)
Patient-Reported Impact of Spasticity Measure (PRISM)
Penn Spasm Frequency Scale (PSFS)
Quantitative Sensory Testing (QST)
Rating Scale for Resistance to Passive Movement (REPAS)
Revised 1992 International Standards for Neurological Classification of Spinal Cord Injury (ISNCSCI92)
Scale for Evaluation of Spinal Cord Injury
Spinal Cord Assessment Tool for Spastic Reflexes (SCATS)
Spinal Cord Injury Ability Realization Measurement Index (SCI-ARMI)
Spinal Cord Injury Spasticity Evaluation Tool (SCI-SET)
University of Miami Neuro-Spinal Index (UMNI)
Valutazione Funzionale Mielolesi (VFM)
Wartenberg Pendulum Test (WPT)

Table 6 Scale, test, or questionnaire for nursing or clinical evaluation in people with spinal cord injury

Name of the scale, test, or questionnaire (acronym)
Barthel Index
Brief Pain Inventory (BPI)
Fatigability Index (FI)
Fatigue Severity Scale (FSS)
Graded Chronic Pain (GCP) Disability Scale
International Spinal Cord Injury Basic Pain Data Set Items (ISCIBPDS:B) (Version 1.1)
International Spinal Cord Injury Basic Pain Data Set Items (ISCIBPDS:B) (Version 1.1) Self Report
International Spinal Cord Injury Basic Pain Data Set Items (ISCIBPDS:B) (Version 2.0)
International Spinal Cord Injury Bowel Function Basic and Extended Data Sets
International Spinal Cord Injury Pain (ISCIP)
International Spinal Cord Injury Pain Extended Data Set (ISCIPEDS) (Version 1.0)
Modified Barthel Index (MBI)
Modified Fatigue Scale Spinal Cord Injury (MFIS-SCI)
Multidimensional Pain Inventory (MPI)
Multidimensional Pain Readiness to Change Questionnaire (MPRCQ)
Multidimensional Pain Readiness to Change Questionnaire 2 (MPRCQ2)
Needs and Provision Complexity Scale (NPCS)
Needs Assessment Checklist (NAC)
Neurogenic Bowel Dysfunction (NBD) Score
Neuropathic Pain Symptom Inventory (NPSI)
Northwick Park Dependency Score (NPDS)
Numerical Rating Scale (NRS) Pain
Pain Medication Questionnaire (PMQ)
Paindetect Questionnaire (PD-Q)
Patient Categorization Tool (PCAT)
Patient Participation In Rehabilitation Questionnaire (PPRQ)
Perceived Manageability Scale (PMNAC)
Performing Pressure—Relief for Pressure Ulcer (PrU)
Pregnancy and Motherhood Evaluation Questionnaire (PMEQ)
Revised Skin Management Needs Assessment Checklist (Revised SMNAC)
Self-Care Assessment Tool (SCAT)
Skin Care Belief Scale (SCBS)
Skin Management Needs Assessment Checklist (SMNAC)
Spinal Cord Impairment Pressure Ulcers Monitoring Tool (SCI-PUMT)
Spinal Cord Injury (SCI) Sacral Sparing Self-Report Questionnaire
Spinal Cord Injury Pain Instrument (SCIPI)

Table 6 (continued)

Name of the scale, test, or questionnaire (acronym)
Spinal Cord Injury Patient Reported Outcome Measure of Bowel Function and Evacuation (SCIPROBE)
Spinal Cord Injury Pressure Ulcers Scale (SCIPUS)
Spinal Cord Injury Secondary Condition Scale (SCI-SCS)

Table 7 Scale, test, or questionnaire measuring pediatric spinal cord injury in people with spinal cord injury

Name of the scale, test, or questionnaire (acronym)
Capabilities of Upper Extremity Test (CUE)
Child Needs Assessment Checklist (ChNAC)
Graded Redefined Assessment of Strength, Sensibility, and Prehension (GRASSP)
Grasp and Release Test (GRT)
International Standards for Neurological Classification of Spinal Cord Injury (ISNCSCI)
Moorong Self-Efficacy Scale (MSES)
Pediatric Neuromuscular Recovery Scale (NRS)
Pediatric Quality of Life Recovery (Peds QL)
Pediatric Spinal Cord Injury Activity Measure (PEDI-SCI AM)
Screening Tool for the Assessment of Malnutrition in Pediatrics (STAMP)
Segmental Assessment of Trunk Control (SATCo)
Shriners Pediatric Instruments For Neuromuscular Scoliosis (SPINS)
Spinal Cord Independence Measure (SCIM) Indoor Mobility Item [12]
Spinal Cord Independence Measure (SCIM) III Self-Report
Walking Index for Spinal Cord Injury (WISCI II)

Table 8 Scale, test, or questionnaire measuring psychological status in people with spinal cord injury

Name of the scale, test, or questionnaire (acronym)
3-Item Loneliness Scale (LS)
Acceptance and Action Questionnaire (AAQ)
Appraisals of Disability: Primary and Secondary Scale (ADAPSS)
Appraisals of Disability: Primary and Secondary Scale Short Version (ADAPSS-SF)
Athletic Identity Measurement Scale (AIMS)
Attachment Style Questionnaire (ASQ)
Brief Symptom Inventory (BSI)
Center For Epidemiologic Studies Depression Scale (CESD)
Community Integration Measure (CIM)

(continued)

Table 8 (continued)

Name of the scale, test, or questionnaire (acronym)
Connor-Davidson Resilience Scale 2 Item (CD-RISC 2)
Connor-Davidson Resilience Scale 25 Item (CD-RISC 25)
Connor-Davidson Resilience Scale 5 Item (CD-RISC 5)
Coping Strategies Questionnaire 24 (CSQ24)
Core Self-Evaluations Scale (CSES)
Depression Anxiety Stress Scales-21 (DASS-21)
Flourishing Scale (FS)
General Handicapped Attitude Scale (GHAS)
General Health Questionnaire-28 (GHQ-28)
General Self-Efficacy Scale (GSES)
Hamilton Depression Rating Scale (HAM-D)
Hopkins Rehabilitation Engagement Rating Scale (HRERS)
Hopkins Symptom Checklist-20 (HSCL-20)
Hospital Anxiety and Depression Scale (HADS)
Loss Inventory (LS)
Medically Based Emotional Distress Scale (MEDS)
Minnesota Multiphasic Personality Inventory-2 (MMPI-2)
Multidimensional Acceptance to Loss Scale (MALS)
Nottingham Health Profile (NHP)
Patient Health Questionnaire-2 (PHQ-2)
Patient Health Questionnaire-9 (PHQ-9)
Patient-Reported Outcome Measurement Information System 8B Short Form (PROMIS-D-8)
Physical Disability Stress Scale (PDSS)
Psychological Evaluation Tool for Spinal Cord Stimulation Candidacy (PETSCSC)
Readiness for Hospital Discharge Scale (RHDS)
Sickness Impact Profile 68 (SIP68)
Spinal Cord Injury—Falls Concern Scale (SCI-FCS)
Spinal Cord Lesion Emotional Wellbeing Questionnaire (SCL-EWQ)
Spinal Cord Lesion Related Coping Strategies Questionnaire (SCL-CSQ)
Stanmore Nursing Assessment of Psychological Status (SNAPS)
Sydney Psychosocial Reintegration Scale (SPRS)
Sydney Psychosocial Reintegration Scale 2 (SPRS-2)
Symptom Checklist-90-R (SCL-90-R)
Trait Hope Scale (THS)
University of Washington Self-Efficacy Scale (UWSES)
Ways of Coping Questionnaire
Work Rehabilitation Questionnaire Self-Report Version (WRQ-SELF)

Table 9 Scale, test, or questionnaire measuring quality of life in people with spinal cord injury

Name of the scale, test, or questionnaire (acronym)
36 Item Short Form Health Survey (SF-36)
36 Item Short Form Health Survey Walk–Wheel (SF-36 WW)
Brief Adaptation to Disability Scale-Revised (B-ADS-R)
Community Integration Questionnaire (CIQ)
Economic QOL-28 Item Scale
Ferrans and Powers Quality of Life Index (QLI)
General Sleep Disturbance Scale (GSDS)
Health Behavioral Questionnaire (HBQ)
International Spinal Cord Injury Quality of Life Basic Data Set (QOL Basic Data Set)
Life Satisfaction Questionnaire (LISAT-9)
Life Situation Questionnaire–Revised (LSQ-R)
Mental Health Subscale (MHS)
Nordic Sleep Questionnaire (NSQ)
Participation ScALE (PS)
Personal Well-Being Index (PWI)
Quality of Life Assessment Tool (Qual-OT)
Quality of Life Profile for Adults With Physical Disabilities (QOLP-PD)
Questionnaire on (Dis)Ability, Impact, and Weighted Score
Rick Hansen Spinal Cord Injury Registry (RHSCIR)
Satisfaction With Life Scale (SWLS)
Sense of Well-Being Inventory (SWBI)
Short Form Health Survey (SF-6D)
Short Form Health Survey Physical Functioning Scale for Veterans (SF-36V)
Spinal Cord Injury Lifestyle Scale (SCILS)
Spinal Cord Injury Quality of Life (SCI-QL)
Utrecht Scale for Evaluation of Rehabilitation–Participation (USER)
World Health Organization Quality of Life 5 (WHOQOL-5)
World Health Organization Quality of Life (WHOQOLBREF)
World Health Organization Quality of Life for Disabilities (WHOQOL-DIS)

Table 10 Scale, test, or questionnaire measuring upper limb function in people with spinal cord injury

Name of the scale, test, or questionnaire (acronym)
AuSpinal
Automated Tools to Quantify Hand and Wrist Motor Function

(continued)

Table 10 (continued)

Name of the scale, test, or questionnaire (acronym)
Capabilities of Upper Extremity Test (CUE-T)
Duruöz Hand Index (DHI)
Functional Standing Test (FST)
Graded Redefined Assessment of Strength, Sensibility, and Prehension (GRASSP)
Graded Redefined Assessment of Strength, Sensibility, and Prehension (GRASSP) Version 2
Handheld Myometer
Intentional Movement Performance Ability (IMPA)
Klein–Bell ADL Scale (K-B Scale)
Motor Capacities Scale (MCS)
Neuromuscular Recovery Scale (NRS) Upper Limb
ReJoyce Automated Hand Function Test (RAHFT)
Swedish Tetraplegia Surgery Satisfaction Questionnaire
Toronto Rehabilitation Institute–Hand Function Test (TRI-HFT)
Van Lieshout Test (VLT)
Wingate Anaerobic Testing (Want)

Table 11 Scale, test, or questionnaire measuring urological aspects in people with spinal cord injury

Name of the scale, test, or questionnaire (acronym)
Incontinence–Activity Participation Scale (I-APS)
Incontinence Quality of Life (I-QOL)
Intermittent Catheterization Acceptance Test (I-CAT)
Intermittent Catheterization Difficulty Questionnaire (ICDQ)
Intermittent Catheterization Satisfaction Questionnaire (InCaSaQ)
Intermittent Self-Catheterization Questionnaire (ISC-Q)
King's Health Questionnaire (KHQ)
Knowledge, Comfort, Approach, and Attitudes Towards Sexuality Scale (KCAASS)
Lower Urinary Track Symptoms Treatments Constraints Assessment (LUTS TCA)
Monitoring Efficacy of Neurogenetic Bowel Dysfunction Treatment on Response (MENTOR)
Multiple Sclerosis Intimacy and Sexuality Questionnaire (MSISQ)
Neurogenic Bladder Symptom Score (NBSS)
Neurogenic Bladder Symptom Score Short Form (NBSS Short Form)
Perceived Sexual Distress Scale–Hindi (PSDS-H)
Qualiveen
Qualiveen–Short Version (SF-Qualiveen)
Self-Report Questionnaire Assessing the Bodily and Physiological Sensations of Orgasm

Table 11 (continued)

Name of the scale, test, or questionnaire (acronym)
Sexual Adjustment Questionnaire (SAQ)
Sexual Attitude and Information Questionnaire (SAIQ)
Urinary Symptom Questionnaire for Individuals With Neuropathic Bladder Using Intermittent Catheterization (USQNB-IC)

References

1. World Health Organization. The ICF: an overview. Geneva: WHO; 2001.
2. Cieza A, Stucki G. Content comparison of health-related quality of life (HRQOL) instruments based on the international classification of functioning, disability and health (ICF). Qual Life Res. 2005. https://doi.org/10.1007/s11136-004-4773-0.
3. Weigl M, Cieza A, Harder M, ct al. Linking osteoarthritis-specific health-status measures to the international classification of functioning, disability, and health (ICF). Osteoarthr Cartil. 2003. https://doi.org/10.1016/S1063-4584(03)00086-4.
4. Kirchberger I, Cieza A, Biering-Sørensen F, et al. ICF Core Sets for individuals with spinal cord injury in the early post-acute context. Spinal Cord. 2010. https://doi.org/10.1038/sc.2009.128.
5. Ballert CS, Stucki G, Biering-Sørensen F, Cieza A. Towards the development of clinical measures for spinal cord injury based on the international classification of functioning, disability and health with Rasch analyses. Arch Phys Med Rehabil. 2014. https://doi.org/10.1016/j.apmr.2014.05.006.
6. Herrmann KH, Kirchberger I, Stucki G, Cieza A. The comprehensive ICF core sets for spinal cord injury from the perspective of occupational therapists: a worldwide validation study using the Delphi technique. Spinal Cord. 2011. https://doi.org/10.1038/sc.2010.168.
7. Herrmann KH, Kirchberger I, Stucki G, Cieza A. The Comprehensive ICF core sets for spinal cord injury from the perspective of physical therapists: a worldwide validation study using the Delphi technique. Spinal Cord. 2011. https://doi.org/10.1038/sc.2010.155.
8. Kirchberger I, Sinnott A, Charlifue S, et al. Functioning and disability in spinal cord injury from the consumer perspective: an international qualitative study using focus groups and the ICF. Spinal Cord. 2010. https://doi.org/10.1038/sc.2009.184.
9. Tomaschek R, Gemperli A, Rupp R, Geng V, Scheel-Sailer A. A systematic review of outcome measures in initial rehabilitation of individuals with newly acquired spinal cord injury: providing evidence for clinical practice guidelines. Eur J Phys Rehabil Med. 2019. https://doi.org/10.23736/S1973-9087.19.05676-4.

10. Dawson J, Shamley D, Jamous MA. A structured review of outcome measures used for the assessment of rehabilitation interventions for spinal cord injury. Spinal Cord. 2008. https://doi.org/10.1038/sc.2008.50.

11. Ioannidis JPA, Greenland S, Hlatky MA, et al. Increasing value and reducing waste in research design, conduct, and analysis. Lancet. 2014. https://doi.org/10.1016/S0140-6736(13)62227-8.

12. Prinsen CAC, Mokkink LB, Bouter LM, et al. COSMIN guideline for systematic reviews of patient-reported outcome measures. Qual Life Res. 2018. https://doi.org/10.1007/s11136-018-1798-3.

13. Mokkink LB, de Vet HCW, Prinsen CAC, et al. COSMIN risk of bias checklist for systematic reviews of patient-reported outcome measures. Qual Life Res. 2018. https://doi.org/10.1007/s11136-017-1765-4.

14. Terwee CB, Prinsen CAC, Chiarotto A, et al. COSMIN methodology for evaluating the content validity of patient-reported outcome measures: a Delphi study. Qual Life Res. 2018. https://doi.org/10.1007/s11136-018-1829-0.

15. Castelnuovo G, Giusti EM, Manzoni GM, et al. What is the role of the placebo effect for pain relief in neurorehabilitation? Clinical implications from the Italian consensus conference on pain in neurorehabilitation. Front Neurol. 2018. https://doi.org/10.3389/fneur.2018.00310.

16. Marquez MA, De Santis R, Ammendola V, et al. Cross-cultural adaptation and validation of the "spinal Cord Injury-Falls Concern Scale" in the Italian population. Spinal Cord. 2018;56(7):712–8. https://doi.org/10.1038/s41393-018-0070-6.

17. Berardi A, De Santis R, Tofani M, et al. The Wheelchair Use Confidence Scale: Italian translation, adaptation, and validation of the short form. Disabil Rehabil Assist Technol. 2018;13(4):i. https://doi.org/10.1080/17483107.2017.1357053.

18. Anna B, Giovanni G, Marco T, et al. The validity of rasterstereography as a technological tool for the objectification of postural assessment in the clinical and educational fields: pilot study. In: Advances in intelligent systems and computing; 2020. https://doi.org/10.1007/978-3-030-23884-1_8.

19. Panuccio F, Berardi A, Marquez MA, et al. Development of the Pregnancy and Motherhood Evaluation Questionnaire (PMEQ) for evaluating and measuring the impact of physical disability on pregnancy and the management of motherhood: a pilot study. Disabil Rehabil. 2020;2020:1–7. https://doi.org/10.1080/09638288.2020.1802520.

20. Amedoro A, Berardi A, Conte A, et al. The effect of aquatic physical therapy on patients with multiple sclerosis: A systematic review and meta-analysis. Mult Scler Relat Disord. 2020. https://doi.org/10.1016/j.msard.2020.102022.

21. Dattoli S, Colucci M, Soave MG, et al. Evaluation of pelvis postural systems in spinal cord injury patients: outcome research. J Spinal Cord Med. 2018;43:185–92.

22. Berardi A, Galeoto G, Guarino D, et al. Construct validity, test-retest reliability, and the ability to detect change of the Canadian Occupational Performance Measure in a spinal cord injury population. Spinal cord Ser cases. 2019. https://doi.org/10.1038/s41394-019-0196-6.

23. Ponti A, Berardi A, Galeoto G, Marchegiani L, Spandonaro C, Marquez MA. Quality of life, concern of falling and satisfaction of the sit-ski aid in sit-skiers with spinal cord injury: observational study. Spinal Cord Ser Cases. 2020. https://doi.org/10.1038/s41394-020-0257-x.

24. Panuccio F, Galeoto G, Marquez MA, et al. General Sleep Disturbance Scale (GSDS-IT) in people with spinal cord injury: a psychometric study. Spinal Cord. 2020; https://doi.org/10.1038/s41393-020-0500-0.

25. Monti M, Marquez MA, Berardi A, Tofani M, Valente D, Galeoto G. The Multiple Sclerosis Intimacy and Sexuality Questionnaire (MSISQ-15): validation of the Italian version for individuals with spinal cord injury. Spinal Cord. 2020. https://doi.org/10.1038/s41393-020-0469-8.

26. Galeoto G, Colucci M, Guarino D, et al. Exploring validity, reliability, and factor analysis of the Quebec user evaluation of satisfaction with assistive technology in an Italian population: a cross-sectional study. Occup Ther Heal Care. 2018. https://doi.org/10.1080/07380577.2018.1522682.

27. Colucci M, Tofani M, Trioschi D, Guarino D, Berardi A, Galeoto G. Reliability and validity of the Italian version of Quebec User Evaluation of Satisfaction with Assistive Technology 2.0 (QUEST-IT 2.0) with users of mobility assistive device. Disabil Rehabil Assist Technol. 2019. https://doi.org/10.1080/17483107.2019.1668975.

28. Berardi A, Galeoto G, Lucibello L, Panuccio F, Valente D, Tofani M. Athletes with disability' satisfaction with sport wheelchairs: an Italian cross sectional study. Disabil Rehabil Assist Technol. 2020. https://doi.org/10.1080/17483107.2020.1800114.

29. Liberati A, Altman DG, Tetzlaff J, et al. The PRISMA statement for reporting systematic reviews and meta-analyses of studies that evaluate health care interventions: explanation and elaboration. J Clin Epidemiol. 2009. https://doi.org/10.1016/j.jclinepi.2009.06.006.

30. Higgins JP. Cochrane handbook for systematic reviews of interventions. Version 5.1. 0 [updated March 2011]. The Cochrane Collaboration. 2011. www.cochrane-handbook.org.

Measuring Neurological Status in Spinal Cord Injury

Anna Berardi, Marco Tofani, Filippo Camerota, Claudia Celletti, Giovanni Fabbrini, and Giovanni Galeoto

1   Introduction

Spinal cord injury (SCI) is one of the most severe and arduous conditions that can affect people and cause disability. For this reason, it is important to underline that SCI isn't a disease but a "new condition" with which SCI individuals have to learn to live. The spinal cord is a part of central nervous system and it organizes the pulse conduction, both ascending and descending. It allows body movements, muscle contractions, and skin sensitivity. So, spinal cord injury causes a loss of these functions, deterioration of motor, sensory and autonomic functions, with consequent profound effects on physical performance. The most evident consequence of motion neuron death is plegia, which is the impossibility of voluntary movements. SCI is a complicated condition, and for this reason, clinicians have to evaluate a person with SCI in a global way. They must evaluate the neurological status that includes the level of SCI. The spinal cord injury level is defined as the lowest spinal cord segment with intact sensory and motor function. This level is determined when the patient is first seen and is used for all subsequent evaluations. Clinicians also have to evaluate all consequences of the level like voluntary muscle contraction and skin sensitivity.

This study aims to describe and evaluate the assessment tools on neurological status in people with SCI through a systematic review of cross-sectional studies.

2   Materials and Methods

This systematic review was conducted by a research group comprised of rehabilitation professionals and medical doctors from the "Sapienza" University of Rome and from "Rehabilitation & Outcome Measure Assessment" (R.O.M.A.) association. R.O. M.A. association in the last few years has dealt with several systematic reviews and the validation of many outcome measures in Italy. This chapter describes all assessment tools regarding neurological status resulted from a systematic review conducted on Pubmed, Scopus, and web of science. For specific details, see chapter "Methodological Approach to Identifying Outcome Measures in Spinal Cord

A. Berardi (✉) · G. Galeoto
Department of Human Neurosciences, Sapienza University of Rome, Rome, Italy
e-mail: anna.berardi@uniroma1.it

M. Tofani
Department of Neurorehabilitation and Robotics, Bambino Gesù Paediatric Hospital, Rome, Italy

F. Camerota · C. Celletti
Physical Medicine and Rehabilitation Division, Umberto I University Hospital of Rome, Rome, Italy

G. Fabbrini
Department of Human Neurosciences, Sapienza University of Rome, Rome, Italy

IRCSS Neuromed, Pozzilli, Italy

Injury." Eligibility criteria for considering studies for this chapter were: validation studies and cross-cultural adaptation studies, studies about the quality of life, studies about tests, questionnaires, and self-reported and performance-based outcome measures, studies with a population of people of SCI and population ≥18 years old. Study selection: selection of studies was conducted in accordance with the 27-item PRISM Statement for Reporting Systematic Reviews [1]. For the data collection, authors followed the recommendations from the COnsensus-based Standards for the selection of health Measurement Instruments (COSMIN) initiative [2]. Study quality and risk of bias were assessed using COSMIN checklist [3].

3   Results

For this chapter, 32 papers were considered. Authors found 19 assessment tools that evaluate the neurological area in persons with SCI. In Fig. 1, a flow chart of included studies is reported [3, 4].

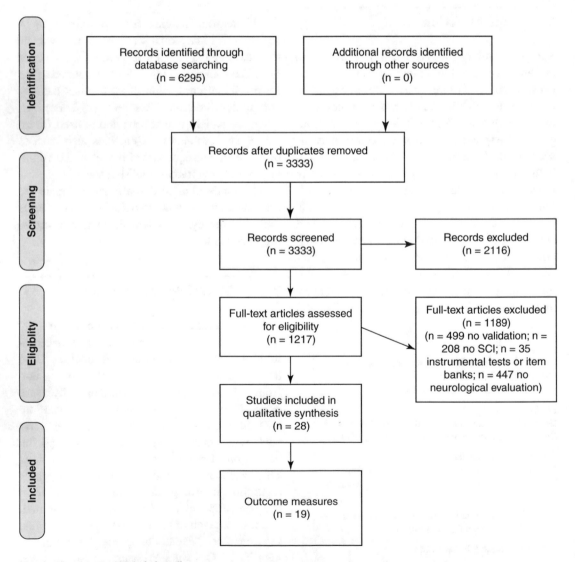

Fig. 1 Flow chart of included studies

3.1 American Spinal Cord Injury Association (ASIA)

Published in 1982, the ASIA "Standards for Neurological Classification of Spinal Injury Patients" have been widely accepted by clinical researchers for use in outcome studies. The original standards included the following definitions and areas of classification: neurologic level of injury, zone of injury, functional grades based on the Frankel classification system, a classification system of incomplete spinal injury syndromes using an anatomic description, definition of sensory level based on a dermatomal map, definition of motor level based on myotomes using key muscles, and the motor index score. In 1989, the ASIA revised the standards by making a number of significant changes and clarifications. These included the use of key areas with anatomic landmarks to define sensory levels rather than relying on the use of a dermatome chart, and redefining the zone of injury as "the zone of partial preservation of sensory and/or motor function." The ASIA revisions provided clarification of muscle grading for determining motor levels with incomplete injuries and clarification of the Frankel classification on the degree of incompleteness [5, 6]. The ASIA assessment protocol consists of two sensory examinations, a motor examination and a classification framework (the impairment scale) to quantify the severity of the SCI. Table 1 summarizes the papers' authors and languages and Table 2 shows the quality of their studies.

3.2 Spinal Cord Injury Ability Realization Measurement Index (SCI-ARMI)

SCI-ARMI was developed at the spinal department of Loewenstein Rehabilitation Hospital in Israel. Then it was also validated in Italy, Spain, United Kingdom, United States, France, and Portugal. SCI-ARMI is a measure to assess disability to be weighted by identifying the neurological deficit level in people with SCI, irrespective of completeness, or incompleteness of injury. It is an index derived from a statistical algorithm capable of measuring the percentage of skill achieved by a patient with spinal cord injury compared to the maximum possible skill for that level and severity. The index is applicable to spinal cord injury cases. The index can evaluate the skill gain achieved concerning the whole optimum, net of the spontaneous neurological recovery that took place between the different measurements [7, 8]. Table 3 summarizes the papers' authors and languages and Table 4 shows the quality of their studies.

3.3 Quantitative Sensory Testing (QST)

In 1999, Andrei Krassioukov et al. worked in Canada to examine the utility of QST to characterize sensory dysfunction in patients with SCI. QST has been used extensively to assess the

Table 1 Characteristics of the studies validating ASIA scale

Authors	Language	n	Age mean (SD, range) year	Gender % Female
Priebe et al. [5]	English	n.a.	n.a.	n.a.
Graves et al. [6]	English	6116	36 (16.53)	1223 (20)

n number of participants of the study, *n.a.* not available

Table 2 Evaluation of quality and risk of bias

Authors	Item of COSMIN checklist									
	1	2	3	4	5	6	7	8	9	10
Priebe et al. [5]	?	?	–	–	–	+	–	–	–	–
Graves et al. [6]	?	?	–	–	–	–	–	+	+	–

Item1 PROM development, *Item 2* content validity, *Item 3* structural validity, *Item 4* internal consistency, *Item 5* cross-cultural validity/measurement invariance, *Item 6* reliability, *Item 7* measurement error, *Item8,* criterion validity, *Item 9,* hypothesis testing for construct validity, *Item 10* responsiveness, + sufficient, – insufficient, ? indeterminate

Table 3 Characteristics of the studies validating SCI-ARMI

Authors	Language	n	Age mean (SD, range) year	Gender % Female
Catz et al. [7]	Hebrew	79	46 (18)	n.a.
	Italian	661	n.a.	n.a.
	English			
	Hebrew			
	Spanish			
	English			
	Portuguese			
Scivoletto et al. [8]	Indian			

N number of participants of the study, *n.a.* not available

Table 4 Evaluation of quality and risk of bias

Authors	Item of COSMIN checklist									
	1	2	3	4	5	6	7	8	9	10
Catz et al. [7]	+	+	–	–	–	+	–	+	+	–
Scivoletto et al. [8]	–	+	–	–	–	–	–	–	–	–

Item1 PROM development, *Item 2* content validity, *Item 3* structural validity, *Item 4* internal consistency, *Item 5* cross-cultural validity/measurement invariance, *Item 6* reliability, *Item 7* measurement error, *Item8* criterion validity, *Item 9* hypothesis testing for construct validity, *Item 10*: responsiveness, + sufficient, – insufficient, ? indeterminate

Table 5 Characteristics of the studies validating QST

Authors	Language	n	Age mean (SD, range) year	Gender % Female
Krassioukov et al. [9]	English (Canadian)	21	n.a.	6 (28.6)
Felix et al. [10]	English (American)	22	41.7 (15.5)	3 (13.6)

N number of participants of the study, *n.a.* not available

Table 6 Evaluation of quality and risk of bias

Authors	Item of COSMIN checklist									
	1	2	3	4	5	6	7	8	9	10
Krassioukov et al. [9]	+	+	–	–	–	+	–	+	+	–
Felix et al. [10]	–	+	–	–	–	–	–	–	–	–

Item1 PROM development, *Item 2* content validity, *Item 3* structural validity, *Item 4* internal consistency, *Item 5* cross-cultural validity/measurement invariance, *Item 6* reliability, *Item 7* measurement error, *Item8* criterion validity, *Item 9* hypothesis testing for construct validity, *Item 10* responsiveness, + sufficient, – insufficient, ? indeterminate

functional integrity of the somatosensory system in a number of patient populations, including persons with diabetic neuropathy, herpes zoster, complex regional pain syndrome, and SCI. QST was validated in the United States and Canada. QST consists of the presentation of four stimuli in the following fixed order: cold sensation (CS), warm sensation (WS), cold pain (CP), and vibra-tion sensation (VS). Using QST as a diagnostic and/or outcome measurement strategy may provide a valuable adjunct for assessing clinical pain and may help determine the underlying mechanisms responsible for specific pain types in SCI [9, 10]. Table 5 summarizes the papers' authors and languages, and Table 6 shows the quality of their studies.

3.4 Knee-Up Test

In 2015, Itaru Yugué et al. worked to prospectively investigate the usefulness of the "knee-up test" to detect postoperative motor deficits in Japan easily. In 2017, Itaru Yugué proposed this useful and simple clinical method to help classify patients with acute cervical spinal cord injury. The "knee-up test" was developed to assess postoperative deficits before endotracheal estuation easily. The patient is placed supine on a bed, and the surgeon flexes the patient's hip to near 90° with the knee maximally flexed with the foot of the flexed leg on the table. When the patient's knee is passively lifted up, and the patient can maintain this position in both legs, the result is negative. In contrast, when the patient cannot maintain the knee in an upright position for one or both legs, the result is positive. The presently accepted criterion for a new-onset postoperative neurologic motor deficit is motor weakness leading to a decrease in function of at least two grades in more than one muscle function within 12 h of spinal surgery, as evaluated by the Manual Muscle Testing [11, 12]. Table 7 summarizes the papers' authors and languages, and Table 8 shows the quality of their studies.

3.5 Ashworth Scale (AS)

The AS was developed by Ashworth in 1964, modified in 1987 by Bohannen and Smith, and validated for SCI population in 1996 [13]. Both scales ask the examiner to move a limb through its full range of movement then rate the amount of resistance felt. The original Ashworth scale ranges from 0 to 4, in which 0: "no increase in muscle tone"; 1: "slight increase in muscle tone giving a catch when the limb is moved"; 2: "more marked increase in tone but limb is easily moved considerable increase in tone-passive movement difficult and 4: "limb rigid in flexion or extension (abduction/adduction)." The Modified Ashworth scale (MAS) also ranges from 0 to 4.

Then, the MAS uses a five-point ordinal scale to subjectively assess muscle tone, and also validate SCI patients, in English [14, 15], Danish [16], and Turkish [17]. In 2016, Mishra et al. in India validated the Modified modified Ashworth Scale (MMAS) in SCI which measures spasticity 0 = no increase in muscle tone; 1 = slight increase in muscle tone, manifested by a catch and release or by minimal resistance at the end of the range of motion when the affected part(s) is moved in flexion or extension; 2 = marked increase in muscle tone, manifested by a catch in the middle range and resistance throughout the remainder of the range of motion, but affected part(s) easily moved; 3 = considerable increase in muscle tone, passive movement difficult; and 4 = affected part(s) rigid in flexion or extension [18]. Table 9 summarizes papers' authors and languages, and Table 10 shows the quality of their studies.

Table 7 Characteristics of the studies validating knee-up test

Authors	Language	n	Age mean (SD, range) year	Gender % Female
Yugué et al. [11]	Japanese	200	62.4 (15.4)	34 (17)
Yugué et al. [12]	Japanese	544	n.a.	n.a.

N number of participants of the study, *n.a.* not available

Table 8 Evaluation of quality and risk of bias

Authors	Item of COSMIN checklist									
	1	2	3	4	5	6	7	8	9	10
Yugué et al. [11]	−	+	−	−	+	−	−	−	−	−
Yugué et al. [12]	−	+	−	−	+	−	−	−	−	−

Item1 PROM development, *Item 2* content validity, *Item 3* structural validity, *Item 4* internal consistency, *Item 5* cross-cultural validity/measurement invariance, *Item 6* reliability, *Item 7* measurement error, *Item8* criterion validity, *Item 9* hypothesis testing for construct validity, *Item 10* responsiveness, + sufficient, − insufficient, ? indeterminate

Table 9 Characteristics of the studies validating AS, MAS, and MMAS

Scale	Authors	Language	n	Age mean (SD, range) year	Gender % Female
AS	Haas et al. [13]	English	24	40.3 (17–72)	6 (26)
MAS	Haas et al. [13]	English	24	40.3 (17–72)	6 (26)
	Smith et al. [15]	English	22	33.4 (12.5, 16–33)	2 (9.1)
	Craven et al. [14]	English	20	38.9 (13.6, 16–67)	3 (15)
	Baunsgaard et al. [16]	Danish	31	48.3 (20.2, 15–88)	11 (35)
	Akpinar et al. [17]	Turkish	65	44 (14, 18–88)	21 (36)
MMAS	Mishra et al. [18]	Hindi	38	31.94 (12.63, 20–62)	6 (15.8)

N number of participants of the study, *n.a.* not available

Table 10 Evaluation of quality and risk of bias

Authors	Item of COSMIN checklist									
	1	2	3	4	5	6	7	8	9	10
Haas et al. [13]	?	?	−	−	−	+	−	+	+	−
Haas et al. [13]	?	?	−	−	−	+	−	+	+	−
Smith et al. [15]	?	?	+	−	−	+	−	−	−	−
Craven et al. [14]	?	?	−	−	−	+	−	−	−	−
Baunsgaard et al. [16]	?	+	−	−	−	+	−	+	+	−
Akpinar et al. [17]	?	+	−	−	−	+	−	+	+	−
Mishra et al. [18]	?	+	−	−	−	+	−	−	−	−

Item1 PROM development, *Item 2* content validity, *Item 3*: structural validity, *Item 4* internal consistency, *Item 5* cross-cultural validity/measurement invariance, *Item 6* reliability, *Item 7* measurement error, *Item8* criterion validity, *Item 9* hypothesis testing for construct validity, *Item 10* responsiveness, + sufficient, −: insufficient, ? indeterminate

Table 11 Characteristics of the studies validating SCI-SET

Authors	Language	n	Age mean (SD, range) year	Gender % Female
Adams et al. [19]	English	61	41.9 (12.6)	16 (26)
Akpinar et al. [17]	Turkish	66	44.06 (14.47, 18–88)	40 (60.6)
Ansari et al. [21]	Persian	100	39.0 (11.0, 20–69)	42 (100)
Sweatman et al. [20]	English	1239	n.a.	396 (32)

N number of participants of the study *n.a.* not available

3.6 Spinal Cord Injury Spasticity Evaluation Tool (SCI-SET)

SCI-SET was developed by Adams et al. in 2007 [19, 20] to measure the impact of spasticity on daily life in patients with SCI in Canada. SCI-SET was validated in Persian [21] and Turkish [17]. SCI-SET considers both the problematic and the useful effects of spasticity and fills a need for a valid and reliable self-report measure of spasticity in SCI patients. It is a self-reported measure consisting of 35 questions to assess the degree to which spasticity has affected patient life activities with SCI over the past 7 days.

Patients were asked to recall their past 7 days when rating spasticity. Responses were on a seven-point scale that ranges from +3 (extremely helpful) to −3 (extremely problematic). The SCI-SET total score was computed by summing all the responses from the applicable items and then dividing the sum by the number of applicable items. SCI-SET was interviewer-administered or self-administered, and it takes ∼10 min to complete the questionnaire. It was created to be comprehensive, but easy to understand for patients. Table 11 summarizes the papers' authors and languages and Table 12 shows the quality of their studies.

Table 12 Evaluation of quality and risk of bias

Authors	Item of COSMIN checklist									
	1	2	3	4	5	6	7	8	9	10
Adams et al. [19]	+	+	–	+	–	–		+	+	–
Akpinar et al. [17]	?	+	–	+	+	+	–	+	+	–
Ansari et al. [21]	?	+	+	+	+	+	+	+	+	–
Sweatman et al. [20]	?	?	+	–	+	–	–	+	+	–

Item1 PROM development, *Item 2* content validity, *Item 3* structural validity, *Item 4* internal consistency, *Item 5* cross-cultural validity/measurement invariance, *Item 6*: reliability, *Item 7* measurement error, *Item8* criterion validity, *Item 9* hypothesis testing for construct validity, *Item 10* responsiveness, + sufficient, – insufficient, ? indeterminate

Table 13 Characteristics of the studies validating SCATS

Authors	Language	n	Age mean (SD, range) year	Gender % Female
Benz et al. [22]	English	27	n.a.	n.a.
Akpinar et al. [23]	Turkish	47	44.19 (14.52)	17 (36.2)

N number of participants of the study, *n.a.* not available

Table 14 Evaluation of quality and risk of bias

Authors	Item of COSMIN checklist									
	1	2	3	4	5	6	7	8	9	10
Benz et al. [22]	?	?	–	–	–	–	–	+	+	–
Akpinar et al. [23]	?	+	–	–	–	+	–	+	+	–

Item1 PROM development, *Item 2* content validity, *Item 3* structural validity, *Item 4* internal consistency, *Item 5* cross-cultural validity/measurement invariance, *Item 6* reliability, *Item 7* measurement error, *Item8* criterion validity, *Item 9* hypothesis testing for construct validity, *Item 10* responsiveness, + sufficient, – insufficient, ? indeterminate

3.7 Spinal Cord Assessment Tool for Spastic Reflexes (SCATS)

The development of the SCATS was based on previous clinical measures of spastic hypertonia that use a physical examination to assess involuntary motor behaviors, as well as recent laboratory measurements of clonus, flexor, and extensor spasms. Specific techniques for the measurement of these spasms follow. It was validated in English [22] and Turkish language [23]. Table 13 summarizes the papers' authors and languages, and Table 14 shows the quality of their studies.

3.8 Patient-Reported Impact of Spasticity Measure (PRISM)

The PRISM is a new instrument that standardizes the collection of self-report information relevant to the clinical assessment of abnormal muscle control or involuntary muscle movement (AMC/IMM). The PRISM subscales assess the impact of altered motor control concerning social avoidance and anxiety, psychological agitation, daily activities, need for assistance or positioning, need for interventions, social embarrassment, and the positive impact of altered motor control. It was validated in the English language [20, 24]. Table 15

Table 15 Characteristics of the studies validating PRISM

Authors	Language	n	Age mean (SD, range) year	Gender % Female
Cook et al. [24]	English	180	52 (12)	n.a.
Sweatman et al. [20]	English	1239	n.a.	396 (32)

N number of participants of the study, *n.a.* not available

Table 16 Evaluation of quality and risk of bias

Authors	Item of COSMIN checklist									
	1	2	3	4	5	6	7	8	9	10
Cook et al. [24]	+	+	+	+	+	+	−	−	−	−
Sweatman et al. [20]	?	?	+	−	+	−	−	+	+	−

Item1 PROM development, *Item 2* content validity, *Item 3* structural validity, *Item 4* internal consistency, *Item 5* cross-cultural validity/measurement invariance, *Item 6* reliability, *Item 7* measurement error, *Item 8* criterion validity, *Item 9* hypothesis testing for construct validity, *Item 10* responsiveness, + sufficient, − insufficient, ? indeterminate

Table 17 Characteristics of the studies of scale, test, or questionnaire with less than two validations

Scale, test, or questionnaire	Authors	Language	n	Age mean (SD, range) year	Gender % Female
ISNCSCI92	Jonsson et al. [25]	Sweden	23	n.a.	8 (34.8)
UMNI	Klose et al. [26]	English	50	n.a.	n.a.
VFM	Taricco et al. [27]	Italian	n.a.	n.a.	n.a.
CSIRPS	Kumar et al. [28]	Hindi	60	41	18 (30)
Scale for evaluation of spinal cord injury	Chehrazi et al. [29]	English	n.a.	n.a.	n.a.
WPT	Joghtaei et al. [30]	Persian	15	34.6 (9.2)	7 (46.7)
MTS	Akpinar et al. [17]	Turkish	65	44 (14, 18–88)	21 (36)
REPAS	Platz et al. [31]	German	3	n.a.	n.a.
PSFS	Mills et al. [32]	English	61	44.1 (12.3)	49 (80.3)

N number of participants of the study, *n.a* not available

summarizes the papers' authors and languages, and Table 16 shows the quality of their studies.

3.9 Revised 1992 International Standards for Neurological and Functional Classification of Spinal Cord Injury (ISCSCI-92)

The ISNCSCI was developed in 1982 by the ASIA. The ISNCSCI examination and classification provide a common language describing the extent of motor and sensory dysfunction due to SCI. The ISCSCI-92 was validated in 2000 in Swedish language [25]. Table 17 summarizes the papers' authors and languages, and Table 18 shows the quality of their studies.

3.10 University of Miami Neuro-Spinal Index (UMNI)

In 1980, K. J. Klose et al. developed a quantitative scale for assessing spinal cord function at the University of Miami. UMNI is composed of a sensory and motor scale, which is sensitive to small changes. The UMNI is composed of two subscale, the sensory scale, and the motor scale. Scale scores are indicators of overall spinal cord functional capacity within the sensory and motor modalities. The total score range on the index 0-460 where "0" represents no detectable function, and "460" indicates normal function. This total score is the sum of the motor and sensory scales. The motor scale scoring system is based on muscle testing. The representative muscle groups were chosen

Table 18 Evaluation of quality and risk of bias

Authors	Item of COSMIN checklist									
	1	2	3	4	5	6	7	8	9	10
Jonsson et al. [25]	?	+	–	–	+	+	–	–	–	–
Klose et al. [26]	+	+	–	–	–	–	–	–	–	–
Taricco et al. [27]	+	+	–	–	–	–	–	+	+	–
Kumar et al. [28]	–	+	–	–	–	–	–	–	–	–
Chehrazi et al. [29]	+	+	–	–	–	–	–	–	–	–
Joghtaei et al. [30]	–	+	–	–	+	–	–	–	–	–
Akpinar et al. [17]	?	+	–	–	–	+	–	+	+	–
Platz et al. [31]	+	+	–	+	–	+	–	+	+	–
Mills et al. [32]	?	?	–	–	–	–	+	–	–	–

Item1 PROM development, *Item 2* content validity, *Item 3* structural validity, *Item 4* internal consistency, *Item 5* cross-cultural validity/measurement invariance, *Item 6* reliability, *Item 7* measurement error, *Item 8* criterion validity, *Item 9* hypothesis testing for construct validity, *Item 10* responsiveness, + sufficient, – insufficient, ? indeterminate

based on functional significance as it correlates to the level of injury. Each muscle group is scored on a 0–5 scale, where: 0 = no function and 5 = normal power. The sensory scale score is an index of total body sensation. Items score are assigned as follows: 0 = absent; 1 = present, not abnormal; 2 = normal. Sensory indices range from 0 = no detectable to 240 = total normal body sensation. The motor and sensory subscale scores can be summed to yield an overall neuro-spinal functional capacity rating [26]. Table 17 summarizes the papers' authors and languages, and Table 18 shows the quality of their studies.

3.11 Valutazione Funzionale Mielolesi (VFM)

In 2000, M. Taricco et al. validated a new function assessment scale for SCI patients in Italy. The VFM was developed for SCI patients to describe and assess functional status when patients are in stable medical conditions. VFM can be administered at regular intervals by a physical or occupational therapist or a physiatrist. The test requires 30–50 min and can be used in different settings (i.e., home, outpatient). It includes eight functional domains with a different number of tasks. The score, ranging from 1 to 5, has to be assigned for each task after direct observation of patient performance [27]. Table 17

summarizes the papers' authors and languages, and Table 18 shows the quality of their studies.

3.12 Cervical Spine Injury Recovery Prediction Scale (CSIRPS)

CSIRPS was developed by Ramesh Kumar et al. in India (2011) to predict outcomes for patients with acute sub axial cervical spine injury (CSI). It is a scale for predicting cervical spine recovery. They developed CSIRPS using the combined correlation of five predictors of neural recovery. They included (1) the American Spinal Injury Association (ASIA) impairment scale, (2) maximum cord compression, (3) maximum canal compromise, and (4) magnetic resonance imaging (MRI) signal intensity pattern in the cord, and (5) the Cervical Spine Injury Severity Score (CSISS) for stability on radiographs or computed tomography (CT) [28]. Table 17 summarizes the paper's authors and languages, and Table 18 shows the quality of their studies.

3.13 Scale for Evaluation of Spinal Cord Injury

In 1981, B. Chehrazi et al. developed a scale for evaluating spinal cord injury in New Haven, Connecticut, USA. The scale has been developed to assess the severity of spinal cord injury and the prognosis for recovery. Based on neurological examination, this scale employs numerical grading of selected functions below the injury level. The score assigned to each patient is determined by grading the strength of selected muscles and the intactness of specific sensory modalities below the level of injury with overall motor strength and sensory function, each having a maximum value of 5. Ten muscles were selected for possible examination. These ten muscles were selected because of the ease with which their strength can be measured, the spectrum of spinal cord segments they represent, and their functional significance. In each patient, the strength of the selected muscles innervated by segments located below the injury level is tested separately and graded from 0 to 5. By dividing the sum of the graded muscle strengths by the number of muscles tested then rounded off to the nearest tenth, an average is obtained. The sensory modalities of superficial pain, position sense, and deep pain are evaluated independently. Response to pinprick is graded between 0 and 2, with 0 indicating no sensation, 1 decreased or abnormal sensation, and 2 intact sensations. The average is obtained by dividing the sum of the dermatomes' responses below the injury level by the number of dermatomes tested and correcting to the nearest tenth [29]. Table 17 summarizes the papers' authors and languages, and Table 18 shows the quality of their studies.

3.14   Wartenberg Pendulum Test (WPT)

In 2015, Mahmoud Joghtaei et al. worked on studying the WPT, in Iran. Passive pendulum testing is a mean, so acquiring passive viscous–elastic parameters of the knee. The subject was placed in a semi-upright sitting position (45°) with the lower legs hanging over the chair's edge. The thigh is tightened with a strap to make it stays in a stationary condition. A plastic ankle foot orthosis is used to keep the ankle at 90°, to avoid any modification to the passive characteristic of the knee due to ankle movements. The sub-

ject's shank is raised and held by the examiner with the knee in maximum extension until the knee muscle was completely relaxed. This takes about 10–15 seconds. Then the subject's leg was released and allowed to swing and oscillate freely between flexion and extension. The leg movement was recorded until the shank reached its final resting position and stopped. The joint and surrounding tissues' viscous–elastic properties, together with the mass of the moving foot and leg, caused the leg to come to rest close to the vertical position. Using a flexible twin axis electronic goniometer (Model: SG110/A, Biometrics Ltd, Newport, UK), leg movements were recorded during a passive pendulum test. During the testing procedure, the subject's eyes are kept close using sleep masks. Performed three times the mean value of three measurements was taken for the analysis [30]. Table 17 summarizes the papers' authors and languages, and Table 18 shows the quality of their studies.

3.15   Modified Tardieu Scale (MTS)

The Tardieu Scale (TS), which quantifies muscle tone at specified velocities, has been suggested as superior to the Ashworth Scale to assess neural versus peripheral contributions of spasticity. In 1999, it was modified by standardizing limb placement conditions and the speeds as slow and fast, to produce the version presently known as the Modified Tardieu Scale (MTS). MTS was validated for SCI patients in Turkey [17]. A standard 0–5 scale was used for the qualitative rating of reaction to fast movements. A score of 0 represents no resistance throughout the course of the passive movement. A score of 1 represents a slight resistance throughout the course of stretching without a clear catch at any angle. A score of 2 represents a clear catch occurring at a precise angle, interrupting the passive movement and followed by a release. A score of 3 represents a fatigable clonus (o10 s, when maintaining the pressure). A score of 4 represents an indefatigable clonus (410 s, when maintaining the pressure) occurring at a precise angle. A score of 5 represents an immovable joint. Only one stretch was used at each speed. Table 17 summarizes the papers' authors and languages, and Table 18 shows the quality of their studies.

3.16 REsistance to PASsive Movement (REPAS)

REPAS is a summary rating scale for a passive movement resistance, used for validating people with SCI in Germany [31]. REPAS contains 52 items, each rated according to the Ashworth scale (0 = "no increase in tone" to 4 = "limb rigid in flexion or extension"), and it has a total score and regional body subtest scores. REPAS evaluates shoulder (external rotation, internal rotation, flexion, extension, abduction, adduction); elbow (flexion and extension); forearm (pronation and supination); wrist (flexion and extension); finger (flexion and extension); hip (abduction, adduction, external rotation, internal rotation, flexion, extension); knee (flexion and extension); foot (inversion/supination, eversion/pronation, plantar flexion, and dorsiflexion). General instructions and instructions for individual joint motions are included. Scoring is based on the original Ashworth scores. Table 17 summarizes the papers' authors and languages, and Table 18 shows the quality of their studies.

3.17 Penn Spasm Frequency Scale (PSFS)

The PSFS is a self-report measure composed of two parts. For Part 1, participants are asked to rate their spasm frequency during the past 7 days on a five-level scale ranging from 0 = no spasms to 4 = spasms occurring more than ten times per hour. If the participant indicates no spasms in Part 1, then they do not proceed to Part 2. Part 2 of the PSFS is a three-level scale assessing the severity of spasms. The PSFS was administered over the phone to minimize participant burden using this outcome measure in potential future studies. It was validated in SCI population [32]. Table 17 summarizes the papers' authors and languages, and Table 18 shows the quality of their studies.

4 Conclusion

This chapter reports all assessment tools described in the literature to assess neurological status in people with SCI. Among the 19 tools included in this chapter resulted that most scales evaluate spasticity and spasms. The most used tools are Modified Ashworth Scale (MAS), which assesses the subjectivity of muscle tone, and the Spinal Cord Injury Spasticity Evaluation Tool (SCI-SET), a self-report scale consisting of 35 questions to assess the degree to which spasticity affects life activities for patients with SCI over 7 days.

References

1. Moher D, Shamseer L, Clarke M, et al. Preferred reporting items for systematic review and meta-analysis protocols (PRISMA-P) 2015 statement. Rev Esp Nutr Human Diet. 2016. https://doi.org/10.1186/2046-4053-4-1
2. Mokkink LB, Terwee CB, Patrick DL, et al. The COSMIN study reached international consensus on taxonomy, terminology, and definitions of measurement properties for health-related patient-reported outcomes. J Clin Epidemiol. 2010. https://doi.org/10.1016/j.jclinepi.2010.02.006.
3. Mokkink LB, de Vet HCW, Prinsen CAC, et al. COSMIN risk of bias checklist for systematic reviews of patient-reported outcome measures. Qual Life Res. 2018. https://doi.org/10.1007/s11136-017-1765-4.
4. Terwee CB, Prinsen CAC, Chiarotto A, et al. COSMIN methodology for evaluating the content validity of patient-reported outcome measures: a Delphi study. Qual Life Res. 2018. https://doi.org/10.1007/s11136-018-1829-0.
5. Priebe MM, Waring WP. The interobserver reliability of the revised American Spinal Injury Association standards for neurological classification of spinal injury patients. Am J Phys Med Rehabil. 1991. https://doi.org/10.1097/00002060-199110000-00007.
6. Graves DE, Frankiewicz RG, Donovan WH. Construct validity and dimensional structure of the ASIA motor scale. J Spinal Cord Med. 2006. https://doi.org/10.1080/10790268.2006.11753855.
7. Catz A, Greenberg E, Itzkovich M, Bluvshtein V, Ronen J, Gelernter I. A new instrument for outcome assessment in rehabilitation medicine: spinal cord injury ability realization measurement index. Arch Phys Med Rehabil. 2004. https://doi.org/10.1016/S0003-9993(03)00475-1.
8. Scivoletto G, Glass C, Anderson KD, et al. An international age- and gender-controlled model for the spinal cord injury ability realization measurement index

(SCI-ARMI). Neurorehabil Neural Repair. 2015. https://doi.org/10.1177/1545968314524631.

9. Krassioukov A, Wolfe DL, Hsieh JTC, Hayes KC, Durham CE. Quantitative sensory testing in patients with incomplete spinal cord injury. Arch Phys Med Rehabil. 1999;80(10):1258–63. https://doi.org/10.1016/S0003-9993(99)90026-6.

10. Felix ER, Widerström-Noga EG. Reliability and validity of quantitative sensory testing in persons with spinal cord injury and neuropathic pain. J Rehabil Res Dev. 2009. https://doi.org/10.1682/JRRD.2008.04.0058.

11. Yugué I, Okada S, Masuda M, Ueta T, Maeda T, Shiba K. "Knee-up test" for easy detection of postoperative motor deficits following spinal surgery. Spine J. 2016. https://doi.org/10.1016/j.spinee.2016.08.015.

12. Yugué I, Okada S, Maeda T, Ueta T, Shiba K. Sensitivity and specificity of the "knee-up test" for estimation of the American spinal injury association impairment scale in patients with acute motor incomplete cervical spinal cord injury. Spinal Cord. 2018. https://doi.org/10.1038/s41393-017-0046-y.

13. Haas BM, Bergström E, Jamous A, Bennie A. The inter rater reliability of the original and of the modified Ashworth scale for the assessment of spasticity in patients with spinal cord injury. Spinal Cord. 1996. https://doi.org/10.1038/sc.1996.100.

14. Craven BC, Morris AR. Modified Ashworth scale reliability for measurement of lower extremity spasticity among patients with SCI. Spinal Cord. 2010. https://doi.org/10.1038/sc.2009.107.

15. Smith AW, Jamshidi M, Lo SK. Clinical measurement of muscle tone using a velocity-corrected modified Ashworth scale. Am J Phys Med Rehabil. 2002. https://doi.org/10.1097/00002060-200203000-00008.

16. Baunsgaard CB, Nissen UV, Christensen KB, Biering-Sørensen F. Modified Ashworth scale and spasm frequency score in spinal cord injury: reliability and correlation. Spinal Cord. 2016. https://doi.org/10.1038/sc.2015.230.

17. Akpinar P, Atici A, Kurt KN, Ozkan FU, Aktas I, Kulcu DG. Reliability and cross-cultural adaptation of the Turkish version of the spinal cord injury spasticity evaluation tool. Int J Rehabil Res. 2017. https://doi.org/10.1097/MRR.0000000000000223.

18. Mishra C, Ganesh GS. Inter-Rater reliability of modified modified Ashworth scale in the assessment of plantar flexor muscle spasticity in patients with spinal cord injury. Physiother Res Int. 2014. https://doi.org/10.1002/pri.1588.

19. Adams MM, Ginis KAM, Hicks AL. The spinal cord injury spasticity evaluation tool: development and evaluation. Arch Phys Med Rehabil. 2007. https://doi.org/10.1016/j.apmr.2007.06.012.

20. Sweatman WM, Heinemann AW, Furbish CL, Field-Fote EC. Modified PRISM and SCI-SET spasticity measures for persons with traumatic spinal cord injury: results of a Rasch analyses. Arch

Phys Med Rehabil. 2020. https://doi.org/10.1016/j.apmr.2020.05.012.

21. Ansari NN, Kashi M, Naghdi S. The spinal cord injury spasticity evaluation tool: a Persian adaptation and validation study. J Spinal Cord Med. 2017. https://doi.org/10.1080/10790268.2016.1195941.

22. Benz EN, Hornby TG, Bode RK, Scheidt RA, Schmit BD. A physiologically based clinical measure for spastic reflexes in spinal cord injury. Arch Phys Med Rehabil. 2005. https://doi.org/10.1016/j.apmr.2004.01.033.

23. Akpinar P, Atici A, Ozkan FU, Aktas I, Kulcu DG, Kurt KN. Reliability of the spinal cord assessment tool for spastic reflexes. Arch Phys Med Rehabil. 2017. https://doi.org/10.1016/j.apmr.2016.09.119.

24. Cook KF, Teal CR, Engebretson JC, et al. Development and validation of patient reported impact of spasticity measure (PRISM). J Rehabil Res Dev. 2007. https://doi.org/10.1682/JRRD.2006.04.0036.

25. Jonsson M, Tollbäck A, Gonzales H, Borg J. Inter-rater reliability of the 1992 international standards for neurological and functional classification of incomplete spinal cord injury. Spinal Cord. 2000. https://doi.org/10.1038/sj.sc.3101067.

26. Klose KJ, Green BA, Smith RS, Adkins RH, MacDonald AM. University of Miami neuro-spinal index (UMNI): a quantitative method for determining spinal cord function. Spinal Cord. 1980;18(5):331–6. https://doi.org/10.1038/sc.1980.60.

27. Taricco M, Apolone G, Colombo C, Filardo G, Telaro E, Liberati A. Functional status in patients with spinal cord injury: a new standardized measurement scale. Arch Phys Med Rehabil. 2000. https://doi.org/10.1053/apmr.2000.7161.

28. Kumar R, Arora S, Mohapatra D. Cervical spine injury recovery prediction scale: a means of predicting neurological recovery in patients with acute subaxial cervical spine injury. J Orthop Surg (Hong Kong). 2011. https://doi.org/10.1177/230949901101900106.

29. Chehrazi B, Wagner FC, Collins WF, Freeman DH. A scale for evaluation of spinal cord injury. J Neurosurg. 1981;54(3):310–5. https://doi.org/10.3171/jns.1981.54.3.0310.

30. Joghtaei M, Arab AM, Hashemi-Nasl H, Joghataei MT, Tokhi MO. Assessment of passive knee stiffness and viscosity in individuals with spinal cord injury using pendulum test. J Spinal Cord Med. 2015. https://doi.org/10.1179/2045772314Y.0000000265.

31. Platz T, Vuadens P, Eickhof C, Arnold P, Van Kaick S, Heise K. REPAS, a summary rating scale for resistance to passive movement: item selection, reliability and validity. Disabil Rehabil. 2008. https://doi.org/10.1080/09638280701191743.

32. Mills PB, Vakil AP, Phillips C, Kei L, Kwon BK. Intra-rater and inter-rater reliability of the Penn spasm frequency scale in people with chronic traumatic spinal cord injury. Spinal Cord. 2018. https://doi.org/10.1038/s41393-018-0063-5.

Psychological Evaluation in Spinal Cord Injury

Maria Auxiliadora Marquez,
Jeronimo Gonzàlez-Bernal, Giulia Grieco,
Marina D'Angelo, Antonella Conte,
and Francescaroberta Panuccio

1   Introduction

Spinal cord injury (SCI) is a health condition with severe consequences on a physical, social, and psychological level. These difficulties represent huge challenges for the affected persons and may severely impact daily activities and participation [1].

Adjustment after an SCI presents a formidable challenge. While the primary emphasis on adjustment is with physical function, psychological adjustment presents an ancillary challenge. Depression following SCI is common and is the most frequently cited psychological issue in SCI populations. Depression following SCI is concerning because of its negative influence on the rehabilitation process, increased hospitalization, decreased longevity, increased suicide rates, restricted community participation and reduced health, and daily functioning are all plausible consequences. The incidence of anxiety and depression in SCI exceeds that of the general population, with psychological morbidity or psychological distress estimates ranging between 20 and 30%, suggesting the need for appropriate screening tools in these patients. Therefore, accurate assessment is important for interventions aimed at reducing morbidity and mortality in SCI [2].

This chapter aims to describe and evaluate assessment tools on psychology in people with SCI through a systematic review.

2   Materials and Methods

This study was conducted by a research group composed of medical doctors and health professionals from the "Sapienza" University of Rome and the "Rehabilitation & Outcome Measure Assessment" (R.O.M.A.) association. Within the last few years, R.O.M.A. has been involved in conducting several studies and validating many outcome measures for the Italian Spinal Cord Injury population [3–16].

This chapter describes all assessment tools regarding the quality of life resulting from a systematic review conducted on Pubmed, Scopus, and web of science. For specific details on the methodology, see chapter "Methodological

M. Auxiliadora Marquez
Universidad Fernando Pessoa-Canarias,
Las Palmas, Spain

J. Gonzàlez-Bernal
Health Sciences, University of Burgos, Burgos, Spain

G. Grieco · M. D'Angelo · F. Panuccio (✉)
R.O.M.A. Rehabilitation Outcome Measures
Assessment, Non-Profit Organization, Rome, Italy

A. Conte
Department of Human Neurosciences, Sapienza
University of Rome, Rome, Italy

IRCSS Neuromed, Pozzilli, Italy

approach to identifying outcome measures in Spinal Cord Injury." The eligibility criteria for consideration of studies for this chapter were validation studies and cross-cultural adaptation studies, studies about the psychological area, studies about tests, questionnaires, self-reported and performance-based outcome measures, studies with a population of people with SCI and population ≥18 years old. Study selection: the study selection was conducted following the 27-item PRISM Statement for Reporting Systematic Reviews [17]. For the data collection, the authors followed recommendations from the

COnsensus-based Standards for the selection of health Measurement Instruments (COSMIN) initiative [18]. Study quality and risk of bias were assessed using COSMIN checklist [19, 20].

3   Results

For this chapter, 77 papers were considered. The authors found 46 assessment tools that evaluate the psychological area in persons with SCI. In Fig. 1, a flow chart of included studies is reported.

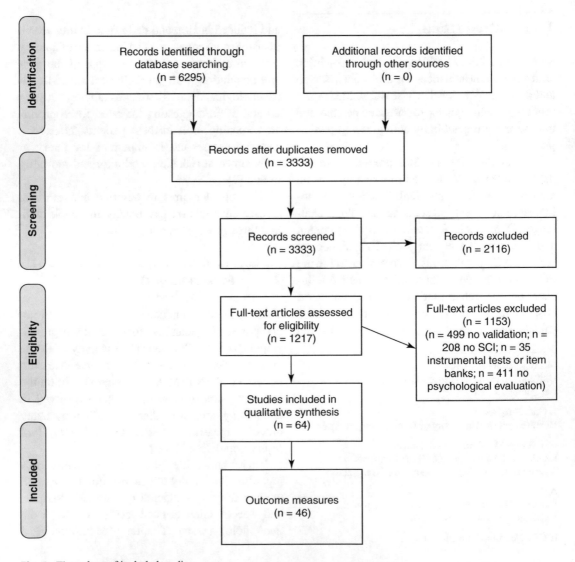

Fig. 1 Flow chart of included studies

3.1 Center for Epidemiologic Studies Depression Scale (CESD)

The CESD was originally developed to screen for the frequency of symptoms of depression in the general population. It was validated for people with SCI in English [2, 21]. The questions for this tool were generated by selecting items from previously validated tools. Its components cover elements related to depressed mood, feelings of guilt and worthlessness, helplessness and hopelessness, psychomotor retardation, appetite loss, and sleep disturbance. Responses capture the frequency of feelings and behaviors over the past 7 days and are rated on a 4-point scale ranging from 0 (rarely or none of the time) to 3 (most or all of the time). Items numbered 4, 8, 12, and 16 are scored in reverse. Once assembled, an aggregate score is calculated by summing the scores with higher scores suggesting greater levels of depressive symptoms. Reported scores of over 15 indicate depression in the general population based on DSM III criteria. Table 1 summarizes the papers' authors and languages and Table 2 shows the quality of the studies.

Table 1 Characteristics of the studies validating CESD

Authors	Language	n	Age mean (SD, range) year	Gender % Female
Miller et al. [2]	English	47	40.6 (12.6)	17 (36)
Chung et al. [21]	English	238	47.3(14.1)	98 (38.7)

n number of participants of the study, *n.a.* not available

Table 2 Evaluation of quality and risk of bias

Authors	Item of COSMIN checklist									
	1	2	3	4	5	6	7	8	9	10
Miller et al. [2]	?	+	−	+	+	+	−	+	+	−
Chung et al. [21]	?	?	+	−	−	−	−	+	+	−

Item 1 PROM development, *Item 2* content validity, *Item 3* structural validity, *Item 4* internal consistency, *Item 5* cross-cultural validity/measurement invariance, Item 6 reliability, *Item 7* measurement error, *Item 8* criterion validity, *Item 9* hypothesis testing for construct validity, *Item 10* responsiveness, + sufficient, − insufficient, ? indeterminate

3.2 Patient Health Questionnaire-9 (PHQ-9)

Spitzer, Kroenke, Williams developed the PHQ-9 in 1999. It was validated in English [21–29], Arabic (Lebanon) [30], and Luganda [31]. It is a self-report depression measure that asks subject to show often they have been bothered by the following problems within the past 2 weeks: (1) little pleasure or interest in doing things; (2) feeling down, depressed, or hopeless; (3) sleeping too little or too much; (4) feeling tired or having little energy; (5) poor appetite or overeating; (6) feelings of worth lessness or guilt; (7) concentration problems; (8) psychomotor retardation or agitation; and (9) thoughts of suicide. Subjects rate how often each symptom occurred: 0 (not at all), 1 (several days), 2 (more than half the days), or 3 (nearly every day). The PHQ-9 has excellent internal and test–retest reliability and a criterion and construct validity in medical samples. It also has been validated for administration over the telephone. The PHQ-9 score has a range between 0 and 27. Classifieds between 5 and 9 recommendations for the severity of depression. The cutoff score of 10 is optimal for highlighting depression of clinical relevance. There are several versions of this instrument: 12 items (PHQ-12, validated in Italian by Piccinelli, Bisoffi et al, 1993), 8 items (PHQ-8), 2 items (PHQ-2). The PHQ-2 is also validated for the SCI population in Luganda [31]. Table 3 summarizes the papers' authors and languages and Table 4 shows the quality of the studies.

3.3 Appraisals of Disability: Primary and Secondary Scale (ADAPSS)

The ADAPSS, created [32] and validated for people with SCI in English [33, 34], consists of 33 items rated on a six-point Likert-type scale, ranging from "strongly disagree" to "strongly agree." Using principal-component factor analysis, the authors identified six independent appraisal factors, including (1) fearful despondency, (2) overwhelming disbelief, (3) determined

Table 3 Characteristics of the studies validating PHQ-9 and PHQ-2

Scale, test or Questionnaire	Authors	Language	n	Age mean (SD, range) year	Gender % Female
PHQ-9	Kalpakjian et al. [22]	English	1168	41 (13.1)	585 (50.1)
	Williams et al. [29]	English	202	42.6 (13.9, 18-80)	67 (33)
	Richardson and Richards [28]	English	682	38.66 (15.32)	147 (21)
	Chung et al. [21]	English	3694	40.4 (16)	858 (23.23)
	Poritz et al. [23]	English	116	56 (12.4)	4 (3.4)
	Summaka et al. [30]	Arabic (Lebanon)	51	37.2 (12.6)	51 (100)
	Bombardier et al. [24]	English	142	42.2 (16.6, 18–88)	31 (21.8)
	Krause et al. [25]	English	7296	n.a.	n.a.
	Krause et al. [27]	English	584	32.4 (11.9)	123 (21)
	Williams et al. [26]	English	133	40 (11)	34 (26)
	Nakku et al. [31]	Luganda	n.a.	n.a.	n.a.
PHQ-2	Nakku et al. [31]	Luganda	n.a.	n.a.	n.a.

n number of participants of the study, *n.a.* not available

Table 4 Evaluation of quality and risk of bias

	Item of COSMIN checklist									
Authors	1	2	3	4	5	6	7	8	9	10
Kalpakjian et al. [22]	?	?	+	−	+	−	−	−	−	−
Williams et al. [29]	?	?	+	−	−	−	−	−	−	−
Richardson and Richards [28]	?	?	+	−	+	−	−	−	−	−
Chung et al. [21]	?	?	+	−	−	−	−	+	+	−
Poritz et al. [23]	?	?	+	−	−	−	−	+	+	−
Summaka et al. [30]	?	?	+	+	+	+	−	+	+	−
Bombardier et al. [24]	?	?	−	−	+	−	−	+	+	−
Krause et al. [25]	?	?	+	−	−	−	−	−	−	−
Krause et al. [27]	?	?	+	−	+	−	−	+	+	+
Williams et al. [26]	?	+	−	−	+	−	−	+	+	+
Nakku et al. [31]	?	+	+	−	+	−	−	−	−	−
Nakku et al. [31]	?	+	+	−	−	−	−	−	−	−

Item 1 PROM development, *Item 2* content validity, *Item 3* structural validity, *Item 4* internal consistency, *Item 5* cross-cultural validity/measurement invariance, *Item 6* reliability, *Item 7* measurement error, *Item 8* criterion validity, *Item 9* hypothesis testing for construct validity, *Item 10* responsiveness, + sufficient, − insufficient, ? indeterminate

resolve, (4) growth and resilience, (5) negative perceptions of disability, and (6) personal agency. Second-order factor analysis of those six factors revealed two broader appraisal patterns, namely, "determined resilience" (comprising the determined resolve, growth and resilience, and personal agency factors) and "catastrophic negativity" (comprising the fearful despondency, overwhelming disbelief, and negative perceptions of disability factors). Whereas catastrophic negativity may be similar to primary appraisals and perceptions of loss and threat, determined resilience may reflect

secondary appraisals of coping and resource. The short version (ADAPSS-SF) is a 6-item measure. Higher scores indicate more negative appraisals, which are indicative of negative adjustment and maladaptive coping strategies. Resilience items "determined resolve," "growth and resilience," and "personal agency" are reverse-coded; therefore, individuals obtain a lower score by endorsing positive appraisals. It was validated in English for SCI people in 2018 [35, 36]. Table 5 summarizes the papers' authors and languages and Table 6 shows the quality of the studies.

Table 5 Characteristics of the studies validating ADPSS and ADAPSS-SF

Scale, test, or questionnaire	Authors	Language	n	Age mean (SD, range) year	Gender % Female
ADAPSS	Dean and Kennedy [32]	English	237	47 (18–81)	76 (32)
	Mignogna et al. [33]	English	98	56.17 (12.9)	4 (4)
	Mcdonald et al. [34]	English	262	57.94 (13.12, 24–90)	11 (4.2)
ADAPSS-SF	Eaton et al. [35]	English	371	53 (15–91)	110 (30)
	Deane et al. [36]	English	115	37.44 (7.85)	48 (41.7)
	Russel et al. [37]	English	90	n.a.	4 (4.4)

n number of participants of the study, *n.a.* not available

Table 6 Evaluation of quality and risk of bias

Authors	Item of COSMIN checklist									
	1	2	3	4	5	6	7	8	9	10
Dean and Kennedy [32]	+	+	+	+	+	+	−	+	+	−
Mignogna et al. [33]	?	?	+	−	+	−	−	+	+	−
Mcdonald et al. [34]	?	?	+	−	+	−	−	+	+	−
Eaton et al. [35]	?	+	+	−	−	−	−	+	+	−
Deane et al. [36]	?	+	+	−	+	−	−	−	−	−
Russel (2020)	?	?	−	−	+	−	−	+	+	−

Item 1 PROM development, *Item 2* content validity, *Item 3* structural validity, *Item 4* internal consistency, *Item 5* cross-cultural validity/measurement invariance, *Item 6* reliability, *Item 7* measurement error, *Item 8* criterion validity, *Item 9* hypothesis testing for construct validity, *Item 10* responsiveness, + sufficient, − insufficient, ? indeterminate

Table 7 Characteristics of the studies validating BSI

Authors	Language	n	Age mean (SD, range) year	Gender % Female
Tate [38]	English	288	31.33 (12.3, 18–65)	55 (20)
Heintich and Tate [39]	English	215	35.2 (14.3, 18–70)	45 (21)

n number of participants of the study, *n.a.* not available

ber of symptoms (PST); the average intensity of positive symptoms (PDSI), and the average item response (GSI). Table 7 summarizes the papers' authors and languages and Table 8 shows the quality of the studies.

3.4 Brief Symptom Inventory (BSI)

The BSI was validated in the United States for people with SCI in 1994 [39]. It is a self-report inventory designed to assess overall distress and/or adjustment. The BSI is an abbreviated version of the Symptom Checklist 90 containing 53 items distributed across nine subscales of distress (somatization; obsessive-compulsive; interpersonal sensitivity; depression; anxiety; hostility; phobic anxiety; paranoid ideation; and psychoticism). Patients are asked to rate how much each symptom or problem has been distressful during the past week, using a Likert-type scale. The test also provides global indices of distress and psychological dysfunction: the total num-

3.5 Hospital Anxiety and Depression Scale (HADS)

The HADS has been developed to measure anxiety and depression disorders among patients in nonpsychiatric hospital clinics. The German version was validated in individuals with SCI in 2012 [40]. The HADS focuses on affective and cognitive rather than somatic aspects. Therefore, it can be used in health conditions accompanied by problems similar to the symptoms of depression, such as loss of appetite, fatigue, or sleep disturbance. The HADS was reliable and valid in assessing the symptom severity and caseness of anxiety disorder and depression in somatic, psychiatric, primary care, and general populations. It is also frequently used in SCI. The HADS is a self-report questionnaire comprising of 14 items, which can be summed to provide a total score (HADS-T) as well as two subscales with 7 items

Table 8 Evaluation of quality and risk of bias

Authors	Item of COSMIN checklist									
	1	2	3	4	5	6	7	8	9	10
Tate (1994)	?	?	–	–	+	–	–	–	–	–
Heintich and Tate [39]	?	?	+	–	+	–	–	+	+	–

Item 1 PROM development, *Item 2* content validity, *Item 3* structural validity, *Item 4* internal consistency, *Item 5* cross-cultural validity/measurement invariance, *Item 6* reliability, *Item 7* measurement error, *Item 8* criterion validity, *Item 9* hypothesis testing for construct validity, *Item 10* responsiveness, + sufficient, – insufficient, ? indeterminate

Table 9 Characteristics of the studies validating HAND

Authors	Language	n	Age mean (SD, range) year	Gender % Female
Tasiemski and Brewer [42]	Poland	1034	35.93 (10.03	173 (16.7)
Müller et al. [40]	German	102	56.5 (16.7)	26 (25.5)
Woolrich et al. [41]	English	936	n.a.	n.a.

n number of participants of the study, *n.a.* not available

Table 10 Evaluation of quality and risk of bias

Authors	Item of COSMIN checklist									
	1	2	3	4	5	6	7	8	9	10
Tasiemski and Brewer [42]	?	+	+	+	+	–	–	+	+	–
Müller et al. [40]	?	?	+	–	+	–	–	+	+	–
Woolrich et al. [41]	?	+	+	–	+	–	–	–	–	–

Item 1 PROM development, *Item 2* content validity, *Item 3* structural validity, *Item 4* internal consistency, *Item 5* cross-cultural validity/measurement invariance, *Item 6* reliability, *Item 7* measurement error, *Item 8* criterion validity, *Item 9* hypothesis testing for construct validity, *Item 10* responsiveness, + sufficient, – insufficient, ? indeterminate

each, assessing anxiety (HADS-A) and depression (HADS-D). Patients are asked to rate how they felt during the past week. Responses are given on a 0–3 Likert-type scale. Higher scores indicate more distress. Scores between 8 and 10 are considered mild cases, 11–15 moderate cases, and 16 or above severe cases [41, 42]. Table 9 summarizes the papers' authors and languages and Table 10 shows the quality of the studies.

3.6 Spinal Cord Lesion-Related Coping Strategies Questionnaire (SCL CSQ)

The SCL CSQ is a specific scale developed to evaluate the coping strategies of persons with SCI [43]. SCL CSQ was translated and validated in English [44, 45], Turkish [46], Spanish [47], Persian [48], and German [45]. The SCL CSQ provides a succinct indication of condition-specific coping mechanisms of acceptance, fighting spirit, and social reliance employed by respondents. Acceptance measures the extent of revaluation of life values, fighting spirit measures efforts to behave independently, and social reliance measures the tendency toward dependent behavior. The scale consists of 12 items mirroring three strategies: acceptance consists of 4 items characterized by the injured person's reforming of life values. It can be rendered as their acceptance of the disease, reinterpretation of life, and attempts to replace the values withheld from their capability because of the lesion. Fighting spirit that consists of 5 items and reflects the effort to conduct independent behavior. The fighting spirit strategy expresses individual efforts to find new goals to lessen the effects of the injury. Social reliance with a 3-item negative strategy is used for the manner of psychologically dependent behavior on others. A four-point scale is used for the assessment: 1. Completely disagree; 2. Somewhat disagree; 3. Agree; 4. Strongly agree. Total score ranges from 1 to 4 points. High scores indicate more utilization of the related strategy. Table 11 summarizes the papers' authors and languages and Table 12 shows the quality of the studies.

Table 11 Characteristics of the studies validating SCI CSQ

Authors	Language	n	Age mean (SD, range) year	Gender % Female
Elfström et al. [43]	German	274	40 (16–95)	70 (25.5)
Elfström et al. [45]	German English	335	49 (12, 20–76)	74 (20.8)
Migliorini et al. [44]	English	443	51.78 (18–86)	97 (22)
Paker et al. [46]	Turkish	100	40.83 (16.21, 17–75)	26 (26)
Sauri et al. (2014)	Spanish	511	49.36 (14.37)	n.a.
Saffari et al. [48]	Persian	220	58.18 (10.32)	56 (25.5)
Elfström et al. [43]	German	274	40 (16–95)	70 (25.5)

n number of participants of the study, *n.a.* not available

Table 12 Evaluation of quality and risk of bias

Authors	Item of COSMIN checklist									
	1	2	3	4	5	6	7	8	9	10
Elfström et al. [43]	+	+	+	–	+	–	–	–	–	–
Elfström et al. [45]	?	+	–	+	+	–	–	+	+	–
Migliorini et al. [44]	?	+	+	–	+	–	–	–	–	–
Paker et al. [46]	?	+	+	+	–	+	–	+	+	–
Sauri et al. [47]	?	+	+	–	+	–	–	+	+	–
Saffari et al. [48]	?	+	+	+	+	–	–	+	+	–

Item 1 PROM development, *Item 2* content validity, *Item 3* structural validity, *Item 4* internal consistency, *Item 5* cross-cultural validity/measurement invariance, *Item 6* reliability, *Item 7* measurement error, *Item 8* criterion validity, *Item 9* hypothesis testing for construct validity, *Item 10* responsiveness, + sufficient, – insufficient, *?* indeterminate

3.7 Nottingham Health Profile (NHP)

NHP Part I was developed in the seventies. It was validated for people with SCI in Dutch in 2001 [49, 50]. The NHP Part I contains 38 questions in six scales measuring physical mobility, pain, emotional reactions, sleep, social isolation, and energy. The number of items in each scale range from 3 to 9. All items are statements concerning health or other problems that are scored dichotomously. In the original version item, scores were weighted for the importance of the item. In the authorized Dutch translation, these item weights have been omitted. For each "yes" answer, one point is added to the raw scale score, and this raw score is transformed to a score between 0 (no quality of life problems) and 100 (very poor quality of life). The NHP contains several questions about mobility impairments that are not suited for wheelchair users. All questions are statements, and only "yes" (applies to my situation) or "no" (does not apply to my situation) answers are allowed. Table 13 summarizes the papers' authors and languages and Table 14 shows the quality of the studies.

Table 13 Characteristics of the studies validating NHP

Authors	Language	n	Age mean (SD, range) year	Gender % Female
Post et al. [49]	Dutch	32	38.2	12 (37.5)
Post et al. [50]	Dutch	33	38.3	13 (37.5)

n number of participants of the study, *n.a.* not available

Table 14 Evaluation of quality and risk of bias

Authors	Item of COSMIN checklist									
	1	2	3	4	5	6	7	8	9	10
Post et al. [49]	?	?	+	–	+	–	–	+	+	–
Post et al. [50]	?	+	–	+	+	–	–	+	+	–

Item 1 PROM development, *Item 2* content validity, *Item 3* structural validity, *Item 4* internal consistency, *Item 5* cross-cultural validity/measurement invariance, *Item 6* reliability, *Item 7* measurement error, *Item 8* criterion validity, *Item 9* hypothesis testing for construct validity, *Item 10* responsiveness, + sufficient, – insufficient, *?* indeterminate

3.8 Sickness Impact Profile 68 (SIP)

The final version of the original SIP was published in 1981. It was validated for people with SCI in Dutch in 1996 [49, 51]. The SIP measures health status by assessing the way health problems change daily activities and behavior, which can be reliably reported and can be verified by observation. The SIP, taking 20–30 min to complete, has been considered to be an obstacle to its routine use. The SIP68 is an abbreviated generic version of the SIP. It consists of selecting 68 SIP items on six new scales, measuring physical, mental, and social aspects of health-related functioning: Somatic Autonomy, Mobility Control, Mobility Range, Social Behavior, Emotional Stability, and Psychological Autonomy and Communication. The SIP68 was judged useful in various rehabilitation groups, like chronic pain or whiplash, traumatic brain injury, and spinal cord injury. For each item of the SIP68, respondents are asked whether, at the moment of the interview, a certain "sickness impact" exists. All items are scored dichotomously (no = 0, yes = 1) and the number of confirmed sickness impacts make up the scale scores and the total scores. The instrument has five domains: (1) access, (2) perceptions and attitudes of others, (3) social and sexual relationships, (4) physical health, and (5) adjustment and loss of independence. The instrument includes 40 items with 7–9 items under each domain. In completing the questionnaire, participants are asked to think about the disability-specific situations mentioned in the items and to indicate how stressful these situations are for them on a scale of 1–5 (1, not at all; 2, slightly; 3, moderately; 4, considerably; 5, highly). Participants are also given the option of circling NA (not applicable) for situations they have not experienced. Table 15 summarizes the papers' authors and languages and Table 16 shows the quality of the studies.

3.9 Sydney Psychosocial Reintegration Scale (SPRS) and SPRS-2

The SPRS was validated for people with SCI in Australia [52]. SPRS is a 12-item question-

Table 15 Characteristics of the studies validating SIP

Authors	Language	n	Age mean (SD, range) year	Gender % Female
Post et al. [51]	Dutch	315	39.4 (12.4, 18–65)	76 (24.6)
Post et al. [49]	Dutch	32	38.2	12 (37.5)

n number of participants of the study, *n.a.* not available

Table 16 Evaluation of quality and risk of bias

Authors	Item of COSMIN checklist									
	1	2	3	4	5	6	7	8	9	10
Post et al. [51]	+	+	+	+	−	−	−	−	−	−
Post et al. [49]	?	?	+	−	+	−	−	+	+	−

Item 1 PROM development, *Item 2* content validity, *Item 3* structural validity, *Item 4* internal consistency, *Item 5* cross-cultural validity/measurement invariance, *Item 6* reliability, *Item 7* measurement error, *Item 8* criterion validity, *Item 9* hypothesis testing for construct validity, *Item 10* responsiveness, + sufficient, − insufficient, ? indeterminate

naire, with 4 items in each domain: Occupation, Relationships, and Living Skills. There are two formats for the SPRS that differ by question phrasing: Form A measures change from the pre-injury level, and Form B measures the current competency level. This measure can be completed by the person who sustained the injury, a clinician, or a significant other. The current article utilized self-rated Form B. Ratings are made on a 7-point scale from "very good" to "very poor." The SPRS results in three domain scores (range: 0–24) and a total score (range: 0–72), with higher scores indicating better psychosocial functioning. In 2012, the second version in English was validated [53]. Table 17 summarizes the papers' authors and languages and Table 18 shows the quality of the studies.

3.10 University of Washington Self-Efficacy Scale (UWSES)

In 2012, Amtmann et al. developed a self-efficacy scale for people living with multiple sclerosis (MS) and SCI, in the United States [54]. In 2012, M.W.M. Post et al. validated and translated

Table 17 Characteristics of the studies validating SPRS and SPRS-2

Scale, test, or questionnaire	Authors	Language	n	Age mean (SD, range) year	Gender % Female
SPRS	De Wolf et al. [52]	English	58	35.3 (15.2)	13 (22)
SPRS-2	Tate et al. [53]	English	50	37.22 (14.93)	11 (22)

n number of participants of the study, *n.a.* not available

Table 18 Evaluation of quality and risk of bias

Authors	Item of COSMIN checklist									
	1	2	3	4	5	6	7	8	9	10
De Wolf et al. [52]	+	+	+	+	+	+	−	+	+	−
Tate et al. [53]	?	?	+	−	+	−	−	+	+	−

Item 1 PROM development, *Item 2* content validity, *Item 3* structural validity, *Item 4* internal consistency, *Item 5* cross-cultural validity/measurement invariance, *Item 6* reliability, *Item 7* measurement error, *Item 8* criterion validity, *Item 9* hypothesis testing for construct validity, *Item 10* responsiveness, + sufficient, − insufficient, *?* indeterminate

Table 19 Characteristics of the studies validating UWSES

Authors	Language	n	Age mean (SD, range) year	Gender % Female
Amtmann et al. [54]	English	253	47.1 (14.3, 18-85)	94 (37.2)
Post et al. [55]	Dutch	261	48.5 (8.8)	70 (26.4)

n number of participants of the study, *n.a.* not available

Table 20 Evaluation of quality and risk of bias

Authors	Item of COSMIN checklist									
	1	2	3	4	5	6	7	8	9	10
Amtmann et al. [54]	+	+	+	+	+	−	−	+	+	−
Post et al. [55]	?	?	+	−	+	−	−	−	−	−

Item 1 PROM development, *Item 2* content validity, *Item 3* structural validity, *Item 4* internal consistency, *Item 5* cross-cultural validity/measurement invariance, *Item 6* reliability, *Item 7* measurement error, *Item 8* criterion validity, *Item 9* hypothesis testing for construct validity, *Item 10* responsiveness, + sufficient, − insufficient, *?* indeterminate

the UWSES into Dutch [55]. The UWSES consists of 17 items, but UW also developed a short form with only 6 items. Table 19 summarizes the papers' authors and languages and Table 20 shows the quality of the studies.

3.11 Spinal Cord Injury–Falls Concern Scale (SCI-FCS)

The SCI-FCS assesses the degree of attention concerning falls in a wheelchair by people with SCI while carrying out daily activities. CL Boswell-Ruys developed the scale in English in 2010 [56]. It was validated in Italy [57] and Sweden [58], Norway [59], and Thailand [60]. The SCI-FCS is an extremely useful tool for determining the degree of comparison with falls but also for determining the weak points in functional mobility training carried out within the spinal area. It is a questionnaire that is self-administered. It contains 16 items. An ordinal scale of four categories is applied to the questionnaire (1 = "not worried at all," 2 = "a little worried," 3 = "quite worried," 4 = "very worried"). Minimum score 16, maximum score 64. Table 21 summarizes the papers' authors and languages and Table 22 shows the quality of the studies.

3.12 Connor–Davidson Resilience Scale (CD-RISC)

The original CD-RISC comprises 25 statements on how one has felt over the past month. The response scale has a 5-point range: 0 (not true at all), 1 (rarely true), 2 (sometimes true), 3 (often true), and 4 (true nearly all of the time). Scores are added up to a maximum score of 100, meaning high revsilience. The shortened version CD-RISC 10 includes 10 items that scored best on salient loadings on the "hardiness" and "persistence" factors, with a maximum overall score of 40. The 2-item CD-RISC 2 includes only statement 1 ("Able to adapt to change") and statement 8 ("Tend to bounce back after illness or hardship") with a maximum score of 8 [61]. Table 23 summarizes the papers' authors and languages and Table 24 shows the quality of the studies.

Table 21 Characteristics of the studies validating SCI-FCS

Authors	Language	n	Age mean (SD, range) year	Gender % Female
Boswell-Ruys et al. [56]	English	125	41 (14)	24 (19.2)
Roaldsen et al. [59]	Norwegian	54	(20–92)	9 (16.6)
Butler Forslund et al. [58]	Swedish	87	(18–79)	12 (13.8)
Marquez et al. [4]	Italian	124	46.2 (15)	24 (19)
Pramod-hyakul and Pramod-hyakul [60]	Thai	54	31.8 (9.5, 18–56)	11 (20)

n number of participants of the study, *n.a.* not available

Table 22 Evaluation of quality and risk of bias

Authors	Item of COSMIN checklist									
	1	2	3	4	5	6	7	8	9	10
Boswell-Ruys et al. [56]	+	+	−	+	+	+	−	+	+	−
Roaldsen et al. [59]	?	+	−	+	−	+	+	−	−	−
Butler Forslund et al. [58]	?	+	+	−	+	−	−	+	+	−
Marquez et al. [4]	?	+	−	+	−	+	−	+	+	−
Pramod-hyakul and Pramod-hyakul [60]	?	+	−	+	+	+	−	−	−	−

Item 1 PROM development, *Item 2* content validity, *Item 3* structural validity, *Item 4* internal consistency, *Item 5* cross-cultural validity/measurement invariance, *Item 6* reliability, *Item 7* measurement error, *Item 8* criterion validity, *Item 9* hypothesis testing for construct validity, *Item 10* responsiveness, + sufficient, − insufficient, ? indeterminate

Table 23 Characteristics of the studies validating CD-RISC

Scale, test or Questionnaire	Authors	Language	n	Age mean (SD, range) year	Gender % Female
CD-RISC 25	Kuiper et al. [61]	English	74	55.8 (17.9)	28 (37.8)
CD-RISC 5	Kuiper et al. [61]	English	74	55.8 (17.9)	28 (37.8)
CD-RISC 2	Kuiper et al. [61]	English	74	55.8 (17.9)	28 (37.8)

n number of participants of the study, *n.a.* not available

Table 24 Evaluation of quality and risk of bias

Authors	Item of COSMIN checklist									
	1	2	3	4	5	6	7	8	9	10
Kuiper et al. [61]	?	+	−	+	−	−	−	+	+	−
Kuiper et al. [61]	?	+	−	+	−	−	−	+	+	−
Kuiper et al. [61]	?	+	−	+	−	−	−	+	+	−

Item 1 PROM development, *Item 2* content validity, *Item 3* structural validity, *Item 4* internal consistency, *Item 5* cross-cultural validity/measurement invariance, *Item 6* reliability, *Item 7* measurement error, *Item 8* criterion validity, *Item 9* hypothesis testing for construct validity, *Item 10* responsiveness, + sufficient, − insufficient, ? indeterminate

3.13 Symptom Checklist-90-R (SCL-90-R)

The SCL-90 was validated in English for individuals with SCI in 1988 [62]. This measure includes 90 symptoms of distress rated from 0, representing "not at all," to 4, indicating "extremely." Subjects were instructed to indicate the amount bothered by each of the symptoms. Each subscale total is divided by the number of items in the scale, yielding a total average scale score of 0–4. Scales included in the SCL-90-R are somatization, obsessive-compulsive, interpersonal sensitivity, depression, anxiety, hostility, phobic anxiety, paranoid ideation, and psychoticism. Table 25 summarizes the papers' authors and languages and Table 26 shows the quality of the studies.

3.14 General Self-Efficacy Scale (GSES)

Schwarzer and Jerusalem introduced the GSES in 1995. It was validated for the SCI population in Switzerland [1]. It has been translated into 30 languages and has been extensively used in health research. The GSES consists of 10 items assessing a general belief in one's own ability. For example, item 4 is phrased "I am confident that I could deal efficiently with unexpected events." Items are assessed on a 4-point response scale with 1 = not at all true and 4 = exactly true. All 10 items' responses are summarized to form a total score, ranging from 10 to 40 points, where a higher score indicates higher self-efficacy. Table 25 summarizes the papers' authors and languages and Table 26 shows the quality of the studies.

Table 25 Characteristics of the studies of scale, test, or questionnaire with less than two validations

Scale, test, or questionnaire	Authors	Language	N	Age mean (SD, range) year	Gender % Female
SCL-90-R	Buckelew et al. [62]	English	52	30	8 (15.4)
GSES	Peter et al. [1]	Swiss	101	56.3	25 (24.8)
DASS-21	Mitchell et al. [63]	English	51	(19–82)	10 (19.6)
WRQ-SELF	Bergamaschi [64]	Swiss	9	29.2 (11.7, 18–52)	2 (22.2)
FS	Perera et al. [65]	English	472	53.7 (15.2, 19–93)	89 (18.9)
HRERS	Kortte et al. [66]	English	206	56.7 (17.5, 18–91)	93 (45.1)
HSCL-20	Williams et al. [26]	English	133	40 (11)	34 (26)
PROMIS-D-8	Chung et al. [21]	English	292	49.2 (13.4)	96 (33)
LS	Robinson-Whelen et al. [67]	English	175	49.5 (1.9)	40 (22.9)
CIM	De Wolf et al. [52]	English	58	35.3 (15.2)	13 (22)
CSES	Smedema et al. [68]	English	247	(20-72)	123 (49)
GHQ-28	Griffiths et al. [69]	English	60	33.8 (27-47)	14 (23)
PDSS	Furlong and Connor [70]	English	41	n.a.	n.a.
PETSCSC	Prabhala et al. [71]	Albanian	34	54.71 (14.2)	15 (44.12)
SCL-EWQ	Migliorini et al. [44]	English	443	51.78 (18–86)	97 (22)
CQW	Margaret Wineman et al. [72]	English	690	46 (13, 19–82)	379 (55)
GHAS	Bermond [73]	Dutch	44	34.6 (10.8, 19–64)	
SNAPS	Smyth et al. [74]	English	80	50.2 (15.9, 19–89)	21 (26.25)
MMPI-2	Barncord and Wanlass [75]	English	17	41.7 (18–77)	5 (29.4)
MEDS	Overholser et al. [76]	English	81	36.1 (14.5)	18 (19.8)
AIMS	Tasiemski and Brewer [42]	Poland	1034	35.93 (10.03	173 (16.7)
CSQ24	Harland and Georgieff [77]	English	214	48.6 (12.6)	117 (56.1)
HAM-D	Williams et al. [26]	English	133	40 (11)	34 (26)
THS	Smedema et al. [78]	English	242	44.6 (13.2, 18–81)	82 (33.9)
AAQ	Kortte et al. [79]	English	n.a.	n.a.	n.a.
ASQ	Iwanaga et al. [81]	English	108	49.8 (11.8, 21–69)	34 (31.5)
MALS	Ferrin et al. [82]	English	161	46.9 (15.15)	37 (23)
LS	Niemeier et al. [83]	English	34	n.a.	n.a.
RHDS	De Lange et al. [84]	English South Africa	50	n.a.	20 (30)

n number of participants of the study, *n.a.* not available

Table 26 Evaluation of quality and risk of bias

Authors	Item of COSMIN checklist									
	1	2	3	4	5	6	7	8	9	10
Buckelew et al. [62]	?	?	−	+	+	−	−	+	+	−
Peter et al. [1]	?	?	+	−	−	−	−	−	−	−
Mitchell et al. [63]	?	?	−	−	+	−	−	+	+	−
Bergamaschi [64]	?	?	−	−	+	−	−	+	+	−
Perera et al. [65]	?	?	+	+	−	−	−	+	+	−
Kortte et al. [66]	+	+	+	+	+	+	−	+	+	−
Williams et al. [26]	?	+	−	−	+	−	−	+	+	+
Chung et al. [21]	?	?	+	−	−	−	−	+	+	−
Robinson-Whelen et al. [67]	?	?	+	−	+	−	−	−	−	−
De Wolf et al. [52]	?	+	−	+	+	+	+	+	+	+
Smedema et al. [68]	?	?	+	−	−	−	−	+	+	−
Griffiths et al. [69]	?	?	−	−	+	−	−	+	+	−
Furlong and Connor [70]	?	?	+	−	−	−	−	−	−	−
Prabhala et al. [71]	?	?	−	−	+	−	−	+	+	−
M−igliorini et al. [44]	?	+	+	−	+	−	−	−	−	−
Margaret Wineman et al. [72]	?	?	+	−	−	−	−	−	−	−
Bermond [73]	?	?	−	−	+	−	−	−	−	−
Smyth et al. [74]	+	+	−	+	−	+	−	−	−	−
Barncord and Wanlass [75]	+	+	−	−	+	−	−	−	−	−
Overholser et al. [76]	+	+	−	+	+	−	−	−	+	−
Tasiemski and Brewer [42]	?	+	+	+	+	−	−	+	+	−
Harland and Georgieff [77]	+	+	+	−	−	−	−	−	−	−
Williams et al. [26]	?	+	−	−	+	−	−	+	+	+
Smedema et al. [78]	?	+	+	+	+	+	−	+	+	−
Kortte et al. [79]	?	?	+	+	−	−	−	+	+	−
Iwanaga et al. [81]	+	+	−	−	−	−	−	+	+	−
Ferrin et al. [82]	?	?	+	+	−	−	−	−	−	−
Niemeier et al. [83]	?	?	−	−	+	−	−	+	+	−
De Lange et al. [84]	?	+	−	+	−	−	−	+	+	−

Item 1 PROM development, *Item 2* content validity, *Item 3* structural validity, *Item 4* internal consistency, *Item 5* cross-cultural validity/measurement invariance, *Item 6* reliability, *Item 7* measurement error, *Item 8* criterion validity, *Item 9* hypothesis testing for construct validity, *Item 10* responsiveness, + sufficient, − insufficient, ? indeterminate

3.15 Depression Anxiety Stress Scale-21 (DASS-21)

The DASS-21 was validated for people with SCI in Australia [63]. It is a 21-item questionnaire with three 7-item subscales: Depression, Anxiety, and Stress. Items consist of statements referring to the past week, and each item is scored on a 4-point scale (0 = "Did not apply to me at all," to 3¼ "Applied to me very much, or most of the time"). Subscale scores are calculated as the sum of the responses to the 7 items from each subscale multiplied by 2. DASS-21 is derived from DASS, which is a 42-item measure of the same three constructs. DASS-21 factor structure is similar to DASS but has lower factor intercorrelations. Higher mean loadings and fewer cross loadings DASS-21 is quick and easy to administer, requiring less than 10 min complete, and excludes many somatic items that may not be relevant to those with SCI. Table 25 summarizes the papers' authors and languages and Table 26 shows the quality of the studies.

3.16 Work Rehabilitation Questionnaire Self-Report Version (WORQ-SELF)

The WORK-SEFL was validated for people with SCI in Switzerland [64]. The initial version of WORQ was interview-administered. Its psychometric properties (test–retest reliability, internal consistency, construct/content validity, and feasibility) were established in a population of patients with various health conditions participating in a return to work program. A self-reported version (WORQ-SELF) containing 40 functioning questions and 18 sociodemographic and work-related questions representing 46 ICF categories was developed to promote better practicability and feasibility in the clinical setting. Table 25 summarizes the papers' authors and languages and Table 26 shows the quality of the studies.

3.17 Flourishing Scale (FS)

The FS was validated in the United States for the SCI population [65]. It is one of few comprehensive and brief measurement instruments available to capture Eudaimonic well-being that is not condition-specific. The FS has 8 items, each measuring core aspects of social psychological functioning: purpose and meaning, supportive relationships engagement, contribution to the well-being of others, competence, self-acceptance, optimism, and feeling respected. The FS is composed of 8 items on a 7-point scale ranging from 1 (strongly disagree) to 7 (strongly agree). Total scores range from 8 to 56. Higher scores indicate that respondents view themselves in positive terms in diverse areas of human functioning. Table 25 summarizes the papers' authors and languages and Table 26 shows the quality of the studies.

3.18 Hopkins Rehabilitation Engagement Rating Scale (HRERS)

Kortte, Johnson-Greene, Wegener introduced HRERS, and it was validated in the United States

for people with SCI [66]. It is a clinician-rated measure that quantifies a patient's engagement in rehabilitation activities through behavioral observations. The HRERS is a 5-item scale for use in rating behavioral observations of patients during acute in-patient rehabilitation. The HRERS items rate to evaluate the elements of engagement in rehabilitation activities, including the following: levels of attendance at therapy sessions, attitudes expressed by the patient toward his/her therapy, the need for verbal or physical prompts to facilitate initiation or maintenance of engagement within the therapy session, the patient's acknowledgment of the need for therapy, and the patient's level of active participation in the therapy. The behavioral observations made by a therapist are rated on a 6-point scale, ranging from "never" to "always." Each patient was rated by one physical therapist and one occupational therapist; each was instructed to rate the patient's participation in his/her portion of the rehabilitation program. The ratings were completed at the time of discharge and represented a summary of the therapist's observations during the patient's rehabilitation stay. Table 25 summarizes the papers' authors and languages and Table 26 shows the quality of the studies.

3.19 Patient-Reported Outcome Measurement Information System (PROMIS-D-8)

The PROMIS-D-8 (8b short form) was validated for people with SCI in English (United States) [21]. It consists of 8 items derived from an item bank scored using item response theory that measures cognitive and affective symptoms. The time frame for PROMIS depression is the past 7 days, and scores for each item range from 1 to 5 (1 = never; 2 = rarely; 3 = sometimes; 4 = often; and 5 = always). Higher scores indicate more depressive symptoms. Test–retest reliability has been reported to range from .66 to .78. Table 25 summarizes the papers' authors and languages and Table 26 shows the quality of the studies.

3.20   3-Item Loneliness Scale (LS)

S. Robinson-Whelen et al. worked in Houston, TX, USA, to examine a measure of loneliness and its correlates in people with spinal cord injury [67]. Loneliness was measured using the 3-item Loneliness Scale, an abbreviated version of the 20-item Revised UCLA Loneliness Scale. The 3-item Loneliness Scale has been shown to have satisfactory reliability and concurrent and discriminant validity in a large U.S. Population. The scale asks how often respondents feel they lack companionship, feel left out, and feel isolated from others. Rated from 1 (hardly ever) to 3 (often), items are averages to a score ranging from 3 to 9, with higher scores reflecting greater loneliness. Table 25 summarizes the papers' authors and languages and Table 26 shows the quality of the studies.

3.21   Community Integration Measure (CIM)

The CIM was validated for people with SCI in Australia [52]. The CIM is a client-centered 10-item scale of participation and measures a person's sense of belonging in the community. The CIM is based on a theoretical model empirically derived from interviews with individuals with moderate to severe brain injuries living in the community. Responses are made on a 5-point rating scale from "always agree" to "always disagree." The CIM results in a single summary score (range 10–50), which is the unweighted sum of the 10 items, with higher scores indicating better integration. Table 25 summarizes the papers' authors and languages and Table 26 shows the quality of the studies.

3.22   Core Self-Evaluations Scale (CSES)

The CSES was validated in the United States in 2015 for people with SCI [68]. CSES is a 12-item instrument rated on a 5-point Likert-type scale (1¼ strongly disagree to 5¼ strongly

agree). Items were designed to assess self-esteem (e.g., "I wish I could have more self-respect"), locus of control (e.g., "I do not feel in control of my success in my career"), self-efficacy (e.g., "I am capable of coping with most of my problems"), and emotional stability/neuroticism (e.g., "There are times when things look pretty bleak and hopeless to me"). Since the CSES is attempting to measure the higher order of the CSE construct rather than individual traits, it also includes items that encompass multiple traits. For example, "I determine what will happen in my life" could be considered to reflect both locus of control and self-efficacy. Furthermore, items on the CSES were selected based on the strength of their relationship with job satisfaction, life satisfaction, and job performance. Table 25 summarizes the papers' authors and languages and Table 26 shows the quality of the studies.

3.23   General Health Questionnaire-28 (GHQ-28)

The GHQ-28, in its several variants, has been extensively used to detect minor, or perhaps more accurately, a nonpsychotic psychiatric disorder in a variety of populations and settings. In 1993, T. C. Griffiths et al. examine the usefulness of the GHQ scaled version Q, both as a measure of the severity of the minor psychiatric disorder in the spinally injured and as a screening instrument to detect psychiatric cases in this population, in Shrewsbury, England [69]. Table 25 summarizes the papers' authors and languages and Table 26 shows the quality of the studies.

3.24   Physical Disability Stress Scale (PDSS)

Furlong developed, in 2007, the PDSS [70] for wheelchair users, including people with SCI, to measure disability-related stress in Brisbane, Australia. "Disability-related stress" is defined as the unique stress experienced by wheelchair users who have an acquired physical disability.

The instrument would provide further insight and awareness into the intensity of the stress experienced by wheelchair users. It would allow pre- and post-assessments of individual or group interventions and rehabilitation, aiming to decrease stress through a greater adjustment to disability factors. On an individual level, high scores on a particular factor(s) may help clinicians modify therapy to a client's particular needs or stress areas. For the administration of the instruments, the PDSS was administrated with other measures. Other measures included the General Health Questionnaire-28 (GHQ-28) and the WHO Quality of Life (WHOQOLBREF), Australian version. Table 25 summarizes the papers' authors and languages and Table 26 shows the quality of the studies.

3.25   Psychological Evaluation Tool for Spinal Cord Stimulation Candidacy (PETSCSC)

Prabhala et al. developed the PETSCSC in Albanian [71] to assess all psychological factors that have a significant correlation with spinal cord stimulation (SCS) outcome, including negative emotive tendencies, aberrant negative thoughts, substance abuse, depression, and presence of concomitant and untreated psychiatric disorders. PETSCSC was divided into subsets. The first section of PETSCSC (questions 1–7) centered on patterns of negative emotions and thoughts, along with maladaptive coping responses, and was referred to as the "emotive" subset. The second section (questions 8–10) consisted of evaluating depression, including that which could benefit from intervention, and was classified as the "depression" subset. The third section (questions 11–14) noted if patients had a personality disorder, other psychiatric disorder, or posttraumatic stress disorder, referred to as the "other disorder" subset. The fourth section (questions 15–18) assesses if patients could derive benefit from medication evaluation, psychotherapy, or a support group, and was classified as the "therapy" subset. A selection of Y (Yes) in the PETSCSC scale indicates 1 point in the PETSCSC score,

and a selection of N (No) indicates 0 points. The total score was added following completion of the examination and used as the total PETSCS score. Table 25 summarizes the papers' authors and languages and Table 26 shows the quality of the studies.

3.26   Spinal Cord Lesion Emotional Well-Being Questionnaire (SCL EWQ)

The SCL EWQ was validated in English in 2008 [44]. SCL EWQ provides a succinct indication of the emotional consequences to personal growth and the negative outcomes of helplessness and intrusion of an SCI: personal growth determines the current positive change in attitude stemming from the life crisis; helplessness determines the level of perplexity (out of control and low self-esteem); and intrusion determines the level of bitterness and brooding. Table 25 summarizes the papers' authors and languages and Table 26 shows the quality of the studies.

3.27   Ways of Coping Questionnaire

Folkman and Lazarus designed the WCQ instrument in 1988 to measure coping behaviors residing in a community residential population. The English version was validated for people with spinal cord injury in 1994 [72]. It includes 66 items measure in a 4-point Likert-type format. Potential responses included 0 (does not apply and/or not used), 1 (used somewhat), 2 (used quite a bit), and 3 (used a great deal). Table 25 summarizes the papers' authors and languages and Table 26 shows the quality of the studies.

3.28   General Handicapped Attitude Scale (GHAS)

GHAS was developed in 1986. The Dutch version was validated for people with SCI in 1987 [73]. Measuring various psychological consequences of the handicap, it consists of a subscale: acceptance (the extent to which a person has accepted to be handicapped), independent help (the extent to which the disabled person finds it frustrating to depend on help), social consequences (the extent to which the disabled person notes a poor understanding of disabled people), and the bottom (the psychic substrate: the person's emotional disposition to come to terms with his or her being disabled). The gash includes 36 statements, nine for each scale, with the score for each statement on a 5-point scale to the extent that I agree or disagree. Table 25 summarizes the papers' authors and languages and Table 26 shows the quality of the studies.

3.29 Stanmore Nursing Assessment of Psychological Status (SNAPS)

In 2016, Smyth et al. developed a brief, reliable instrument to enable nurses to accurately assess, record, and respond to spinal cord injury patients' psychological status in London, United Kingdom [74]. It is designed for nurses to use on all adult patients with SCI daily from their admission throughout their rehabilitation. When using SNAPS, patients are routinely rated in the morning from 0 to 2 against each of the eight domains (motivation, anxiety, sadness, weight of disability, relationship with family, relationship with staff, irritability, and isolation). A score of 0 indicates a non-concerning psychological status for each item, a score of 1 is suggestive of some concern about psychological status, and a score of 2 indicates cause for major concern regarding psychological status. If a patient is rated 1 or 2 on any item in the morning (am), the assessment should be repeated in the evening (pm). If the patient is still scoring 2 in the evening, they are referred immediately to the nurse in charge. The nursing staff monitors patients scoring 1 on any item. Table 25 summarizes the papers' authors and languages and Table 26 shows the quality of the studies.

3.30 Minnesota Multiphasic Personality Inventory 2 (MMPI-2)

The Minnesota Multiphasic Personality Inventory (MMPI) and updated MMPI-A and MMPI-2 are among the most widely employed instruments for measuring personality factors, with literally thousands of research reports published in the scientific literature. The physical disease has been linked to changes in MMPI and MMPI-2 profiles, and SCI significantly moderates MMPI scores. It was validated in English [75]. Table 25 summarizes the papers' authors and languages and Table 26 shows the quality of the studies.

3.31 Medically Based Emotional Distress Scale (MEDS)

The Medically Based Emotional Distress Scale was designed to quantify the type and severity of emotional distress following a physical illness, injury, or disability. The MEDS includes seven subscales measuring Dysphoria (8 items), Irritability (9 items), Anhedonia (11 items), Social Withdrawal (9 items), Ruminations over Past Events (6 items), Cognitive Perspective in the Present (8 items), and Expectations for the Future (9 items). Some items were rated on a 5-point scale to quantify the frequency of different emotional reactions (ranging from never to always present). Other items were rated for the intensity of emotion that occurred (ranging from not present at all to very much present). It was validated in 1993 in English language [76]. Table 25 summarizes the papers' authors and languages and Table 26 shows the quality of the studies.

3.32 Athletic Identity Measurement Scale (AIMS)

The Athletic Identity Measurement Scale (AIMS) is used to assess athletic identity. The AIMS, which was designed as a measure of the athletic portion of a multidimensional self-concept, features 7 items pertaining to affective, behavioral, and cognitive aspects of identification with the athlete role. Respondents rate the extent to which they agree with each of the items on a scale from 1 (strongly disagree) to 7 (strongly agree) [42]. Table 25 summarizes the papers' authors and languages and Table 26 shows the quality of the studies.

3.33 Coping Strategies Questionnaire 24 (CSQ-24)

Harland NJ et al. validated for the SCI population a 24-item version of the CSQ, designed to assess coping strategies and the effectiveness of those strategies to control and decrease pain [77]. Table 25 summarizes the papers' authors and languages and Table 26 shows the quality of the studies.

3.34 Hopkins Symptom Checklist-20 (HSCL-20)

The HSCL-20 version B is a hybrid depression measure created by Katon and colleagues, consisting of 14 items from the Hopkins Symptom Checklist-90 depression scale and the Hopkins Symptom Checklist-90 revised 29 plus six items derived from the Hopkins Symptom Checklist-90 anxiety and obsessive/compulsive dimensions and items based on DSM-IV symptoms. It was validated in 2016 in the SCI population in English [26]. Table 25 summarizes the papers' authors and languages and Table 26 shows the quality of the studies.

3.35 Hamilton Depression Rating Scale (HAM-D)

For many years, the HAM-D has been the criterion standard measure of depression severity for clinical trials. Clinicians or trained research staff rate participants' symptom severity over the past week using rating scales unique to each item.

Using a structured interview guide, the scores on the 17-item version demonstrate good test–retest reliability. It was validated in 2016 in SCI population in English [26]. Table 25 summarizes the papers' authors and languages and Table 26 shows the quality of the studies.

3.36 Trait Hope Scale (THS)

Snyder et al. developed the THS in 1991 to operationally define and measure the construct of dispositional hope. Four agency items on the scale, four pathway items, and four distractor items are not included in the scoring. The agency subscale consists of statements such as "I energetically pursue my goals"; the pathway scale consists of statements such as "There are lots of ways around any problem"; Items are rated on an 8-point Likert-type agreement scale (1 5 definitely false to 8 5 definitely true). It was validated in the SCI population [78]. Table 25 summarizes the papers' authors and languages and Table 26 shows the quality of the studies.

3.37 Acceptance and Action Questionnaire (AAQ)

The AAQ includes nine statements that represent various aspects of avoidance (e.g., "I'm not afraid of my feelings" and "When I compare myself to other people, it seems that most of them are handling their lives better than I am"). Respondents rate each statement on a scale of 1 (never true) to 7 (always true) as it applies to them in the time since the medical event occurred. Several items are reverse scored. It was validated in English [79, 80]. Table 25 summarizes the papers' authors and languages and Table 26 shows the quality of the studies.

3.38 Attachment Style Questionnaire (ASQ)

The ASQ 40-item, self-report measures three subscales: (a) secure attachment, (b) avoidant attachment, and (c) anxious attachment. Respondents rate each item using a 6-point Likert-type agreement scale ranging from 1 (totally disagree) to 6 (totally agree). It was validated in English [81]. Table 25 summarizes the papers' authors and languages and Table 26 shows the quality of the studies.

3.39 Multidimensional Acceptance of Loss Scale (MALS)

Development of the Multidimensional Acceptance of Loss Scale was the primary focus of the present study. Multidimensional Acceptance of Loss Scale items was developed based on a comprehensive review of Wright's disability acceptance theory, the psychosocial adjustment literature, in consultation with Beatrice Wright. The draft of Multidimensional Acceptance of Loss Scale items was reviewed by Disability acceptance Beatrice Wright and a panel of seven experts who have published extensively in the areas of psychosocial adjustment to chronic illness and disability. Based on the expert panel's recommendations, 6 items were deleted, and several items were rewritten for clarity and style. The instrument's final draft comprised 60 items with an equal number of items for each of the four value changes. Items were rated on a 4-point Likert-type rating scale (1 = strongly disagree, 2 = disagree, 3 = agree, and 4 = strongly agree) [82]. Table 25 summarizes the papers' authors and languages and Table 26 shows the quality of the studies.

3.40 Loss Inventory (LI)

The LI is a 30-item self-report scale. Each subject is asked to read 30 declarative sentences describing feelings or reactions to the losses. The patient is then asked to indicate whether he or she has the feeling or reaction "Never," "Rarely," "Sometimes," "Often," or "Always." Values assigned to each response choice are on a 5-point scale and are as follows: Never—1, rarely = 2, sometimes = always, often = 4, and always = 5. A summative score is derived from totaling the values for each item. It was validated in 2004 in English [83]. Table 25 summarizes the papers' authors and languages and Table 26 shows the quality of the studies.

3.41 Readiness for Hospital Discharge Scale (RHDS)

The Readiness for Hospital Discharge Scale (RHDS) measures if patients perceive themselves ready to be discharged from the hospital and manage their care needs in a home setting (Weiss & Piacentine 2006). The RHDS also measures variables related to discharge readiness by nurses, clinical specialists, and managers in adult care, maternal–neonatal, and pediatric care. It was validated in 2020 in English (South Africa) [84]. Table 25 summarizes the papers' authors and languages, and Table 26 shows the quality of their studies.

4 Conclusions

This chapter reports all assessment tools described in the literature to assess psychological aspects in people with SCI. Among the 46 tools included in this chapter resulted that most scales evaluate anxiety and depression, self-efficacy, and coping strategies. The most common assessment tools are the Patient Health Questionnaire-9 (PHQ-9), which is a self-report measure that asks subjects how often they have been bothered by the problems such as feeling depressed, feeling tired, poor appetite, feelings of guilt, or thoughts of suicide; the Spinal Cord Lesion Related Coping Strategies Questionnaire (SCL-CSQ) which is a specific scale developed to evaluate the coping strategies of persons with SCI; and, the Spinal Cord Injury–Falls Concern Scale (SCI-FCS) which is a scale that assesses the degree of attention concerning falls in a wheelchair while carrying out their activities daily.

References

1. Peter C, Cieza A, Geyh S. Rasch analysis of the general self-efficacy scale in spinal cord injury. J Health Psychol. 2014. https://doi.org/10.1177/1359105313475897.

2. Miller WC, Anton HA, Townson AF. Measurement properties of the CESD scale among individuals with spinal cord injury. Spinal Cord. 2008. https://doi.org/10.1038/sj.sc.3102127.

3. Castelnuovo G, Giusti EM, Manzoni GM, et al. What is the role of the placebo effect for pain relief in neurorehabilitation? Clinical implications from the Italian consensus conference on pain in neurorehabilitation. Front Neurol. 2018. https://doi.org/10.3389/fneur.2018.00310.

4. Marquez MA, De Santis R, Ammendola V, et al. Cross-cultural adaptation and validation of the "spinal cord injury-falls concern scale" in the Italian population. Spinal Cord. 2018;56(7):712–8. https://doi.org/10.1038/s41393-018-0070-6.

5. Berardi A, De Santis R, Tofani M, et al. The Wheelchair Use Confidence Scale: Italian translation, adaptation, and validation of the short form. Disabil Rehabil Assist Technol. 2018;13(4):i. https://doi.org/10.1080/17483107.2017.1357053.

6. Anna B, Giovanni G, Marco T, et al. The validity of rasterstereography as a technological tool for the objectification of postural assessment in the clinical and educational fields: pilot study. In: Advances in intelligent systems and computing. 2020. https://doi.org/10.1007/978-3-030-23884-1_8.

7. Panuccio F, Berardi A, Marquez MA, et al. Development of the pregnancy and motherhood evaluation questionnaire (PMEQ) for evaluating and measuring the impact of physical disability on pregnancy and the management of motherhood: a pilot study. Disabil Rehabil. 2020;2020:1–7. https://doi.org/10.1080/09638288.2020.1802520.

8. Amedoro A, Berardi A, Conte A, et al. The effect of aquatic physical therapy on patients with multiple sclerosis: a systematic review and meta-analysis. Mult Scler Relat Disord. 2020. https://doi.org/10.1016/j.msard.2020.102022.

9. Dattoli S, Colucci M, Soave MG, et al. Evaluation of pelvis postural systems in spinal cord injury patients: outcome research. J Spinal Cord Med. 2018;43:185–92.

10. Berardi A, Galeoto G, Guarino D, et al. Construct validity, test-retest reliability, and the ability to detect change of the Canadian occupational performance measure in a spinal cord injury population. Spinal Cord Ser Cases. 2019. https://doi.org/10.1038/s41394-019-0196-6.

11. Ponti A, Berardi A, Galeoto G, Marchegiani L, Spandonaro C, Marquez MA. Quality of life, concern of falling and satisfaction of the sit-ski aid in sit-skiers with spinal cord injury: observational study. Spinal Cord Ser Cases. 2020. https://doi.org/10.1038/s41394-020-0257-x.

12. Panuccio F, Galeoto G, Marquez MA, et al. General sleep disturbance scale (GSDS-IT) in people with spinal cord injury: a psychometric study. Spinal Cord. 2020. https://doi.org/10.1038/s41393-020-0500-0.

13. Monti M, Marquez MA, Berardi A, Tofani M, Valente D, Galeoto G. The multiple sclerosis intimacy and sexuality questionnaire (MSISQ-15): validation of the Italian version for individuals with spinal cord injury. Spinal Cord. 2020. https://doi.org/10.1038/s41393-020-0469-8.

14. Galeoto G, Colucci M, Guarino D, et al. Exploring validity, reliability, and factor analysis of the Quebec user evaluation of satisfaction with assistive technology in an Italian population: a cross-sectional study. Occup Ther Heal Care. 2018. https://doi.org/10.1080/07380577.2018.1522682.

15. Colucci M, Tofani M, Trioschi D, Guarino D, Berardi A, Galeoto G. Reliability and validity of the Italian version of Quebec user evaluation of satisfaction with assistive technology 2.0 (QUEST-IT 2.0) with users of mobility assistive device. Disabil Rehabil Assist Technol. 2019. https://doi.org/10.1080/17483107.2019.1668975.

16. Berardi A, Galeoto G, Lucibello L, Panuccio F, Valente D, Tofani M. Athletes with disability' satisfaction with sport wheelchairs: an Italian cross sectional study. Disabil Rehabil Assist Technol. 2020; https://doi.org/10.1080/17483107.2020.1800114.

17. Moher D, Shamseer L, Clarke M, et al. Preferred reporting items for systematic review and meta-analysis protocols (PRISMA-P) 2015 statement. Rev Esp Nutr Human Diet. 2016. https://doi.org/10.1186/2046-4053-4-1.

18. Mokkink LB, Terwee CB, Patrick DL, et al. The COSMIN study reached international consensus on taxonomy, terminology, and definitions of measurement properties for health-related patient-reported outcomes. J Clin Epidemiol. 2010. https://doi.org/10.1016/j.jclinepi.2010.02.006.

19. Terwee CB, Prinsen CAC, Chiarotto A, et al. COSMIN methodology for evaluating the content validity of patient-reported outcome measures: a Delphi study. Qual Life Res. 2018. https://doi.org/10.1007/s11136-018-1829-0.

20. Mokkink LB, de Vet HCW, Prinsen CAC, et al. COSMIN risk of bias checklist for systematic reviews of patient-reported outcome measures. Qual Life Res. 2018. https://doi.org/10.1007/s11136-017-1765-4.

21. Chung H, Kim J, Askew RL, Jones SMW, Cook KF, Amtmann D. Assessing measurement invariance of three depression scales between neurologic samples and community samples. Qual Life Res. 2015. https://doi.org/10.1007/s11136-015-0927-5.

22. Kalpakjian CZ, Toussaint LL, Albright KJ, Bombardier CH, Krause JK, Tate DG. Patient health questionnaire-9 in spinal cord injury: an examination of

factor structure as related to gender. J Spinal Cord Med. 2009. https://doi.org/10.1080/10790268.2009. 11760766.

23. Poritz JMP, Mignogna J, Christie AJ, Holmes SA, Ames H. The patient health questionnaire depression screener in spinal cord injury. J Spinal Cord Med. 2018. https://doi.org/10.1080/10790268.2017. 1294301.

24. Bombardier CH, Kalpakjian CZ, Graves DE, Dyer JR, Tate DG, Fann JR. Validity of the patient health questionnaire-9 in assessing major depressive disorder during inpatient spinal cord injury rehabilitation. Arch Phys Med Rehabil. 2012. https://doi.org/10.1016/j.apmr.2012.04.019.

25. Krause JS, Saunders LL, Bombardier C, Kalpakjian C. Confirmatory factor analysis of the patient health Questionnaire-9: a study of the participants from the spinal cord injury model systems. PM R. 2011. https://doi.org/10.1016/j.pmrj.2011.03.003.

26. Williams RT, Heinemann AW, Neumann HD, et al. Evaluating the psychometric properties and responsiveness to change of 3 depression measures in a sample of persons with traumatic spinal cord injury and major depressive disorder. Arch Phys Med Rehabil. 2016. https://doi.org/10.1016/j.apmr.2016.01.017.

27. Krause JS, Reed KS, McArdle JJ. Factor structure and predictive validity of somatic and nonsomatic symptoms from the patient health Questionnaire-9: a longitudinal study after spinal cord injury. Arch Phys Med Rehabil. 2010;91(8):1218–24. https://doi.org/10.1016/j.apmr.2010.04.015.

28. Richardson EJ, Richards JS. Factor structure of the PHQ-9 screen for depression across time since injury among persons with spinal cord injury. Rehabil Psychol. 2008. https://doi.org/10.1037/0090-5550.53.2.243.

29. Williams RT, Heinemann AW, Bode RK, et al. Improving measurement properties of the patient health Questionnaire-9 with rating scale analysis. Rehabil Psychol. 2009. https://doi.org/10.1037/a0015529.

30. Summaka M, Zein H, Abbas LA, et al. Validity and reliability of the Arabic patient health Questionnaire-9 in patients with spinal cord injury in Lebanon. World Neurosurg. 2019. https://doi.org/10.1016/j.wneu.2019.01.234.

31. Nakku JEM, Rathod SD, Kizza D, et al. Validity and diagnostic accuracy of the Luganda version of the 9-item and 2-item patient health questionnaire for detecting major depressive disorder in rural Uganda. Glob Ment Heal. 2016. https://doi.org/10.1017/gmh.2016.14.

32. Dean RE, Kennedy P. Measuring appraisals following acquired spinal cord injury: a preliminary psychometric analysis of the appraisals of disability. Rehabil Psychol. 2009. https://doi.org/10.1037/a0015581.

33. Mignogna J, Christie AJ, Holmes SA, Ames H. Measuring disability-associated appraisals for veterans with spinal cord injury. Rehabil Psychol. 2015. https://doi.org/10.1037/rep0000022.

34. McDonald SD, Goldberg-Looney LD, Mickens MN, Ellwood MS, Mutchler BJ, Perrin PB. Appraisals of DisAbility primary and secondary scale—short form (ADAPSS−sf): psychometrics and association with mental health among U.S. military veterans with spinal cord injury. Rehabil Psychol. 2018;63(3):372–382. https://doi.org/10.1037/rep0000230.

35. Eaton R, Jones K, Duff J. Cognitive appraisals and emotional status following a spinal cord injury in post-acute rehabilitation. Spinal Cord. 2018. https://doi.org/10.1038/s41393-018-0151-6.

36. Deane KC, Chlan KM, Vogel LC, Zebracki K. Use of appraisals of DisAbility primary and secondary scale-short form (ADAPSS-sf) in individuals with pediatric-onset spinal cord injury. Spinal Cord. 2020. https://doi.org/10.1038/s41393-019-0375-0.

37. Russell M, Ames H, Dunn C, Beckwith S, Holmes SA. Appraisals of disability and psychological adjustment in veterans with spinal cord injuries. J Spinal Cord Med. 2020;14:1–8. https://doi.org/10.1080/10790268.2020.1754650. Epub ahead of print. PMID: 32406809.

38. Tate DG, Heinrich RK, Maynard F, Buckelew SP. Moderator-variable effect on the Brief Symptom Inventory test-item endorsements of spinal cord injury patients. Paraplegia. 1994;32(7):473–9. https://doi.org/10.1038/sc.1994.75. PMID: 7970849.

39. Heinrich RK, Tate DG. Latent variable structure of the brief symptom inventory in a sample of persons with spinal cord injuries. Rehabil Psychol. 1996. https://doi.org/10.1037//0090-5550.41.2.131.

40. Müller R, Cieza A, Geyh S. Rasch analysis of the hospital anxiety and depression scale in spinal cord injury. Rehabil Psychol. 2012. https://doi.org/10.1037/a0029287.

41. Woolrich RA, Kennedy P, Tasiemski T. A preliminary psychometric evaluation of the hospital anxiety and depression scale (HADS) in 963 people living with a spinal cord injury. Psychol Health Med. 2006;11(1):80–90. https://doi.org/10.1080/13548500500294211.

42. Tasiemski T, Brewer BW. Athletic identity, sport participation, and psychological adjustment in people with spinal cord injury. Adapt Phys Act Q. 2011. https://doi.org/10.1123/apaq.28.3.233.

43. Elfström ML, Rydén A, Kreuter M, Persson LO, Sullivan M. Linkages between coping and psychological outcome in the spinal cord lesioned: development of SCL-related measures. Spinal Cord. 2002. https://doi.org/10.1038/sj.sc.3101238.

44. Migliorini CE, Elfström ML, Tonge BJ. Translation and Australian validation of the spinal cord lesion-related coping strategies and emotional well-being questionnaires. Spinal Cord. 2008. https://doi.org/10.1038/sc.2008.22.

45. Elfström ML, Kennedy P, Lude P, Taylor N. Condition-related coping strategies in persons with spinal cord lesion: a cross-national validation of the spinal cord lesion-related coping strategies questionnaire in four

community samples. Spinal Cord. 2007. https://doi.org/10.1038/sj.sc.3102003.

46. Paker N, Bugdayci D, Kesiktas N, Sahin M, Elfström ML. Reliability and validity of the Turkish version of spinal cord lesion-related coping strategies. Spinal Cord. 2014. https://doi.org/10.1038/sc.2013.142.

47. Saurí J, Umana MC, Chamarro A, Soler MD, Gilabert A, Elfström ML. Adaptation and validation of the Spanish version of the spinal cord lesion-related coping strategies questionnaire (SCL CSQ-S). Spinal Cord. 2014. https://doi.org/10.1038/sc.2014.44.

48. Saffari M, Pakpour AH, Yaghobidoot M, Al Zaben F, Koenige HG. Cross-cultural adaptation of the spinal cord lesion-related coping strategies questionnaire for use in Iran. Injury. 2015. https://doi.org/10.1016/j.injury.2015.04.035.

49. Post MWM, Gerritsen J, Diederiks JPM, De Witte LP. Measuring health status of people who are wheelchair-dependent: validity of the sickness impact profile 68 and the Nottingham health profile. Disabil Rehabil. 2001. https://doi.org/10.1080/096382801750110874.

50. Post MWM, Gerritsen J, Van Leusen NDM, Paping MA, Prevo AJH. Adapting the Nottingham health profile for use in people with severe physical disabilities. Clin Rehabil. 2001. https://doi.org/10.1191/026921501672698006.

51. Post MWM, de Bruin A, de Witte L, Schrijvers A. The SIP68: a measure of health-related functional status in rehabilitation medicine. Arch Phys Med Rehabil. 1996;77(5):440–5. https://doi.org/10.1016/S0003-9993(96)90031-3.

52. De Wolf A, Lane-Brown A, Tate RL, Middleton J, Cameron ID. Measuring community integration after spinal cord injury: validation of the Sydney psychosocial reintegration scale and community integration measure. Qual Life Res. 2010. https://doi.org/10.1007/s11136-010-9685-6.

53. Tate R, Simpson G, Lane-Brown A, Soo C, de Wolf A, Whiting D. Sydney psychosocial reintegration scale (SPRS-2): meeting the challenge of measuring participation in neurological conditions. Aust Psychol. 2012. https://doi.org/10.1111/j.1742-9544.2011.00060.x.

54. Amtmann D, Bamer AM, Cook KF, Askew RL, Noonan VK, Brockway JA. University of Washington self-efficacy scale: a new self-efficacy scale for people with disabilities. Arch Phys Med Rehabil. 2012. https://doi.org/10.1016/j.apmr.2012.05.001.

55. Post MWM, Adriaansen JJE, Peter C. Rasch analysis of the University of Washington Self-Efficacy Scale short-form (UW-SES-6) in people with long-standing spinal cord injury. Spinal Cord. 2018. https://doi.org/10.1038/s41393-018-0166-z.

56. Boswell-Ruys CL, Harvey LA, Delbaere K, Lord SR. A falls concern scale for people with spinal cord injury (SCI-FCS). Spinal Cord. 2010. https://doi.org/10.1038/sc.2010.1.

57. Marquez MA, De Santis R, Ammendola V, et al. Cross-cultural adaptation and validation of the "spinal cord injury-falls concern scale" in the Italian population. Spinal Cord. 2018. https://doi.org/10.1038/s41393-018-0070-6.

58. Butler Forslund E, Roaldsen KS, Hultling C, Wahman K, Franzén E. Concerns about falling in wheelchair users with spinal cord injury-validation of the Swedish version of the spinal cord injury falls concern scale. Spinal Cord. 2016. https://doi.org/10.1038/sc.2015.125.

59. Roaldsen KS, Måøy ÅB, Jørgensen V, Stanghelle JK. Test-retest reliability at the item level and total score level of the Norwegian version of the spinal cord injury falls concern scale (SCI-FCS). J Spinal Cord Med. 2016. https://doi.org/10.1080/10790268.2015.1119965.

60. Pramodhyakul N, Pramodhyakul W. Thai translation and cross-cultural adaptation of the spinal cord injury falls concern scale (SCI-FCS). Spinal Cord. 2020. https://doi.org/10.1038/s41393-019-0405-y.

61. Kuiper H, van Leeuwen CCM, Stolwijk-Swüste JM, Post MWM. Measuring resilience with the Connor–Davidson resilience scale (CD-RISC): which version to choose? Spinal Cord. 2019;57(5):360–6. https://doi.org/10.1038/s41393-019-0240-1.

62. Buckelew SP, Burk JP, Brownlee-Duffeck M, Frank RG, et al. Cognitive and somatic aspects of depression among a rehabilitation sample: reliability and validity of SCL-90-R research subscales. Rehabil Psychol. 1988. https://doi.org/10.1037//0090-5550.33.2.67.

63. Mitchell MC, Burns NR, Dorstyn DS. Screening for depression and anxiety in spinal cord injury with DASS-21. Spinal Cord. 2008. https://doi.org/10.1038/sj.sc.3102154.

64. Portmann Bergamaschi R, Escorpizo R, Staubli S, Finger ME. Content validity of the work rehabilitation questionnaire-self-report version WORQ-SELF in a subgroup of spinal cord injury patients. Spinal Cord. 2014. https://doi.org/10.1038/sc.2013.129.

65. Perera MJ, Meade MA, DiPonio L. Use and psychometric properties of the flourishing scale among adults with spinal cord injury. Rehabil Psychol. 2018. https://doi.org/10.1037/rep0000184.

66. Kortte KB, Falk LD, Castillo RC, Johnson-Greene D, Wegener ST. The Hopkins rehabilitation engagement rating scale: development and psychometric properties. Arch Phys Med Rehabil. 2007. https://doi.org/10.1016/j.apmr.2007.03.030.

67. Robinson-Whelen S, Taylor HB, Feltz M, Whelen M. Loneliness among people with spinal cord injury: exploring the psychometric properties of the 3-item loneliness scale. Arch Phys Med Rehabil. 2016. https://doi.org/10.1016/j.apmr.2016.04.008.

68. Smedema SM, Morrison B, Yaghmaian RA, Deangelis J, Aldrich H. Psychometric validation of the Core self-evaluations scale in people with spinal cord injury. Disabil Rehabil. 2016. https://doi.org/10.3109/09638288.2015.1065012.

69. Griffiths TC, Myers DH, Talbot AW. A study of the validity of the scaled version of the general health questionnaire in paralysed spinally injured out-

patients. Psychol Med. 1993. https://doi.org/10.1017/S0033291700028580.

70. Furlong M, Connor JP. The measurement of disability-related stress in wheelchair users. Arch Phys Med Rehabil. 2007. https://doi.org/10.1016/j.apmr.2007.06.763.

71. Prabhala T, Kumar V, Gruenthal E, et al. Use of a psychological evaluation tool as a predictor of spinal cord stimulation outcomes. Neuromodulation. 2019. https://doi.org/10.1111/ner.12884.

72. Margaret Wineman N, Durand EJ, Jan McCuuoch B. Examination of the factor structure of the ways of coping questionnaire with clinical populations. Nurs Res. 1994. https://doi.org/10.1097/00006199-199409000-00003.

73. Bermond B. The general handicapped attitude scale (GHAS). Int J Rehabil Res. 1987;10(1):49–54. https://doi.org/10.1097/00004356-198703000-00005.

74. Smyth C, Spada MM, Coultry-Keane K, Ikkos G. The Stanmore nursing assessment of psychological status: understanding the emotions of patients with spinal cord injury. J Spinal Cord Med. 2016. https://doi.org/10.1080/10790268.2016.1163809.

75. Barncord SW, Wanlass RL. A correction procedure for the Minnesota multiphasic personality inventory-2 for persons with spinal cord injury. Arch Phys Med Rehabil. 2000. https://doi.org/10.1053/apmr.2000.6287.

76. Overholser JC, Schubert DSP, Foliart R, Frost F. Assessment of emotional distress following a spinal cord injury. Rehabil Psychol. 1993. https://doi.org/10.1037//0090-5550.38.3.187.

77. Harland NJ, Georgieff K. Development of the coping strategies questionnaire 24, a clinically utilitarian version of the coping strategies questionnaire.

Rehabil Psychol. 2003. https://doi.org/10.1037/0090-5550.48.4.296.

78. Smedema SM, Pfaller J, Moser E, Tu W-M, Chan F. Measurement structure of the trait Hope scale in persons with spinal cord injury: a confirmatory factor analysis. Rehabil Res Policy Educ. 2013. https://doi.org/10.1891/2168-6653.27.3.206.

79. Kortte KB, Veiel L, Batten SV, Wegener ST. Measuring avoidance in medical rehabilitation. Rehabil Psychol. 2009. https://doi.org/10.1037/a0014703.

80. Kennedy P, Smithson E, Blakey L. Planning and structuring spinal cord injury rehabilitation: the needs assessment checklist. Topics in Spinal Cord Injury Rehabilitation. 2012. https://doi.org/10.1310/sci1802-135.

81. Iwanaga K, Blake J, Yaghmaian R, et al. Preliminary validation of a short-form version of the attachment style questionnaire for use in clinical rehabilitation Counseling research and practice. Rehabil Couns Bull. 2018. https://doi.org/10.1177/0034355217709477.

82. Ferrin JM, Chan F, Chronister J, Chiu CY. Psychometric validation of the multidimensional acceptance of loss scale. Clin Rehabil. 2011. https://doi.org/10.1177/0269215510380836.

83. Niemeier JP, Kennedy RE, McKinley WO, Cifu DX. The loss inventory: preliminary reliability and validity data for a new measure of emotional and cognitive responses to disability. Disabil Rehabil. 2004. https://doi.org/10.1080/09638280410001696692.

84. De Lange JS, Jacobs J, Meiring N, et al. Reliability and validity of the readiness for hospital discharge scale in patients with spinal cord injury. South African J Physiother. 2020;76(1) https://doi.org/10.4102/sajp.v76i1.1400.

Measuring Quality of Life in Spinal Cord Injury

Anna Berardi, Marina D'Angelo, Francescaroberta Panuccio, Giulia Grieco, and Giovanni Galeoto

1 Introduction

People with spinal cord injury (SCI) face limitations in their daily life, including limitations in the functioning of activities in daily life, social and professional participation, and important psychological consequences such as major depression [1].

The barriers identified include the emergence of secondary health conditions and health decline, 2–5 job opportunities reduced, 6–8 limited social support and functioning of the family role, 9 limited access to recreational and leisure activities, 10–12, and lack of accessible means of transport [2]. However, through clinical and rehabilitation practice, it is possible to improve people's quality of life with SCI.

Determining whether improvement has often occurred is based on therapist observations influenced by personal value or the professional value system. For example, a therapist may believe there has been an improvement based on the higher number of times the client requires or an increase in the amount of assistance she needs to get dressed. These changes can represent valid improvements in the quality of life, but only based on the client's belief. Williams et al. [3] encouraged clinicians to systematically measure their patients' quality of life to improve therapeutic judgments and improve the level of communication between patients and doctors [4]. Therefore, instruments are needed to accurately measure this outcome.

The objective of this chapter is to describe and evaluate assessment tools on quality of life in people with SCI through a systematic review.

2 Materials and Methods

This study was conducted by a research group composed of medical doctors and health professionals from the "Sapienza" University of Rome and from "Rehabilitation & Outcome Measure Assessment" (R.O.M.A.) association. R.O.M.A. association in the last few years has dealt with several studies and validation of many outcome measures in Italy for Spinal Cord Injury population [5–18].

This chapter describes all assessment tools regarding the quality of life resulting from a systematic review conducted on Pubmed, Scopus, and web of science. For specific details on methodology, see chapter "Methodological Approach to Identifying Outcome Measures in Spinal Cord Injury." Eligibility criteria for considering studies for this chapter were validation studies and

A. Berardi · G. Galeoto (✉)
Department of Human Neurosciences, Sapienza University of Rome, Rome, Italy
e-mail: giovanni.galeoto@uniroma1.it

M. D'Angelo · F. Panuccio · G. Grieco
R.O.M.A. Rehabilitation Outcome Measures Assessment, Non-Profit Organization, Rome, Italy

cross-cultural adaptation studies, studies about the quality of life, studies about tests, question- naires, and self-reported and performance-based outcome measures, studies with a population of people of SCI and population ≥18 years old. Study selection: the selection of studies was con- ducted in accordance with the 27-item PRISM Statement for Reporting Systematic Reviews [19]. For the data collection, the authors followed the recommendations from the COnsensus- based standards for the selection of the health Measurement Instruments (COSMIN) initiative

[20]. Study quality and risk of bias were assessed using COSMIN checklist [21, 22].

3 Results

For this chapter, 53 papers were considered. The authors found 29 assessment tools that evaluate the Quality of Life (QoL) area in persons with SCI. In Fig. 1, a flow chart of included studies is reported [21, 22]. The assessment tools are described subsequently.

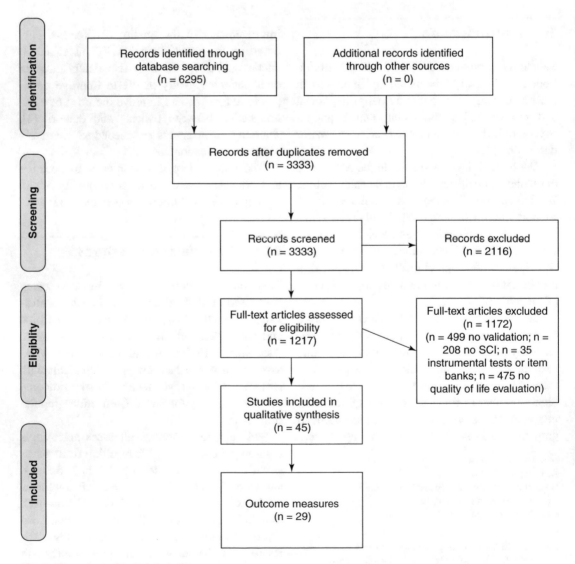

Fig. 1 Flow chart of included studies

3.1 Community Integration Questionnaire (CIQ)

The Community Integration Questionnaire (CIQ), a brief and easy to administer self-report tool developed for individuals with traumatic brain injury (TBI), addresses three central factors of integration: home competency, social integration, and productive activity. It was validated for people with SCI in Spanish [23] and English [24–26]. The CIQ has 15 items and three subscales. The Home Integration subscale has 5 items rated on a 3-point scale that assess household shopping involvement, meal preparation, housework, childcare, and planning social arrangements. The Social Integration subscale has 1 item assessing involvement in home finances, 3 items assessing the monthly frequency of shopping, leisure activities, visiting friends/relatives, 1 item asking about having a best friend, and 1 item about whom one participates leisure activities with. The Productive subscale consists of four questions that assess travel frequency outside the home, current work situation, student status, and volunteer activities. The CIQ [27] has a total scale score range of 0–27, with possible ranges of 0–10 for the Home subscale, 0–12 for the Social subscale, and 0–7 for the Productive subscale. Table 1 summarizes the papers' authors and languages and Table 2 shows the quality of the studies.

Table 1 Characteristics of the studies validating CIQ

Authors	Language	n	Age mean (SD, range) year	Gender % Female
Rintala et al. [23]	Spanish	99	37.5 (13.3, 18–73)	18 (18.2)
Gontkovsky et al. [26]	English	28	42 (17, 15–87)	10 (35)
Hirsh et al. [24]	English	146	n.a.	n.a.
Kratz et al. [25]	English	627	48.28 (13.5, 18–89)	228 (36.5)

n number of participants of the study, *n.a.* not available

Table 2 Evaluation of quality and risk of bias

Authors	Item of COSMIN checklist									
	1	2	3	4	5	6	7	8	9	10
Rintala et al. [23]	?	?	−	+	−	+	−	+	+	−
Gontkovsky et al. [26]	?	+	−	−	+	−	−	+	+	−
Hirsh et al. [24]	?	?	+	+	+	−	−	+	+	−
Kratz et al. [25]	?	?	+	+	+	+	−	−	−	−

Item 1 PROM development, *Item 2* content validity, *Item 3* structural validity, *Item 4* internal consistency, *Item 5* cross-cultural validity/measurement invariance, *Item 6* reliability, *Item 7* measurement error, *Item 8* criterion validity, *Item 9* hypothesis testing for construct validity, *Item 10* responsiveness, + sufficient, − insufficient, ? indeterminate

3.2 Utrecht Scale for Evaluation of Rehabilitation–Participation (USER)

The scale is a newly developed International Classification of Functioning, Disability, and Health (ICF) based participation measure assessing objective and subjective participation. It was developed in Dutch [28, 29] and translated into Swiss [30]. The USER–Participation is a self-report questionnaire of 32 items with three separate scales: Frequency, Restrictions, and Satisfaction. The Frequency scale consists of 11 items, 4 items on vocational activities and 7 items on leisure and social activities. The 4 items on vocational activities address the number of hours spent per week and are scored on a 6-point ordinal scale from 0 (not at all) to 5. The 7 items on leisure and social activities address the frequency in the last 4 weeks scoring from 0 (not at all) to 5. The Restrictions scale consists of 11 items that address activities that may be restricted by their health condition. The perceived difficulty in performing the activity rated on a 4-point scale, ranging from 0 (not possible at all) to 3 (no difficulty at all). If any item is not relevant to the person or the restrictions are not related to the person's health status, the option "not applicable" is available. The Satisfaction scale consists of 10 items on satisfaction with vocational, leisure, and social activities. Items are rated on a scale from 0 (not at all) to 5 (very satisfied). For the items on vocational activities and partner relationship, a "not applicable" option is available. The sum score of each scale is based on all applicable items and is converted to a 0–100 scale, with higher scores indicating better participation (more time spent/higher frequency, fewer restrictions, higher satisfaction). There is no total USER-Participation score aggregating the scores from each scale. Table 3 summarizes the papers' authors and languages and Table 4 shows the quality of the studies.

Table 3 Characteristics of the studies validating USER

Authors	Language	N	Age mean (SD, range) year	Gender % Female
Van Der Zee et al. [29]	Dutch	157	50.6 (10.5)	53 (33.8)
Post et al. [28]	Dutch	341	53.8 (14.9)	144 (42.4)
Mader et al. [30]	Swiss	1549	52.4 (14.8)	422 (28.5)

n number of participants of the study, *n.a.* not available

Table 4 Evaluation of quality and risk of bias

Authors	Item of COSMIN checklist									
	1	2	3	4	5	6	7	8	9	10
Van Der Zee et al. [29]	?	+	–	+	+	+	–	+	+	–
Post et al. [28]	+	+	–	+	–	+	–	+	+	+
Mader et al. [30]	?	+	+	+	+	–	–	–	–	–

Item 1 PROM development, *Item 2* content validity, *Item 3* structural validity, *Item 4* internal consistency, *Item 5* cross-cultural validity/measurement invariance, *Item 6* reliability, *Item 7* measurement error, *Item 8* criterion validity, *Item 9* hypothesis testing for construct validity, *Item 10* responsiveness, + sufficient, – insufficient, ? indeterminate

3.3 World Health Organization Quality of Life (WHOQOLBREF) and World Health Organization Quality of Life for Disabilities (WHOQOL-DIS) and World Health Organization Quality of Life 5 Items (WHOQOL-5)

The WHOQOL Group originally developed a WHOQOL-BREF questionnaire. These facets are categorized into four domains: Physical Capacity (7 items), psychological well-being (6 items), social relationships (3 items), and environment (8 items). All items are rated on a 5-point Likert-type scale, and then domain scores are calculated by multiplying the mean of all facet scores included in each domain by a factor of 4, with a possible range of each raw domain score of 0–16. This scale was validated for the SCI population in Chinese [31], Chinese (Taiwan) [32], Spanish [33], and English [34, 35]. In 2010, the WHO developed a 13-question WHOQOL-DIS module to measure QOL for disabilities. The WHOQOL-DIS was validated in Korean [36]. A new module was added to the WHOQOL-BREF (26 items) 18 to assess the QOL of people with disabilities and comprises a 13-item self-report questionnaire for three sub-domains. Responses to each item were measured on a scale from 1 (not at all) to 5 (yes very much) to calculate the average score of the three categories. A higher score reflected a higher QOL. The WHOQOL-5 validate for people with SCI in English [37] is a selection of five satisfaction items out of the World Health Organization's short health-related quality of life measure, the WHOQOL-BREF. The 5 items cover overall quality of life, satisfaction with health, daily activities, relationships, and living conditions. Table 5 summarizes the papers' authors and languages and Table 6 shows the quality of the studies.

Table 5 Characteristics of the studies validating WHOQOLBREF, WHOQOL-5, and WHOQOL-DIS

Scale, test, or questionnaire	Authors	Language	n	Age mean (SD, range) year	Gender % Female
WHOQOLBREF	Lin et al. [32]	Chinese (Taiwan)	187	n.a.	n.a.
	Miller et al. [35]	English	161	46.88 (15.52)	28 (23)
	Jang et al. [31]	Chinese	111	40 (13)	12 (6)
	Salvador De la Barrera et al. [33]	Spanish	54	45.5 (13.2)	10 (18.5)
WHOQOL-5	Geyh et al. [37]	English	243	41.4 (13.6)	50 (20.6)
WHOQOL-DIS	Lee et al. [36]	Korean	85	48.17(14.13)	22 (25.9)

n number of participants of the study, *n.a.* not available

Table 6 Evaluation of quality and risk of bias

Authors	Item of COSMIN Check List									
	1	2	3	4	5	6	7	8	9	10
Lin et al. [32]	?	+	−	+	+	+	−	+	+	+
Miller et al. [35]	?	?	+	−	−	−	−	−	−	−
Jang et al. [31]	?	+	+	+	+	−	−	−	−	−
Salvador De la Barrera et al. [33]	?	+	+	−	+	−	−	−	−	−
Geyh et al. [37]	?	?	+	−	−	−	−	−	−	−
Lee et al. [36]	?	?	+	+	−	+	−	−	−	−

Item 1 PROM development, *Item 2* content validity, *Item 3* structural validity, *Item 4* internal consistency, *Item 5* cross-cultural validity/measurement invariance, *Item 6* reliability, *Item 7* measurement error, *Item 8* criterion validity, *Item 9* hypothesis testing for construct validity, *Item 10* responsiveness, + sufficient, − insufficient, ? indeterminate

3.4 Ferrans and Powers Quality of Life Index (QLI)

The Ferrans and Powers Quality of Life Index (QLI) affirms and evaluates QoL in importance-weighted life satisfaction. It was validated for people of SCI in Canada [38, 39]. The QLI is composed of two parts: the first measure of satisfaction with the various aspects of life and the second measure of those present. The original QLI is made up of 33 articles for each of the two parts. In the four domain SCI version, there are 36 articles. Three additional articles reflect SCI-specific problems. All items are rated on a 6-point scale and that are reported calculated by weighting the satisfaction unit with the corresponding element of importance. In 2015, Mendes Reis et al. validated the QLI Version III for SCI in Portuguese (Brazil) [40] and Spanish [41]. Table 7 summarizes the papers' authors and languages and Table 8 shows the quality of the studies.

3.5 Sense of Well-being Inventory (SWBI)

The SWBI was developed initially to operationalize the construct of QOL for vocational rehabilitation clients. The SWBI was further validated in a sample of people with SCI in English [34, 42]. The SWBI is composed of 36 items (e.g., "I get frustrated about my disability," "I can afford the medical services I need") with five subscales: physical well-being and associated feelings about self, psychological well-being, family and social well-being, financial well-being, and medical care. Rehabilitation clients indicated the extent to which the SWBI items were descriptive of them, using a 4-point Likert-type rating scale (rating: 1 = Strongly disagree, 4 = Strongly agree). Table 9 summarizes the authors and languages of the papers and Table 10 shows the quality of the studies.

Table 7 Characteristics of the studies validating QLI

Authors	Language	n	Age mean (SD, range) year	Gender % Female
Kovacs et al. [41]	Spanish	77	45.1 (15.6)	29 (37.7)
May and Warren [38]	English	11	33.1 (26–42)	
May and Warren [39]	English	98	45.2 (21–81)	22 (23)
Reis et al. [40]	Portuguese (Brazil)	30	38.4 (14.1)	8 (26.6)

n number of participants of the study, *n.a.* not available

Table 8 Evaluation of quality and risk of bias

Authors	Item of COSMIN checklist									
	1	2	3	4	5	6	7	8	9	10
Kovacs et al. [41]	?	?	–	–	–	+	–	+	+	+
May and Warren [38]	?	+	+	–	–	–	–	–	–	–
May and Warren [39]	?	+	+	–	–	–	–	+	+	–
Reis et al. [40]	?	+	–	–	–	–	–	–	–	–

Item 1 PROM development, *Item 2* content validity, *Item 3* structural validity, *Item 4* internal consistency, *Item 5* cross-cultural validity/measurement invariance, *Item 6* reliability, *Item 7* measurement error, *Item 8* criterion validity, *Item 9* hypothesis testing for construct validity, *Item 10* responsiveness, + sufficient, – insufficient, ? indeterminate

Table 9 Characteristics of the studies validating SWBI

Authors	Language	n	Age mean (SD, range) year	Gender % Female
Catalano et al. [42]	English	413	44.42 (14.09)	120(29)
Chapin et al. [34]	English	132	45.82 (16.67)	44 (23)

n number of participants of the study, *n.a.* not available

3.6 Satisfaction with Life Scale (SWLS)

The SWLS is validated for people with SCI in English [37, 43] and Dutch [44]. The SWLS is a measure of individuals' global judgment of their

Table 10 Evaluation of quality and risk of bias

Authors	Item of COSMIN checklist									
	1	2	3	4	5	6	7	8	9	10
Catalano et al. [42]	?	?	+	–	–	–	–	+	+	–
Chapin et al. [34]	?	?	+	–	–	–	–	+	+	–

Item 1 PROM development, *Item 2* content validity, *Item 3* structural validity, *Item 4* internal consistency, *Item 5* cross-cultural validity/measurement invariance, *Item 6* reliability, *Item 7* measurement error, *Item 8* criterion validity, *Item 9* hypothesis testing for construct validity, *Item 10* responsiveness, + sufficient, – insufficient, ? indeterminate

Table 11 Characteristics of the studies validating SWLS

Authors	Language	n	Age mean (SD, range) year	Gender % Female
Amtmann et al. [43]	English	8566	38.96 (16.94)	1799 [21]
Geyh et al. [37]	English	243	41.4 (13.6)	50 (20.6)
Post et al. [44]	Dutch	145	45.4 (13.7)	41 (28)

n number of participants of the study, *n.a.* not available

Table 12 Evaluation of quality and risk of bias

Authors	Item of COSMIN checklist									
	1	2	3	4	5	6	7	8	9	10
Amtmann et al. [43]	?	?	+	–	–	–	–	+	+	–
Geyh et al. [37]	?	?	+	–	–	–	–	+	+	–
Post et al. [44]	?	?	+	–	–	–	–	+	+	–

Item 1 PROM development, *Item 2* content validity, *Item 3* structural validity, *Item 4* internal consistency, *Item 5* cross-cultural validity/measurement invariance, *Item 6* reliability, *Item 7* measurement error, *Item 8* criterion validity, *Item 9* hypothesis testing for construct validity, *Item 10* responsiveness, + sufficient, – insufficient, ? indeterminate

life. The SWLS consists of five statements, scored on a scale ranging from 1 (completely disagree) to 7 (completely agree). The total score is the sum of the item scores (range, 5–35). SWLS scores have been reported as weakly associated with impairment and disability variables and moderately associated with handicap variables. Table 11 summarizes the papers' authors and languages and Table 12 shows the quality of the studies.

3.7 Economic-QOL 28-Item Bank

The economic-QOL 28-item bank developed in 2015 was translated from English [45] into German and validated for SCI population by Gecht et al. [1]. The German Rasch-based economic-QOL scale represents a suitable instrument to investigate the influences of economic factors on patients' QOL at group and individual levels. The scale can be easily applied in research and practice and maybe administered quickly in combination with other instruments. The short test duration implies a low test burden for patients and a minimum time expenditure by clinicians when evaluating the results. The German economic-QOL-scale has 11 items with a 4-point Likert-type scale scoring ranging from "not at all true" to "totally true" with higher scores indicating a higher agreement with the respective aspect of economic QOL. Table 13 summarizes the papers' authors and languages and Table 14 shows the quality of the studies.

Table 13 Characteristics of the studies validating economic QOL 28-item bank

Authors	Language	n	Age mean (SD, range) year	Gender % Female
Tulsky et al. [45]	English	6	n.a.	n.a.
Gecht et al. [1]	German	325	n.a.	199 (61.2)

n number of participants of the study, *n.a.* not available

Table 14 Evaluation of quality and risk of bias

Authors	Item of COSMIN Check List									
	1	2	3	4	5	6	7	8	9	10
Tulsky et al. [45]	?	?	+	−	−	−	−	+	+	−
Gecht et al. [1]	?	?	+	−	−	−	−	+	+	−

Item 1 PROM development, *Item 2* content validity, *Item 3* structural validity, *Item 4* internal consistency, *Item 5* cross-cultural validity/measurement invariance, *Item 6* reliability, *Item 7* measurement error, *Item 8* criterion validity, *Item 9* hypothesis testing for construct validity, *Item 10* responsiveness, + sufficient, − insufficient, ? indeterminate

3.8 36-Item Short-Form Health Survey (SF-36), 36-Item Short-Form Health Walk-wheel (SF-36 w.w.), Short-Form Health Survey Physical Functioning Scale for Veterans (SF-36V) and Short-Form Health Survey (SF-6D)

The SF-36 was validated in English for people with SCI [46] and also in Chinese (Taiwan) [32]. The SF-36 is one of the most widely used health-related quality of life (HRQL) instruments in the world. The SF-36 dimensions are physical functioning (10 items), role limitations due to physical health problems (4 items), bodily pain (2 items), general health (5 items), vitality (energy/fatigue) (4 items), social functioning (2 items), role limitations due to emotional problems (3 items), and mental health (psychological distress and psychological well-being) (5 items). The eight dimensions are collapsed to create two global components, a physical component score (PCS) and a mental component score (MCSA). The SF-36V version of SF-36 has been designed for use with Veterans Health Administration (VHA) ambulatory care populations. In 2006, Luther et al. worked to develop a valid and reliable SCI-specific physical functioning (PF) scale for veterans with SCI in the United States [47]. Finally, in 2006, Lee et al. determined the feasibility, acceptability, discriminative validity, responsiveness, and "minimal important difference" (MID) of the SF-6D [48, 49] for people with SCIin Australia. The SF-6D is a utility measure, calculated from SF-36, based on six-dimensional state health classifications, and derived from a subset of 11 SF-36 questions covering the dimensions of Physical Functioning, Role Limitation, Social Functioning, Pain, Mental Health, and Vitality. In 2009, Lee et al. validated the modified SF-36 ww with three additional questions, replacing the word walk with wheel for PF questions 9–11 (items 3g–i) of the SF-36. The original questions were also asked, allowing coding to either SF-36 walk-wheel (SF-36ww) or the original SF-36

Table 15 Characteristics of the studies validating SF-36, SF-36 ww, SF-36V, and SF-6D

Scale, test, or questionnaire	Authors	Language	n	Age mean (SD, range) year	Gender % Female
SF-36	Forchheimer et al. [46]	English	215	38.8 (14.5)	46 (21.5)
	Lin et al. [32]	Chinese (Taiwan)	187	n.a.	n.a.
SF-36 ww	Lee et al. [50]	English	305	44	n.a.
SF-36V	Luther et al. [47]	English	392	n.a.	21 (6)
SF-6D	Engel et al. [49]	English	274	43.5 (18.3)	64 (23.3)
	Lee et al. [48]	English	305	n.a.	53 (17)

n number of participants of the study, *n.a.* not available

Table 16 Evaluation of quality and risk of bias

Authors	Item of COSMIN checklist									
	1	2	3	4	5	6	7	8	9	10
Forchheimer et al. [46]	?	?	+	–	–	–	–	+	+	–
Lin et al. [32]	?	?	+	–	–	–	–	+	+	–
Lee et al. [50]	?	?	+	–	–	–	–	+	+	–
Luther et al. [47]	?	?	+	–	–	–	–	+	+	–
Engel et al. [49]	?	?	+	–	–	–	–	+	+	–
Lee et al. [48]	?	?	+	–	–	–	–	+	+	–

Item 1 PROM development, *Item 2* content validity, *Item 3* structural validity, *Item 4* internal consistency, *Item 5* cross-cultural validity/measurement invariance, *Item 6* reliability, *Item 7* measurement error, *Item 8* criterion validity, *Item 9* hypothesis testing for construct validity, *Item 10* responsiveness, + sufficient, – insufficient, ? indeterminate

[50]. Table 15 summarizes the papers' authors and languages and Table 16 shows the quality of the studies.

3.9 Life Satisfaction Questionnaire (LISAT-9)

The LISAT-9 was validated for people with SCI in English [37], Dutch [44], and Polish [51]. The LISAT-9 consists of one question about satisfaction with life as a whole and eight questions about satisfaction with different life domains: self-care ability, leisure time, vocational situation, financial situation, sexual life, partnership relations, fam-

Table 17 Characteristics of the studies validating LISAT-9

Authors	Language	n	Age mean (SD, range) year	Gender % Female
Tasiemski and Brewer [51]	Poland	1034	35.93 (10)	173 (16.7)
Geyh et al. [37]	English	243	41.4 (13.6)	50 (20.6)
Post et al. [44]	Dutch	145	45.4 (13.7)	41 (28)

n number of participants of the study, *n.a.* not available

ily life, and contact with friends. Each question is scored on a 6-point scale (1, very unsatisfied; 6, very satisfied). Item scores can be dichotomized into unsatisfied [1–4] and satisfied [5, 6] to report results on item level, if appropriate. Further, a total score is computed as the mean of the item scores (range, 1–6). The LiSat-9 has been reported as responsive to decreased life satisfaction after experiencing an SCI and increased life satisfaction after a psychosocial activity course. Table 17 summarizes the papers' authors and languages and Table 18 shows the quality of the studies.

3.10 Spinal Cord Injury Lifestyle Scale (SCILS)

Pruitt et al. created the Spinal Cord Injury Lifestyle Scale (SCILS) in 1998 as a new measure to assess health behaviors that delay or prevent secondary impairments in individuals with SCI. In 2017, Shabany et al. validated SCILS in the Persian language. The SCILS evaluates

Table 18 Evaluation of quality and risk of bias

Authors	Item of COSMIN checklist									
	1	2	3	4	5	6	7	8	9	10
Tasiemski and Brewer [51]	?	?	+	–	–	–	–	+	+	–
Geyh et al. [37]	?	?	+	–	–	–	–	+	+	–
Post et al. [44]	?	?	+	–	–	–	–	+	+	–

Item 1 PROM development, *Item 2* content validity, *Item 3* structural validity, *Item 4* internal consistency, *Item 5* cross-cultural validity/measurement invariance, *Item 6* reliability, *Item 7* measurement error, *Item 8* criterion validity, *Item 9* hypothesis testing for construct validity, *Item 10* responsiveness, + sufficient, – insufficient, *?* indeterminate

Table 19 Characteristics of the studies validating SCILS

Authors	Language	n	Age mean (SD, range) year	Gender % Female
Pruitt et al. [53]	English	49	45.54 (13.05, 19–73)	49 (100)
Shabany et al. [52]	Persian	97	36.29 (11.49)	20 (26)

n = number of participants of the study, *n.a.* not available

Table 20 Evaluation of quality and risk of bias

Authors	Item of COSMIN checklist									
	1	2	3	4	5	6	7	8	9	10
Pruitt et al. [53]	?	?	+	–	–	–	–	+	+	–
Shabany et al. [52]	?	?	+	–	–	–	–	+	+	–

Item 1 PROM development, *Item 2* content validity, *Item 3* structural validity, *Item 4* internal consistency, *Item 5* cross-cultural validity/measurement invariance, *Item 6* reliability, *Item 7* measurement error, *Item 8* criterion validity, *Item 9* hypothesis testing for construct validity, *Item 10* responsiveness, + sufficient, – insufficient, *?* indeterminate

health behaviors in person with SCI. The SCILS contains five subscales (skin = 7 items, cardiovascular = 4 items, genitourinary = 4 items, neuromuscular = 8 items, and mental = 2 items), for a total of 25 items, and the scores are based on a Likert-type scale of 0–4 (where 0 = never, 1 = rarely, 2 = sometimes, 3 = often, and 4 = always) [52, 53]. Table 19 summarizes the papers' authors and languages and Table 20 shows the quality of the studies.

3.11 International Spinal Cord Injury Quality of Life Basic Data Set (Basic Data Set)

An international expert committee developed the QoL Basic Data Set. It is based on the definition of subjective QoL as reflecting an individual's overall perception of and satisfaction with how things are in their life. To define "what" to measure, QoL was considered as an umbrella term covering both health and well-being, and it was considered useful to distinguish at least a physical health and a mental health domain. It was validated for the SCI population in 2016 in Dutch [54] and 2020 in Thai [55]. Table 21 summarizes the papers' authors and languages and Table 22 shows the quality of the studies.

3.12 The Brief Adaptation to Disability Scale–Revised (B-ADS-R)

The B-ADS-R is an abbreviated version of the ADS-R originally developed by Groomes and

Table 21 Characteristics of the studies validating Basic Data Set

Authors	Language	n	Age mean (SD, range) year	Gender % Female
Post et al. [54]	Dutch	261	47.9 (8.8, 28–66)	70 (26.8)
Pattanakuhar et al. [55]	Thai	130	43 (13.1)	35 (27)

n number of participants of the study, *n.a.* not available

Table 22 Evaluation of quality and risk of bias

Authors	Item of COSMIN checklist									
	1	2	3	4	5	6	7	8	9	10
Post et al. [54]	?	?	+	–	–	–	–	+	+	–
Pattanakuhar et al. [55]	?	?	+	–	–	–	–	+	+	–

Item 1 PROM development, *Item 2* content validity, *Item 3* structural validity, *Item 4* internal consistency, *Item 5* cross-cultural validity/measurement invariance, *Item 6* reliability, *Item 7* measurement error, *Item 8* criterion validity, *Item 9* hypothesis testing for construct validity, *Item 10* responsiveness, + sufficient, – insufficient, *?* indeterminate

Linkowski (2007). It comprises 12 items and four subscales:

1. Enlarging, 3 items (e.g., "There are many things a person with my disability is able to do")
2. Containing, 3 items (e.g., "My disability affects those aspects of life, which I care most about")
3. Subordinating, 3 items (e.g., "Good physical appearance and physical ability are the most important things in life") and
4. Transforming, 3 items (e.g., "Because of my disability, I have little to offer other people"). Each item is rated on a 4-point Likert-type scale ranging from 1 (strongly agree) to 4 (strongly disagree). It was validated in English in 2013 for persons with SCI [56]. Table 23 summarizes the papers authors and languages and Table 24 shows the quality of the studies.

3.13 The SCIQL-23

The SCIQL-23 was developed to specifically examine the HR QOL in people with spinal cord lesions. It consists of 23 questions. The last question is the question of assessing the global quality of life (GQOL). The remaining 22 items are categorized into three main subscales:

1. Functioning (FUNC): This variable assesses the physical and social limitations in patients with SCI.
2. Mood state (MOOD): It concerns the psychological situation of the patients.
3. Problems related to injury (PROB): This item evaluates the level of independence and other issues relating to injury in SCI people.
4. GQOL: This subscale generally shows the life situation of the patients.

All domains' scores will be transformed to make a scale range of 0–100 and only in the GQOL section; a higher score is representative of a higher QOL. Conversely, in the remaining three sections including FUNC, PROB, and MOOD, higher scores equal the poorer status. It was validated for SCI people in Persian language [57]. Table 23 summarizes the papers' authors and languages and Table 24 shows the quality of the studies.

Table 23 Characteristics of the studies of scale, test, or questionnaire with less than two validations

Scale, test, or questionnaire	Authors	Language	n	Age mean (SD, range) year	Gender % Female
PWI	Geyh et al. [37]	English	243	41.4 (13.6)	50 (20.6)
QOLP-PD	Renwick et al. [58]	English	40	35.85 (9.29, 16–61)	10 (25)
QUESTIONNAIRE ON (DIS)ABILITY, IMPACT, AND WEIGHTED SCORE	Laman and Lankhorst [59]	English	25	38.5 (19–67)	3 (13)
MHS	Van Leeuwen et al. [60]	Dutch	145	45.4 (13.7)	38 (26.2)
Qual-OT	Robnett et al. [4]	English	78		
PS	Van Brakel et al. [61]	Portuguese (Brazil) Hindi Dutch	90		
LSQ-R	Krause et al. [62]	English	1203	44.8	324 (27)
RHSCIR	Noreau et al. [63]	Dutch	50	34.5 (12.4)	15 (30)
HBQ	Shabany et al. [52]	Persian	97	36.29 (11.49)	20 (26)
NSQ	Biering-Sorensen et al. [64]	Danish	32	42 (13, 23–72)	8 (25)
B-ADS-R	Lin et al. [56]	English	154	42.1 (13.2)	43 (27.9)
SCI-QL	Ebrahimzadeh et al. [57]	Persian	43	49.3 (7.9, 38–80)	
GSDS	Panuccio et al. [14]	Italian	57	49 (5.15)	20 (35)

n number of participants of the study, *n.a.* not available

Table 24 Evaluation of quality and risk of bias

| Authors | Item of COSMIN checklist | | | | | | | | | |
	1	2	3	4	5	6	7	8	9	10
Geyh et al. [37]	?	?	+	–	–	–	–	–	–	–
Renwick et al. [58]	?	?	+	–	–	–	–	+	+	–
Laman and Lankhorst [59]	?	?	+	–	–	–	–	+	+	–
Van Leeuwen et al. [60]	?	?	+	–	–	–	–	+	+	–
Robnett et al. [4]	?	?	+	–	–	–	–	+	+	–
Van Brakel et al. [61]	?	?	+	–	–	–	–	+	+	–
Krause et al. [62]	?	?	+	–	–	–	–	+	+	–
Noreau et al. [63]	?	?	+	–	–	–	–	+	+	–
Shabany et al. [52]	?	?	+	–	–	–	–	+	+	–
Biering-Sorensen et al. [64]	?	?	+	–	–	–	–	+	+	–
Lin et al. [56]	?	?	+	–	–	–	–	+	+	–
Ebrahimzadeh et al. [57]	?	?	+	–	–	–	–	+	+	–
Panuccio et al. [14]	?	?	+	–	–	–	–	+	+	–

Item 1 PROM development, *Item 2* content validity, *Item 3* structural validity, *Item 4* internal consistency, *Item 5* cross-cultural validity/measurement invariance, *Item 6* reliability, *Item 7* measurement error, *Item 8* criterion validity, *Item 9* hypothesis testing for construct validity, *Item 10* responsiveness, + sufficient, – insufficient, ? indeterminate

3.14 General Sleep Disturbance Scale (GSDS-IT)

The GSDS-IT is a self-assessment scale (Likert-type) measuring sleep disturbances. It is composed of 21 items divided into six domains related to the frequency during the last week of the following experiences: difficulty getting to sleep (1 item), waking up during sleep (2 items), quality of sleep (3 items), quantity of sleep (2 items), daytime sleepiness (7 items), and the use of substances to help induce sleep (6 items). It was validated in Italian in 2020 [14]. Table 23 summarizes the papers authors and languages and Table 24 shows the quality of the studies.

3.15 The Quality of Life Profile for Adults with Physical Disabilities (QOLP-PD)

QOL-PD was validated in Canada by Rebecca Renwick et al. in 2003 for people with SCI [58]. Designed to offer a new approach to measuring QOL that is grounded and congruent with the perspective and experience of people with disabilities. Based on the Centre for Health Promotion (CHP) QOL model that views QOL as arising out of the ongoing relationship between the person and his/her environment. It is comprised of three domains: being, belonging, becoming. Table 23 summarizes the papers' authors and languages and Table 24 shows the quality of the studies.

3.16 Questionnaire on (Dis)Ability, Impact, and Weighted Score

A questionnaire was developed from a compressed disability list based on WHO's International Classification of Impairments, Disabilities, and Handicaps (ICIDH). The questionnaire is based mainly on the disability code. However, some impairments (pain, disfigurement, incontinence) were added because they have an unmistakable influence on the quality of life in many patients. The items were carefully formulated in (Dutch) layman's terms. The questionnaire consists of 39 items. Each item is rated for the (dis)ability aspect on a 0–10 point scale (0: maximal disability; 10: no disability). Each ability question is followed by asking the respondent to rate the impact or importance of that particular disability (weight), using the same kind of 0–10 point scale (0: not important at all; 10: most important of all)

[59]. Table 23 summarizes the papers' authors and languages and Table 24 shows the quality of the studies.

3.17 Mental Health Subscale (MHS-5)

The MHI-5 was validated in Dutch for people with SCI [60]. It is a mental health subscale of the 36-Item Short-Form Health Survey (SF-36). The MHI-5 has a good specificity and sensitivity for detecting mental health disorders and depression in the general population and persons with various chronic conditions. The MHI-5 consists of 5 items concerning nervousness, sadness, peacefulness, mood, and happiness. Respondents rate the frequency of each item for the previous 4 weeks on a 6-point Likert-type response scale ($1\frac{1}{4}$ all of the time, $2\frac{1}{4}$ most of the time, $3\frac{1}{4}$ a good bit of the time, $4\frac{1}{4}$ some of the time, $5\frac{1}{4}$ a little of the time, $6\frac{1}{4}$ none of the time). For example, "How much of the time, during the last month, have you felt downhearted and blue?" A total score is computed by summing and transforming the 5-item scores into a score between 0 (lowest mental health) and 100 (highest mental health). A cutoff point of 72 or lower refers to mental health problems and 60 or lower refers to severe mental health problems. Table 23 summarizes the papers' authors and languages and Table 24 shows the quality of the studies.

3.18 Quality-of-Life Assessment Tool (Qual-OT)

The Qual-OT was developed in 1995 by Regula H. Robnett, Jeffrey A. in the United States [4]. The Qual-OT is an assessment tool developed to help define the quality of life for occupational therapists. The Qual-OT comprises a series of 80 adjective pairs or phrases on which each participant was to rate himself or herself. Each half of the opposite item pair were placed randomly on either side of a 5-point Likert-type scale. The participants also were asked to pick out any ten adjectives/phrases (from either or both sides) that would be of utmost importance to their quality of life given ideal conditions. This process allowed each participant the opportunity to weigh what quality of life meant to them specifically and personally. Each person was also asked a question of general affect based on Bradburn and Caplovitz's Happiness scale (1965). Table 23 summarizes the papers' authors and languages and Table 24 shows the quality of the studies.

3.19 Participation Scale (PS)

In 2006, W. H. van Brakel et al. developed PS in Nepal, India, and Brazil [61]. The instrument, available in Portuguese (Brazil), Hindi, and Dutch, was created based on the Participation domains of the International Classification of Functioning, Disability, and Health (ICF). The scale has been validated for use with people affected by leprosy, spinal cord injuries, polio, and other disabilities. The Participation Scale contains 18-item that measure perceived problems in major, mainly socioeconomic areas of life, with the response "0" = no restriction, "1" = some restriction, but no problem, "2" = small problem, "3" = medium problem, and "5" = large problem. Table 23 summarizes the papers' authors and languages and Table 24 shows the quality of the studies.

3.20 Life Situation Questionnaire– Revised (LSQ-R)

In 2009, the Medical University of South Carolina, USA, validated the LSQ-R [62]. The questionnaire measures multiple aspects of subjective well-being in adults with SCI. The LSQ-R has two major sets of subjective items that include 20 satisfaction items and 30 problem items. Both the satisfaction and problem items are measured on a 5-point scale, although the anchor points are specific to each set of items. Seven subjective well-being scales were identified by factor analysis of the 50 items: (a) Engagement, (b) Negative Affect, (c) Health Problems, (d) Finances, (e) Career Opportunities, (f) Living Circumstances, and (g) Interpersonal Relations. Both satisfaction and problem items are to be used independently, depending on the study's purpose. Table 23 summarizes the papers' authors and languages of the papers and Table 24 shows the quality of the studies.

3.21 Rick Hansen Spinal Cord Injury Registry (RHSCIR)

The RHSCIR was validated in Canada in 2006 [63]. A comprehensive follow-up questionnaire, referred to as the RHSCIR Community Follow-up Questionnaire Version 2.0 (CFQ-V2.0), includes eight instruments. Four newly developed instruments, with two existing instruments modified, and two previously published instruments were included. Table 23 summarizes the papers' authors and languages and Table 24 shows the quality of the studies.

3.22 Health Behavior Questionnaire (HBQ)

Bloemen-Vrencken (2007) used the spinal cord injury (SCILS) as a basis for creating a new health behavior questionnaire (HBQ), and several items from the original SCILS instrument were adopted. In 2017, M. Shabany et al. validated the HBQ in the Persian language. The HBQ contains 22 items, and scoring is based on a Likert-type scale of 0–3. The questionnaire derived from the SCILS by Bloemen-Vrencken et al. was reduced to 22 items (some new) [52]. Table 23 summarizes the papers' authors and languages and Table 24 shows the quality of the studies.

3.23 Nordic Sleep Questionnaire (NSQ)

The original version of NSQ is in English, and in 1994 it was translated into Danish. The NSQ contains 21 sleep questions. Most of the questions can be answered by a ticking the appropriate box, but some must be answered by inputting the numbers of minutes, hours, years, or by time of day or night. The last question is an open one where sleep problems can be described in free text. The questionnaire generally asks the subject to describe their situation during "the last three months." In addition, there are some introductory questions on the job situation, intake of stimulants (smoking, alcohol, coffee/tea), together with questions on the respondent's height and weight [64]. Table 23 summarizes the papers' authors and languages and Table 24 shows the quality of the studies.

3.24 Personal Well-being Index (PWI)

The PWI has been developed in Australia for national surveys and has been adapted for international use. It was validated for people with SCI in the United States [37]. It consists of 7 items about satisfaction with specific life domains (living standard, health, achievement, relationships, safety, community, future security) and one optional item about overall life satisfaction. Responses follow a 0–10 numeric rating scale with the endpoints "completely dissatisfied" to "completely satisfied." Table 23 summarizes the papers' authors and languages and Table 24 shows the quality of the studies.

4 Conclusions

This chapter reports all assessment tools described in the literature to assess the quality of life in people with SCI. The majority of scales assess participation by persons with SCI, while six scales assess satisfaction. There are several scales, each of which assesses the quality of life in various ways.

References

1. Gecht J, Mainz V, Boecker M, et al. Development of a short scale for assessing economic environmental aspects in patients with spinal diseases using Rasch analysis. Health Qual Life Outcomes. 2017. https://doi.org/10.1186/s12955-017-0767-9.
2. Hitzig SL, Romero Escobar EM, Noreau L, Craven BC. Validation of the reintegration to normal living index for community-dwelling persons with chronic spinal cord injury. Arch Phys Med Rehabil. 2012. https://doi.org/10.1016/j.apmr.2011.07.200.
3. Williams A. Do we really need to measure the quality of life? Br J Hosp Med. 1988;39(3):181.
4. Robnett RH, Gliner JA. Qual-OT: a quality of life assessment tool. Occup Ther J Res. 1995. https://doi.org/10.1177/153944929501500304.
5. Castelnuovo G, Giusti EM, Manzoni GM, et al. What is the role of the placebo effect for pain relief in neurorehabilitation? Clinical implications from the Italian consensus conference on pain in neurorehabilitation. Front Neurol. 2018. https://doi.org/10.3389/fneur.2018.00310.
6. Marquez MA, De Santis R, Ammendola V, et al. Cross-cultural adaptation and validation of the "spinal cord injury-falls concern scale" in the Italian population. Spinal Cord. 2018;56(7):712–8. https://doi.org/10.1038/s41393-018-0070-6.
7. Berardi A, De Santis R, Tofani M, et al. The Wheelchair Use Confidence Scale: Italian translation, adaptation, and validation of the short form. Disabil Rehabil Assist Technol. 2018;13(4):i. https://doi.org/10.1080/17483107.2017.1357053.
8. Anna B, Giovanni G, Marco T, et al. The validity of rasterstereography as a technological tool for the objectification of postural assessment in the clinical and educational fields: pilot study. In: Advances in intelligent systems and computing. 2020. https://doi.org/10.1007/978-3-030-23884-1_8.
9. Panuccio F, Berardi A, Marquez MA, et al. Development of the pregnancy and motherhood evaluation questionnaire (PMEQ) for evaluating and measuring the impact of physical disability on pregnancy and the management of motherhood: a pilot study. Disabil Rehabil. 2020;2020:1–7. https://doi.org/10.1080/09638288.2020.1802520.
10. Amedoro A, Berardi A, Conte A, et al. The effect of aquatic physical therapy on patients with multiple sclerosis: a systematic review and meta-analysis. Mult Scler Relat Disord. 2020. https://doi.org/10.1016/j.msard.2020.102022.
11. Dattoli S, Colucci M, Soave MG, et al. Evaluation of pelvis postural systems in spinal cord injury patients: outcome research. J Spinal Cord Med. 2018;43:185–92.
12. Berardi A, Galeoto G, Guarino D, et al. Construct validity, test-retest reliability, and the ability to detect change of the Canadian occupational performance measure in a spinal cord injury population. Spinal Cord Ser Cases. 2019; https://doi.org/10.1038/s41394-019-0196-6.
13. Ponti A, Berardi A, Galeoto G, Marchegiani L, Spandonaro C, Marquez MA. Quality of life, concern of falling and satisfaction of the sit-ski aid in sit-skiers with spinal cord injury: observational study. Spinal Cord Ser Cases. 2020. https://doi.org/10.1038/s41394-020-0257-x.
14. Panuccio F, Galeoto G, Marquez MA, et al. General sleep disturbance scale (GSDS-IT) in people with spinal cord injury: a psychometric study. Spinal Cord. 2020. https://doi.org/10.1038/s41393-020-0500-0.
15. Monti M, Marquez MA, Berardi A, Tofani M, Valente D, Galeoto G. The multiple sclerosis intimacy and sexuality questionnaire (MSISQ-15): validation of the Italian version for individuals with spinal cord injury. Spinal Cord. 2020. https://doi.org/10.1038/s41393-020-0469-8.
16. Galeoto G, Colucci M, Guarino D, et al. Exploring validity, reliability, and factor analysis of the Quebec user evaluation of satisfaction with assistive technology in an Italian population: a cross-sectional study. Occup Ther Heal Care. 2018. https://doi.org/10.1080/07380577.2018.1522682.
17. Colucci M, Tofani M, Trioschi D, Guarino D, Berardi A, Galeoto G. Reliability and validity of the Italian version of Quebec user evaluation of satisfaction with assistive technology 2.0 (QUEST-IT 2.0) with users of mobility assistive device. Disabil Rehabil Assist Technol. 2019. https://doi.org/10.1080/17483107.2019.1668975.
18. Berardi A, Galeoto G, Lucibello L, Panuccio F, Valente D, Tofani M. Athletes with disability' satisfaction with sport wheelchairs: an Italian cross sectional study. Disabil Rehabil Assist Technol. 2020. https://doi.org/10.1080/17483107.2020.1800114.
19. Moher D, Shamseer L, Clarke M, et al. Preferred reporting items for systematic review and meta-analysis protocols (PRISMA-P) 2015 statement. Rev Esp Nutr Human Diet. 2016. https://doi.org/10.1186/2046-4053-4-1.
20. Mokkink LB, Terwee CB, Patrick DL, et al. The COSMIN study reached international consensus on taxonomy, terminology, and definitions of measurement properties for health-related patient-reported outcomes. J Clin Epidemiol. 2010. https://doi.org/10.1016/j.jclinepi.2010.02.006.
21. Terwee CB, Prinsen CAC, Chiarotto A, et al. COSMIN methodology for evaluating the content validity of patient-reported outcome measures: a Delphi study. Qual Life Res. 2018. https://doi.org/10.1007/s11136-018-1829-0.

22. Mokkink LB, de Vet HCW, Prinsen CAC, et al. COSMIN risk of bias checklist for systematic reviews of patient-reported outcome measures. Qual Life Res. 2018. https://doi.org/10.1007/s11136-017-1765-4.

23. Rintala DH, Novy DM, Garza HM, Young ME, High WM, Chiou-Tan FY. Psychometric properties of a Spanish-language version of the community integration questionnaire (CIQ). Rehabil Psychol. 2002. https://doi.org/10.1037/0090-5550.47.2.144.

24. Hirsh AT, Braden AL, Craggs JG, Jensen MP. Psychometric properties of the community integration questionnaire in a heterogeneous sample of adults with physical disability. Arch Phys Med Rehabil. 2011. https://doi.org/10.1016/j.apmr.2011.05.004.

25. Kratz AL, Chadd E, Jensen MP, Kehn M, Kroll T. An examination of the psychometric properties of the community integration questionnaire (CIQ) in spinal cord injury. J Spinal Cord Med. 2015. https://doi.org/10.1179/2045772313y.0000000182.

26. Gontkovsky ST, Russum P, Stokic DS. Comparison of the CIQ and chart short form in assessing community integration in individuals with chronic spinal cord injury: a pilot study. NeuroRehabilitation. 2009. https://doi.org/10.3233/NRE-2009-0467.

27. Ioncoli M, Berardi A, Tofani M, et al. Crosscultural validation of the community integration questionnaire-revised in an Italian population. Occup Ther Int. 2020. https://doi.org/10.1155/2020/8916541.

28. Post MWM, van de Port IGL, Kap B, Berdenis van Berlekom SH. Development and validation of the Utrecht scale for evaluation of clinical rehabilitation (USER). Clin Rehabil. 2009. https://doi.org/10.1177/0269215509341524.

29. Van Der Zee CH, Post MW, Brinkhof MW, Wagenaar RC. Comparison of the Utrecht scale for evaluation of rehabilitation – participation with the ICF measure of participation and activities screener and the WHO disability assessment schedule ii in persons with spinal cord injury. Arch Phys Med Rehabil. 2014. https://doi.org/10.1016/j.apmr.2013.08.236.

30. Mader L, Post MWM, Ballert CS, Michel G, Stucki G, Brinkhof MWG. Metric properties of the Utrecht scale for evaluation of rehabilitation-participation (user-participation) in persons with spinal cord injury living in Switzerland. J Rehabil Med. 2016. https://doi.org/10.2340/16501977-2010.

31. Jang Y, Hsieh CL, Wang YH, Wu YH. A validity study of the WHOQOL-BREF assessment in persons with traumatic spinal cord injury. Arch Phys Med Rehabil. 2004. https://doi.org/10.1016/j.apmr.2004.02.032.

32. Lin MR, Hwang HF, Chen CY, Chiu WT. Comparisons of the brief form of the world health organization quality of life and short form-36 for persons with spinal cord injuries. Am J Phys Med Rehabil. 2007. https://doi.org/10.1097/01.phm.0000247780.64373.0e.

33. Salvador-De La Barrera S, Mora-Boga R, Ferreiro-Velasco ME, et al. A validity study of the Spanish—World Health Organization quality of life short version instrument in persons with traumatic spinal cord

injury. Spinal Cord. 2018. https://doi.org/10.1038/s41393-018-0139-2.

34. Chapin MH, Miller SM, Ferrins JM, Chan F, Rubin SE. Psychometric validation of a subjective well-being measure for people with spinal cord injuries. Disabil Rehabil. 2004. https://doi.org/10.1080/09638280410001714772.

35. Miller SM, Chan F, Ferrin JM, Lin CP, Chan JYC. Confirmatory factor analysis of the World Health Organization quality of life questionnaire-brief version for individuals with spinal cord injury. Rehabil Couns Bull. 2008. https://doi.org/10.1177/0034355208316806.

36. Lee KJ, Jang HI, Choi H. Korean translation and validation of the WHOQOL-DIS for people with spinal cord injury and stroke. Disabil Health J. 2017. https://doi.org/10.1016/j.dhjo.2016.12.017.

37. Geyh S, Fellinghauer BAG, Kirchberger I, Post MWM. Cross-cultural validity of four quality of life scales in persons with spinal cord injury. Health Qual Life Outcomes. 2010. https://doi.org/10.1186/1477-7525-8-94.

38. May LA, Warren S. Measuring quality of life of persons with spinal cord injury: substantive and structural validation. Qual Life Res. 2001. https://doi.org/10.1023/A:1013027520429.

39. May LA, Warren S. Measuring quality of life of persons with spinal cord injury: external and structural validity. Spinal Cord. 2002. https://doi.org/10.1038/sj.sc.3101311.

40. Reis PAM, Carvalho ZM de F, Darder JJT, Oriá MOB, Studart RMB, Maniva SJC de F. Cross-cultural adaptation of the quality of life index spinal cord injury – version III. Rev da Esc Enferm. 2015. https://doi.org/10.1590/S0080-623420150000300007.

41. Kovacs FM, Barriga A, Royuela A, Seco J, Zamora J. Spanish adaptation of the quality of life index-spinal cord injury version. Spinal Cord. 2016. https://doi.org/10.1038/sc.2015.200.

42. Catalano D, Kim JH, Ditchman NM, uk SH, Lee J, Chan F. The sense of well-being inventory as a quality of life measure for people with spinal cord injury. Aust J Rehabil Couns. 2010. https://doi.org/10.1375/jrc.16.2.57.

43. Amtmann D, Bocell FD, Bamer A, et al. Psychometric properties of the satisfaction with life scale in people with traumatic brain, spinal cord, or burn injury: a National Institute on Disability, Independent Living, and Rehabilitation Research model system study. Assessment. 2019. https://doi.org/10.1177/1073191117693921.

44. Post MW, Van Leeuwen CM, Van Koppenhagen CF, De Groot S. Validity of the life satisfaction questions, the life satisfaction questionnaire, and the satisfaction with life scale in persons with spinal cord injury. Arch Phys Med Rehabil. 2012. https://doi.org/10.1016/j.apmr.2012.03.025.

45. Tulsky DS, Kisala PA, Lai JS, Carlozzi N, Hammel J, Heinemann AW. Developing an item bank to measure economic quality of life for individuals with dis-

abilities. Arch Phys Med Rehabil. 2015. https://doi.org/10.1016/j.apmr.2014.02.030.

46. Forchheimer M, McAweeney M, Tate DG. Use of the SF-36 among persons with spinal cord injury. Am J Phys Med Rehabil. 2004. https://doi.org/10.1097/01.PHM.0000124441.78275.C9.

47. Luther SL, Kromrey J, Powell-Cope G, et al. A pilot study to modify the SF-36V physical functioning scale for use with veterans with spinal cord injury. Arch Phys Med Rehabil. 2006. https://doi.org/10.1016/j.apmr.2006.05.010.

48. Lee BB, King MT, Simpson JM, et al. Validity, responsiveness, and minimal important difference for the SF-6D health utility scale in a spinal cord injured population. Value Heal. 2008. https://doi.org/10.1111/j.1524-4733.2007.00311.x.

49. Engel L, Bryan S, Evers SMAA, Dirksen CD, Noonan VK, Whitehurst DGT. Exploring psychometric properties of the SF-6D, a preference-based health-related quality of life measure, in the context of spinal cord injury. Qual Life Res. 2014. https://doi.org/10.1007/s11136-014-0677-9.

50. Lee BB, Simpson JM, King MT, Haran MJ, Marial O. The SF-36 walk-wheel: a simple modification of the SF-36 physical domain improves its responsiveness for measuring health status change in spinal cord injury. Spinal Cord. 2009. https://doi.org/10.1038/sc.2008.65.

51. Tasiemski T, Brewer BW. Athletic identity, sport participation, and psychological adjustment in people with spinal cord injury. Adapt Phys Act Q. 2011. https://doi.org/10.1123/apaq.28.3.233.

52. Shabany M, Nasrabadi AN, Rahimi-Movaghar V, Mansournia MA, Mohammadi N, Pruitt SD. Reliability and validity of the Persian version of the spinal cord injury lifestyle scale and the health behavior questionnaire in persons with spinal cord injury. Spinal Cord. 2018. https://doi.org/10.1038/s41393-017-0056-9.

53. Pruitt SD, Wahlgren DR, Epping-Jordan JE, Rossi AL. Health behavior in persons with spinal cord injury: development and initial validation of an outcome measure. Spinal Cord. 1998. https://doi.org/10.1038/sj.sc.3100649.

54. Post MWM, Adriaansen JJE, Charlifue S, Biering-Sørensen F, Van Asbeck FWA. Good validity of the international spinal cord injury quality of life basic data set. Spinal Cord. 2016. https://doi.org/10.1038/sc.2015.99.

55. Pattanakuhar S, Suttinoon L, Wongpakaran T, Tongprasert S. The reliability and validity of the international spinal cord injury quality of life basic data set in people with spinal cord injuries from a middle-income country: a psychometric study of the Thai version. Spinal Cord. 2020; https://doi.org/10.1038/s41393-020-0468-9.

56. Lin C-P, Wang C-C, Fujikawa M, et al. Psychometric validation of the brief adaptation to disability scale-revised for persons with spinal cord injury in Taiwan. Rehabil Res Policy, Educ. 2013. https://doi.org/10.1891/2168-6653.27.3.223.

57. Ebrahimzadeh MH, Makhmalbaf H, Soltani-Moghaddas SH, Mazloumi SM. The spinal cord injury quality-of-life-23 questionnaire, Iranian validation study. J Res Med Sci. 2014;19:349–54.

58. Renwick R, Nourhaghighi N, Manns PJ, Rudman DL. Quality of life for people with physical disabilities: a new instrument. Int J Rehabil Res. 2003. https://doi.org/10.1097/00004356-200312000-00005.

59. Laman H, Lankhorst GJ. Subjective weighting of disability: an approach to quality of life assessment in rehabilitation. Disabil Rehabil. 1994. https://doi.org/10.3109/09638289409166613.

60. Van Leeuwen CMC, Van Der Woude LHV, Post MWM. Validity of the mental health subscale of the SF-36 in persons with spinal cord injury. Spinal Cord. 2012. https://doi.org/10.1038/sc.2012.33.

61. Van Brakel WH, Anderson AM, Mutatkar RK, et al. The participation scale: measuring a key concept in public health. Disabil Rehabil. 2006. https://doi.org/10.1080/09638280500192785.

62. Krause JS, Reed KS. Life satisfaction and self-reported problems after spinal cord injury: measurement of underlying dimensions. Rehabil Psychol. 2009. https://doi.org/10.1037/a0016555.

63. Noreau L, Cobb J, Bélanger LM, Dvorak MF, Leblond J, Noonan VK. Development and assessment of a community follow-up questionnaire for the rick Hansen spinal cord injury registry. Arch Phys Med Rehabil. 2013. https://doi.org/10.1016/j.apmr.2013.03.006.

64. Biering-Sørensen F, Biering-Sørensen M, Hilden J. Reproducibility of nordic sleep questionnaire in spinal cord injured. Paraplegia. 1994. https://doi.org/10.1038/sc.1994.124.

Measuring Activity of Daily Living in Spinal Cord Injury

Francescaroberta Panuccio, Giulia Grieco,
Marina D'Angelo, and Maria Auxiliadora Marquez

1 Introduction

Spinal cord injury (SCI) results in a loss of motor and sensory function and autonomic innervation below the level of the injury. As a result, patients suffer limitations in performing daily activities, which causes significant functional impact [1]. The ability in performing activities of daily living (ADLs) is a prerequisite for independent living in the community for SCI patients [2]. It has been shown to have a positive influence on their quality of life. Health professionals and rehabilitation professionals often use a person's ability or inability to perform ADLs to measure their functional status. This focus on rehabilitation after an SCI aims to identify the best treatment methods and routines to help patients return to their previous lives and daily activities. The use of the term "activities of daily living" is familiar to many; however, universal agreement of the concept and definition of ADL has been problematic, with subdivision of ADL into basic or personal ADLS (BADL, PADL) and instrumental or extended ADLs (IADL, EADL). The Medical Dictionary defines ADL as "the things we normally do… such as feeding our-selves, bathing, dressing, grooming, work, home-making, and leisure." Consistent with the Medical Dictionary's definition we have considered ADLs, including basic, personal, instrumental, and extended daily living activities.

Furthermore, ADL corresponds to "participation," defined as involvement in life situations, including being autonomous to some extent, or being able to control one's own life, according to the World Health Organization's International Classification of Functioning, Disability, and Health. Accurately measuring the ADL of SCI patients is essential for appropriate treatment planning, clinical decision-making, long-term prognosis, and outcome measurements. The objective documentation of functional ability after SCI is decisive in interpreting outcomes and evaluating the validity of rehabilitation.

The objective of this study was to describe and evaluate assessment tools on the activity of daily living in people with SCI through a systematic review.

2 Materials and Methods

This study was conducted by a research group composed of medical doctors and health professionals from the "Sapienza" University of Rome and the "Rehabilitation & Outcome Measure Assessment" (R.O.M.A.) association. In the last few years, the R.O.M.A. association has

F. Panuccio (✉) · G. Grieco · M. D'Angelo
R.O.M.A. Rehabilitation Outcome Measures Assessment, Non-Profit Organization, Rome, Italy

M. Auxiliadora Marquez
Universidad Fernando Pessoa-Canarias,
Las Palmas, Spain

engaged several studies and the validation of many outcome measures in Italy for the Spinal Cord Injury population [3–16]. This chapter describes all assessment tools regarding the activity of daily living resulting from a systematic review conducted on PubMed, Scopus, and Web of Science. For specific details on methodology, see chapter "Methodological Approach to Identifying Outcome Measures in Spinal Cord Injury." Eligibility criteria for considering studies for this chapter were validation studies and cross-cultural adaptation studies, studies about the activity of daily living, studies about tests, questionnaires, and self-reported and performance-based outcome measures, studies with a population of people of SCI and population ≥18 years old. Study selection: the selection of studies was conducted in accordance with the 27-item PRISM Statement for Reporting Systematic Reviews [17]. For the data collection, the authors followed the recommendations from the COnsensus-based Standards for the selection of health Measurement Instruments (COSMIN) initiative [18]. Study quality and risk of bias were assessed using COSMIN Checklist [19, 20].

3 Results

For this chapter, 123 papers were considered. The authors found 48 assessment tools that evaluate the neurological area in persons with an SCI. See Fig. 1 a flow chart of included studies.

3.1 The Physical Activity Recall Assessment for People with Spinal Cord Injury (PARA-SCI)

It was developed by Martin Ginis et al. in 2005 in the English language [2, 21, 22]. The PARA-SCI is a valid and reliable instrument administered via a semi-structured interview. The PARA-SCI is a self-report measure of time spent doing mild, moderate, and heavy intensity physical activity

for the 3-day period preceding the interview. Table 1 summarizes the papers' authors and languages and Table 2 shows the quality of the studies.

3.2 Transfer Assessment Instrument (TAI)

The TAI was designed to be used by clinicians to evaluate transfer quality and a patient's adherence to best transfer techniques. It was validated in the United States [23–25] and India [26]. The instrument assesses the conservation of upper limb function, safety, and how well people can direct caregivers to assist them with a transfer. The TAI is made up of two parts. In part 1, a transfer is broken down from start to finish into small components, and the person is evaluated on each small component. Part 2 evaluates the person's global performance on quality, conservation techniques, safety, and direction of care. The tool is intended to be used by clinicians (typically occupational and physical therapists) who instruct full-time wheelchair users on transfer skills and have been trained to use the outcome measure. The TAI contains two parts. Part 1 comprises of 15 items and is scored as follows: "yes", 1 point, "no", 0 points or "not applicable" (N/A), which means a removed item. Part 1 is completed after each transfer, and item scores are averaged to produce a single representative item score. Part one is the summation of each item's score multiplied by 10 and then divided by the number of applicable items, ranging from 0 to 10. The items in part two are completed after all transfers have been performed. The 12 items in part 2 are scored on a Likert-type scale ranging from 0 (strongly disagree) to 4 (strongly agree). The part 2 score is the summation of each item's score multiplied by 2.5 and then divided by the number of applicable items, resulting in a range of scores from 0 to 10. The final score of TAI is the average of parts 1 and 2. Other versions are TAI 3.0 (Tsai et al.) and TAI 4.0. Table 3 summarizes the papers' authors and languages and Table 4 shows the quality of the studies.

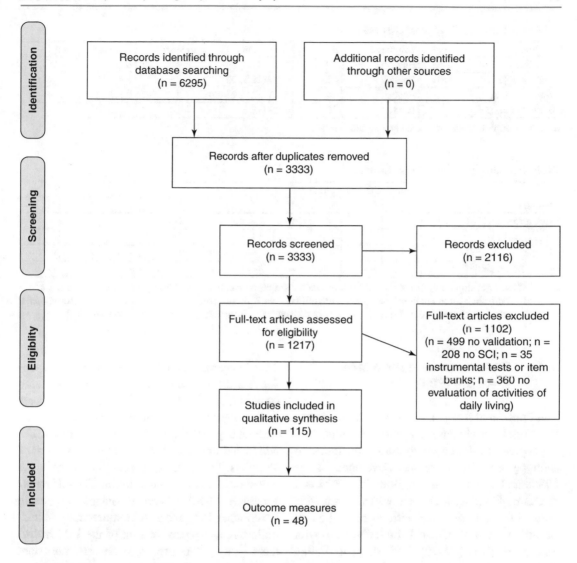

Fig. 1 Flow chart of the included study

Table 1 Characteristics of the studies validating PARA-SCI

Authors	Language	n	Age mean (SD, range) year	Gender % Female
Latimer et al. [21]	English	158	38.47 (11.1)	48 (30.4)
Ginis et al. [22]	English	102	39 (11.2)	30 (29.4)
Latimers et al. [21]	English	73	39 (11.2)	21 (28.8)

n number of participants of the study, *n.a.* not available

Table 2 Evaluation of quality and risk of bias

Authors	Item of COSMIN checklist									
	1	2	3	4	5	6	7	8	9	10
Latimer et al. [21]	?	?	−	−	+	−	−	−	−	−
Ginis et al. [22]	+	+	−	−	+	+	−	+	+	−
Latimer et al. [21]	?	?	+	−	+	−	−	+	+	−

Item 1 PROM development, *Item 2* content validity, *Item 3* structural validity, *Item 4* internal consistency, *Item 5* cross-cultural validity/measurement invariance, *Item 6* reliability, *Item 7* measurement error, *Item 8* criterion validity, *Item 9* hypothesis testing for construct validity, *Item 10* responsiveness, + sufficient, − insufficient, ? indeterminate

Table 3 Characteristics of the studies validating TAI

Authors	Language	n	Age mean (SD, range) year	Gender % Female
McClure et al. [23]	English	40	51.7 (11.3, 27–74)	6 (15)
Tsai et al. [24]	English	41	49.9 (12.7, 23–75)	10 (24)
Worobey et al. [25]	English	44	56.5 (12.7, 25–86)	9 (16.7)
Baghel et al. [26]	Hindi	30	31.9 (12.3)	5 (16.7)

n number of participants of the study, *n.a.* not available

Table 4 Evaluation of quality and risk of bias

Authors	Item of COSMIN checklist									
	1	2	3	4	5	6	7	8	9	10
McClure et al. [23]	?	+	−	+	−	+	−	−	−	−
Tsai et al. [24]	?	?	−	−	−	−	+	−	−	−
Worobey et al. [25]	?	?	−	+	−	+	+	+	+	−
Baghel et al. [26]	?	+	−	−	−	+	+	+	+	−

Item 1 PROM development, *Item 2* content validity, *Item 3* structural validity, *Item 4* internal consistency, *Item 5* cross-cultural validity/measurement invariance, *Item 6* reliability, *Item 7*: measurement error, *Item 8* criterion validity, *Item 9* hypothesis testing for construct validity, *Item 10*: responsiveness, + sufficient, − insufficient, ? indeterminate

3.3 Functional Independence Measure (FIM)

The Functional Independence Measure measures functional capacity and independence, estimating the degree of difficulty or limitation attributed to each person. The scale was developed in the 1980s and was validated in 1986. The FIM is a measure of activity limitation used across a wide range of conditions and various rehabilitation situations. It was validated for individuals with SCI in English [27–29], Turkish [30], Italian [31], Danish [31], Arabic [31], Portuguese (Brazil) [1, 32], Finnish [33], French [34], Swedish [35], and Norwegian [35]. The FIM scale is a multidimensional instrument that evaluates the performance in the motor and cognitive/social domains, considering the aspects: feeding, personal hygiene, bathing, dressing the upper body, dressing the lower body, using the toilet, urine control, fecal control, transfers to the bed, chair and wheelchair, transfer to the toilet, transfer to bath or shower, mobility, mobility on stairs, comprehension, expression, social interaction, problem resolution, and memory. Each item is scored on a scale from 1 to 7, with seven indicating total independence and one indicating total dependence. The intermediate values cover mod-ified independence (score 6), moderate dependence with the need for supervision or preparation (score 5), or with the need for direct help (scores 1–4). Regarding the complete scale, a person without any disability will achieve a score of 126 points and one with total dependency a score of 18 points. The more dependent the patient is, the lower the total score of the FIM is. The self-report version (FIM-SR) has the advantage of reducing the clinician time and effort required for administration. A self-report version of the FIM instrument may therefore provide an important additional tool for assessing patient independence [36, 37]. Middelton et al. validated Five Additional Mobility And Locomotor Items (5-AML items) [38] and included two mobility and three locomotor items. One mobility item assesses patients' ability to get from a supine position to a sitting position on the edge of a plinth. The other mobility item assesses patients' ability to get from the floor back into their wheelchair. The three locomotor items assess patients' ability to propel a manual wheelchair over flat ground, ramps, and curbs. Subjects were assessed in a manual rather than in a motorized wheelchair to validate the 5-AML locomotion items. Table 5 summarizes the papers' authors and languages and Table 6 shows the quality of the studies.

Table 5 Characteristics of the studies validating FIM, FIM-SF, and FIM-5-AML

Scale, test, or questionnaire	Authors	Language	n	Age mean (SD, range) year	Gender % Female
FIM	Grey and Kennedy [27]	English	40	n.a.	n.a.
	Dodds et al. [28]	English	11,102	65	5439 (49)
	Hall et al. [29]	English	3971	n.a.	n.a.
	Ravaud and Alain Yelnik [34]	French (Canada)	2	n.a.	n.a.
	Küçükdeveci et al. [30]	Tuskish	62	32.7	34 (56)
	Lawton et al. [31]	Italian Danish Arabic English	647	46 (11–93)	200 (31)
	Lundgren-Nilsson et al. [35]	Swedish Norwegian	157	n.a.	n.a.
	da Silva et al. [32]	Portuguese (Brazil)	228	n.a.	35 (15.45)
	Barbetta et al. [1]	Portuguese (Brazil)	218	32 (11.6)	25 (11.5)
	Saltychev et al. [33]	Finnish	155	58.7 (15.5)	68 (44)
FIM-SF	Hoenig et al. [37]	English	6361	n.a.	n.a.
	Masedo et al. [36]	English	38	44.58 (11.38)	3 (9)
FIM-5-AML	Middleton et al. [103]	English	39	28	7 (17.9)

n number of participants of the study, *n.a.* not available

Table 6 Evaluation of quality and risk of bias

Authors	Item of COSMIN checklist									
	1	2	3	4	5	6	7	8	9	10
Grey and Kennedy [27]	?	?	–	–	+	–	–	–	–	–
Dodds et al. [28]	?	?	–	+	–	+	–	+	+	+
Hall et al. [29]	?	?	–	–	+	–	–	–	–	–
Ravaud and Alain Yelnik [34]	?	+	–	–	–	–	–	+	+	–
Küçükdeveci et al. [30]	?	+	+	+	+	+	–	+	+	+
Lawton et al. [31]	?	?	–	–	+	–	–	–	–	–
Lundgren-Nilsson et al. [35]	?	?	–	–	+	–	–	–	–	–
da Silva et al. [32]	?	+	–	–	+	–	–	–	–	+
Barbetta et al. [1]	?	+	–	–	+	–	–	–	–	–
Saltychev et al. [33]	?	+	+	+	+	–	–	–	–	+
Hoening et al. [37]	?	+	–	–	+	–	–	+	+	–
Masedo et al. [36]	?	?	–	+	+	+	–	+	+	+
Middleton et al. [103]	+	+	+	–	+	–	–	–	–	–

Item 1 PROM development, *Item 2* content validity, *Item 3* structural validity, *Item 4* internal consistency, *Item 5* cross-cultural validity/measurement invariance, *Item 6* reliability, *Item 7* measurement error, *Item 8* criterion validity, *Item 9* hypothesis testing for construct validity, *Item 10* responsiveness, + sufficient, – insufficient, ? indeterminate

3.4 World Health Organization Disability Assessment Scale (WHODS II)

WHODAS II is an instrument that measures everyday functioning across six domains that cor-respond with the activity and participation components of the International Classification of Functioning, Disability, and Health (ICF; WHO 2001). It was validated in Lettish [39], English (Australian) [40–42], and Chinese (Taiwanese) [43]. It was designed as a generic measure suitable

Table 7 Characteristics of the studies validating WHODS II

Authors	Language	n	Age mean (SD, range) year	Gender % Female
Noonan et al. [41]	English	145	48.7 (17.4, 21–86)	66 (45.5)
Steinerte and Vetra [39]	Lettish	101	43.9 (23.5)	27 (27.6)
De Wolf et al. [40]	English	63	34.7 (14.6)	12 (19)
Chiu et al. [43]	Chinese (Taiwan)	521	51.03 (16.43)	117 (32.8)
Noonan et al. [42]	English	n.a.	n.a.	n.a.

n number of participants of the study, *n.a.* not available

Table 8 Evaluation of quality and risk of bias

Authors	Item of COSMIN checklist									
	1	2	3	4	5	6	7	8	9	10
Noonan et al. [41]	?	+	–	+	+	+	+	+	+	–
Steinerte and Vetra [39]	?	+	–	+	+	–	–	–	–	–
De Wolf et al. [40]	?	+	+	+	+	–	–	+	+	–
Chiu et al. [43]	?	+	+	–	+	–	–	–	–	–
Noonan et al. [42]	n.a.	n.a.	n.a.	n.a.	n.a.	n.a.	n.a.	n.a.	n.a.	n.a.

Item 1 PROM development, *Item 2* content validity, *Item 3* structural validity, *Item 4* internal consistency, *Item 5* cross-cultural validity/measurement invariance, *Item 6* reliability, *Item 7* measurement error, *Item 8* criterion validity, *Item 9* hypothesis testing for construct validity, *Item 10* responsiveness, + *sufficient* – insufficient, *?* indeterminate

for different health conditions in different countries and cultures. It is a 36-item generic measure of disability that examines difficulties in six domains of life during the previous 30 days: understanding and communicating (6 items), getting around (5 items), self-care (4 items), getting along with others (5 items), life activities (8 items), and participation in society (8 items). Each item rates on a 5-point scale, from 1 (no difficulty) to 5 (extreme difficulty/cannot do). The instrument produces a total score (disability index) and six domain scores, ranging from 0 (best) to 100 (worst). The domain scores are transformed from the total raw score (sum of items) of each domain according to the following formula: Transformed score = [(actual raw score − lowest possible raw score)/(possible raw score range)] × 100. Table 7 summarizes the papers' authors and languages and Table 8 shows the quality of the studies.

3.5 Spinal Cord Injury Functional Index (SCI-FI)

Jette et al. developed SCI-FI in 2012 [44–46]. The abbreviated version was also developed (SCI-FI short forms) [47]. The SCI-FI measures activity limitations in five domains: basic mobility (54 items), ambulation (39 items), wheelchair mobility (56 items), self-care (90 items), and fine motor function (36 items). The scale uses five response options to describe the amount of difficulty a person has in performing functions without another person's devices, aids, or help. (i.e., 5 = without difficulty at 1 = unable to pay). The SCI-FI can also be administered through a computer or a touchscreen tablet. The Spinal Cord Injury Functional Index/Assistive Technology (SCI-FI/AT) was developed to complement the SCI-FI version 1.0, providing a measure of functional abilities using AT that was designed specifically for persons with SCI. SCI-FI/AT instructions ask participants to select a response based on their ability to do an activity without help from another person, but using equipment or devices they normally use. With the development of the SCI-FI/AT, we have an instrument to evaluate functional status using AT in the domains of Basic Mobility, Self-Care, Fine Motor Function, and Ambulation (along with a previously designed and calibrated Wheelchair mobility scale and SF) [48]. Table 9 summarizes the papers' authors and languages and Table 10 shows the quality of the studies.

Table 9 Characteristics of the studies validating SCI-FI, SCI-FI SF, and SCI-FI-AT

Scale, test, or questionnaire	Authors	Language	n	Age mean (SD, range) year	Gender % Female
SCI-FI	Tulsky et al. [45]	English	855	43.1 (15.3)	198 (23)
	Jette et al. [44]	English	855	43.1 (15.3)	198 (23)
	Sinha et al. [46]	English	855	43.1 (15.3)	198 (23)
SCI-FI SF	Heinemann et al. [58]	English	n.a.	n.a.	n.a.
SCI-FI-AT	Slavin et al. [48]	English	460	43 (15)	87 (19)

n number of participants of the study, *n.a.* not available

Table 10 Evaluation of quality and risk of bias

Authors	Item of COSMIN checklist									
	1	2	3	4	5	6	7	8	9	10
Tulsky et al. [45]	+	+	–	–	+	–	–	–	–	–
Jette et al. [44]	?	+	–	–	–	–	–	+	+	–
Sinha et al. [46]	?	+	–	–	+	–	–	+	+	–
Heinemann et al. [58]	+	+	–	–	–	–	–	–	–	–
Slavin et al. [48]	+	+	–	+	+	–	–	+	+	–

Item 1 PROM development, *Item 2* content validity, *Item 3* structural validity, *Item 4* internal consistency, *Item 5* cross cultural validity/measurement Invariance, *Item 6* reliability, *Item 7* measurement error, *Item 8* criterion validity, *Item 9* hypothesis testing for construct validity, *Item 10* responsiveness, + sufficient, – insufficient, ? indeterminate

Table 11 Characteristics of the studies validating CHART and CHART SF

Scale, test, or questionnaire	Authors	Language	n	Age mean (SD, range) year	Gender % Female
CHART	Whiteneck et al. [49]	English	135	n.a.	n.a.
	Tozato et al. [50]	Japan	293	38.3 (11.9, 18–60)	47 (16)
	Walker et al. [51]	English	236	n.a.	n.a.
CHART SF	Golhasani-Keshtan et al. [52]	Persian	52	n.a.	n.a.

n number of participants of the study, *n.a.* not available

3.6 Craig Handicap Assessment and Reporting Technique (CHART)

The original CHART was developed in 1992 [49], intended to measure handicap among rehabilitation clients living in the community. CHART was validated for SCI population in Japan [50], and English (United States) [51]. The questionnaire consisted of items regarding a medical condition, motor function, performance in basic activities of daily living (BADL) and instrumental activities of daily living (IADL), and level of handicap. Several demographic questions, such as gender, age at injury, injury level, impairment level, place of residence, education completed, and primary employment/ training status, were included in the same questionnaire. The Craig Handicap Assessment and Reporting Technique (CHART) short form in an Iranian population was validated in 2013 [52]. Table 11 summarizes the papers' authors and languages and Table 12 shows the quality of the studies.

3.7 Craig Hospital Inventory of Environmental Factors (CHIEF)

The CHIEF was validated for the SCI population in the English [53] and Hindi languages [54]. The 25-item self-administered CHIEF developed by Whiteneck et al. is a common tool used to assess

Table 12 Evaluation of quality and risk of bias

Authors	Item of COSMIN checklist									
	1	2	3	4	5	6	7	8	9	10
Whiteneck et al. [49]	+	+	–	–	–	–	–	–	–	–
Tozato et al. [50]	?	+	–	–	+	+	–	–	–	–
Walker et al. [51]	?	+	–	–	+	+	–	–	–	–
Golhasani-Keshtan et al. [52]	?	+	–	+	–	–	–	+	+	–

Item 1 PROM development, *Item 2* content validity, *Item 3* structural validity, *Item 4* internal consistency, *Item 5* cross-cultural validity/measurement Invariance, *Item 6* reliability, *Item 7* measurement error, *Item 8* criterion validity, *Item 9* hypothesis testing for construct validity, *Item 10* responsiveness, + sufficient, – insufficient, ? indeterminate

Table 13 Characteristics of the studies validating CHIEF

Authors	Language	n	Age mean (SD, range) year	Gender % Female
Whiteneck et al. [53]	English	n.a.	n.a.	n.a.
Soni et al. [54]	Hindi	30	31.67 (10.09)	4 (13.3)

n number of participants of the study, *n.a.* not available

Table 14 Evaluation of quality and risk of bias

Authors	Item of COSMIN checklist									
	1	2	3	4	5	6	7	8	9	10
Whiteneck et al. [53]	+	+	+	+	+	+	–	+	+	–
Soni et al. [54]	?	?	–	–	+	–	+	–	–	–

Item 1 PROM development, *Item 2* content validity, *Item 3* structural validity, *Item 4* internal consistency, *Item 5* cross-cultural validity/measurement invariance, *Item 6* reliability, *Item 7* measurement error, *Item 8* criterion validity, *Item 9* hypothesis testing for construct validity, *Item 10* responsiveness, + sufficient, – insufficient, ? indeterminate

environmental barriers in people with spinal cord injury and other disabilities. CHIEF addresses both the frequency and magnitude of the environmental barriers encountered and it covers five different domains (i.e., physical, attitudinal, service, productivity, and policy) of barriers that hinder people from doing what they need and want to do. In contrast to other environmental assessment tools, the CHIEF instrument was designed as a shorter inventory of only environmental barriers, not facilitators. The CHIEF instrument has a shorter version developed from the longer version by retaining 12 questions. The frequency with which barriers encountered are scored on a 5-point scale (0 = never; 1 = less than monthly; 2 = monthly; 3 = weekly; and 4 = daily) and the magnitude of the barrier are scored on 3-point scale (0 = no problem because the barrier was never encountered; 1 = a little problem; and 2 = a big problem). A frequency–magnitude product

score was calculated as the product of the frequency score and the magnitude score. Table 13 summarizes the papers' authors and languages and Table 14 shows the quality of the studies.

3.8 Ghent Participation Scale (GPS)

In 2016, D. Van De Velde et al. developed the Ghent Participation Scale, in Belgium [55]. GPS [56] is a digital, self-administered instrument, which provides a generic, pathology-independent measure of participation. The respondent is asked to prioritize the five most important activities he or she carried out personally and the five most important activities he or she delegated to others during the last week. Consequently, every time a patient completes the Ghent Participation Scale, he starts with a different set of prioritized activi-

Table 15 Characteristics of the studies validating GPS

Authors	Language	n	Age mean (SD, range) year	Gender % Female
Van De Velde et al. [55]	Dutch	11	n.a.	n.a.
Van de Velde et al. [56]	Dutch	26	n.a.	n.a.

n number of participants of the study, *n.a.* not available

Table 16 Evaluation of quality and risk of bias

Authors	Item of COSMIN checklist									
	1	2	3	4	5	6	7	8	9	10
Whiteneck et al. [53]	+	+	+	–	–	–	–	–	–	–
Soni et al. [54]	?	+	+	+	+	+	–	–	–	+

Item 1 PROM development, *Item 2* content validity, *Item 3* structural validity, *Item 4* internal consistency, *Item 5* cross-cultural validity/measurement Invariance, *Item 6* reliability, *Item 7* measurement error, *Item 8* criterion validity, *Item 9* hypothesis testing for construct validity, *Item 10* responsiveness, + sufficient, – insufficient, ? indeterminate

ties. After prioritizing, the respondent has to appraise these activities in terms of 15 different subjective variables. For example, one question asks "Was it entirely your choice to engage in this activity?" All items in the scale score using a Likert scale ranging from 1 ("I totally disagree") to 5 ("I totally agree"). A total score is calculated by summing the mean scores for the three sub-scales. Scores for self-performed activities are weighted according to the time spent doing them, and delegated activities weigh according to the number of delegated activities that the respondent wanted to perform personally. The final score is recalculated as a percentage of participation, with higher values indicating greater perceived participation. Table 15 summarizes the papers' authors and languages and Table 16 shows the quality of the studies.

3.9 International Classification of Functioning (ICF) Core Sets for SCI

In 2010, Kirchberger et al. developed the first ICF core sets to assess SCI people in the early post-acute context and long-term context [57]. In 2011, KH Herrmann et al. worked to validate the International Classification of Functioning, Disability, and Health (ICF) core sets for SCI individuals in Switzerland and Germany. These ICF core sets are selections of ICF categories relevant to persons with SCI, 162 categories for per-

sons in the early post-acute context, and 168 categories for persons in the long-term context. The early post-acute context covers any setting where the first comprehensive rehabilitation after the acute SCI is provided. The long-term context refers to any setting care is provided after ending comprehensive rehabilitation [58]. In 2013, the ICF core set SCI was validated in Spanish [59] and Turkish 2019 [60]. In 2014, Ballert et al. worked to determine whether the International Classification of Functioning, Disability, and Health (ICF) categories relevant to SCI can be integrated into clinical measures and obtain insights to guide their future operationalization. They worked in Switzerland, Germany, and Denmark. A total of 33 ICF categories were included in analyzing the body functions and body structures dimension, and 31 were included in the activities and participation (A&P) dimension [61]. In 2015, Chen et al. developed an ICF core set describing subacute SCI specifically for Taiwanese patients in Taiwan [62]. Table 17 summarizes the papers' authors and languages and Table 18 shows the quality of the studies.

3.10 Physical Activity Scale for Individuals with Physical Disabilities (PASIPD)

In 2002, Washburn et al. developed in the United States the Physical Activity Scale for Individuals with Physical Disabilities (PASIPD) [63], spe-

Table 17 Characteristics of the studies validating (ICF) Core Sets for SCI

Authors	Language	n	Age mean (SD, range) year	Gender % Female
Kirchberger et al. [57]	English	n.a.	n.a.	n.a.
Chen et al. [62]	Chinese (Taiwan)	n.a.	n.a.	n.a.
Herrmann et al. [58]	German	n.a.	n.a.	n.a.
Ballert et al. [61]	German	1048	42.2 (15)	225 (21.5)
Lema et al. [59]	Spanish	100		10 (10)
Tatli et al. [60]	Turkish	120	37.5 (15.7)	35 (29.2)

n number of participants of the study, *n.a.* not available

Table 18 Evaluation of quality and risk of bias

Authors	Item of COSMIN checklist									
	1	2	3	4	5	6	7	8	9	10
Kirchberger et al. [57]	+	+	–	–	–	–	–	–	–	–
Chen et al. [62]	+	+	–	–	–	–	–	–	–	–
Herrmann et al. [58]	+	+	–	–	–	–	–	–	–	–
Ballert et al. [61]	+	+	+	–	+	–	–	–	–	–
Lema et al. [59]	?	+	–	–	+	–	–	+	+	–
Tatli et al. [60]	?	+	–	–	+	–	–	+	+	–

Item 1 PROM development, *Item 2* content validity, *Item 3* structural validity, *Item 4* internal consistency, *Item 5* cross-cultural validity/measurement invariance, *Item 6* reliability, *Item 7* measurement error, *Item 8* criterion validity, *Item 9* hypothesis testing for construct validity, *Item 10* responsiveness, + sufficient, – insufficient, ? indeterminate

Table 19 Characteristics of the studies validating PASIPD

Authors	Language	n	Age mean (SD, range) year	Gender % Female
Mat Rosly et al. [65]	English Malaysian	250	42.6 (14.4)	73 (29.2)
Washburn et al. [63]	English	372	n.a.	145 (39)
Van den Berg-Emons et al. [66]	Dutch	21	40.7 (14.3)	7 (33.3)

n number of participants of the study, *n.a.* not available

cifically for use in epidemiologic studies of physical activity, health, and function of individuals with physical disabilities. The PASIPD is a modification of the Physical Activity Scale for the Elderly (PASE) [64]. The PASIPD is validated for people with SCI in Malaysian [65] and Dutch [66]. The PASIPD is a 13-item 7-day recall questionnaire that solicits information about leisure activities performed for purposes other than exercise, including walking and wheeling outside the home; light, moderate, and strenuous sports and recreation to increase muscle strength and endurance; light and heavy household activity; home repair; lawn work; outdoor gardening; caring for another person; and occupational activity. Respondents were asked to recall the number of days within 7 days that they participated in the

mentioned activities and how many hours they spent on each. Table 19 summarizes the papers' authors and languages and Table 20 shows the quality of the studies.

3.11 Spinal Cord Independence Measure (SCIM)

The Spinal Cord Independence Measure (SCIM) is a disability scale developed by Catz-Itzkovich in Israel in 1997, and validated in English [67], Hebrew [68], Swiss, and Italian [69]. SCIM II was validated in Israel and Swiss [70–74], SCIM III was validated in Hebrew [75–78], English [75–77, 79–82], Italian [75–77, 83], Danish [75–77], German [76, 77] Portuguese (Brazil) [84, 85],

Table 20 Evaluation of quality and risk of bias

Authors	Item of COSMIN checklist									
	1	2	3	4	5	6	7	8	9	10
Mat Rosly et al. [65]	?	+	+	−	+	+	−	−	−	−
Washburn et al. [63]	+	+	+	−	+	−	−	−	−	−
Van den Berg-Emons et al. [66]	?	?	−	−	−	−	−	+	+	−

Item 1 PROM development, *Item 2* content validity, *Item 3* structural validity, *Item 4* internal consistency, *Item 5* cross-cultural validity/measurement invariance, *Item 6* reliability, *Item 7* measurement error, *Item 8* criterion validity, *Item 9* hypothesis testing for construct validity, *Item 10* responsiveness, + sufficient, − insufficient, ? indeterminate

Spanish [86], Greek [87], Turkish [88], Thai [89], Persian [90], and Korean [91]. Also, a Self-report SCIM exists, and it was validated in German [92, 93], Spanish [94], English [95], Greek [95], Italian [93, 96], French [93], and Thai [97]. SCIM is specifically for patients with SCI and includes the following areas of function: self-care, respiration, sphincter management, and mobility. Each area scores according to its proportional weight in these patients' general activity. Self-care with scores ranging from 0 to 20 includes the following tasks: feeding, bathing, dressing, and grooming. Respiration and sphincter management includes respiration, bladder management, bowel management, and use of toilet. Scores for this area range from 0 to 40. Mobility divides into two parts: (1) tasks performed in the room and toilet and (2) tasks performed all over the house (indoors) and outdoors. Mobility in room and toilet includes mobility in bed and action to prevent pressure sores and transfers of bed-wheelchair and wheelchair toilet tub. Mobility indoors and outdoors includes mobility for short, moderate, and long distances, stair management, and wheelchair–car transfer. Scores for this area range from 0 to 40. The final score ranges from 0 to 100. Table 21 summarizes the papers' authors and languages and Table 22 shows the quality of the studies.

3.12 Impact on Participation and Autonomy Questionnaire (IPA)

The IPA was validated for people with SCI in English [41, 42, 98], Swedish [99], and Thai [100]. The IPA evaluates perceived personal impacts of chronic disability on participation and autonomy, comprising 32 items in five domains (autonomy indoors, family role, autonomy outdoors, social life and relationships, and work and education), and 8 items of the experience of problems (mobility, self-care, family role, financial situation, leisure, social relation, work, and education). The participants responded to each item by grading his/her perceived participation and autonomy on a 5-point rating scale (range: very good, 0; very poor, 4). Table 23 summarizes the papers' authors and languages and Table 24 shows the quality of the studies.

3.13 Leisure Time Physical Activity Questionnaire (LTPA)

LTPA is a brief measure of leisure-time physical activity (LTPA) for people with spinal cord injury (SCI). It was validated in English [2] and French (Canadian) [101]. LTPAQ-SCI is an SCI-specific, self-report measure of LTPA that assesses minutes of mild, moderate, and heavy intensity LTPA performed over the previous 7 days. The LTPAQ-SCI takes less than 5 min to complete and can be self-administered. Specifically, for each intensity level, participants recalled the number of days, over the past 7 days, that they performed LTPA at each intensity. Next, they are asked to recall how many minutes they usually spent doing LTPA at that intensity. The scale was scored by calculating the total number of minutes of activity performed at each intensity (number of days of activity and number of minutes of activity), thus yielding the total number of minutes of activity performed over the past week. Table 25 summarizes the papers' authors and languages and Table 26 shows the quality of the studies.

Table 21 Characteristics of the studies validating SCI-FI, SCI-FI SF, and SCI-FI-AT

Scale, test or, questionnaire	Authors	Language	n	Age mean (SD, range) year	Gender % Female
SCIM-I	Catz et al. [67]	English	30	45 (18, 17–76)	8 (26.6)
	Catz et al. [68]	Hebrew	22	48.1 (16.2, 23–76)	5 (22.7)
	Scivoletto et al. [69]	Italian	225	41.9 (18.4)	56 (24.8)
SCIM-II	Catz et al. [70]	Hebrew	28	46 (17, 20–79)	10 (35.7)
	Itzkovich et al. [72]	Hebrew	202	46.78 (18.38)	64 (31.7)
	Itzkovich et al. [71]	Hebrew	28	46 (17, 20–79)	10 (35.7)
	Van Hedel et al. [73]	Swiss	886	n.a.	n.a.
	Catz et al. [74]	Hebrew	n.a.	n.a.	n.a.
SCIM-III	Catz et al. [75]	Hebrew English Italian Danish	425	46.9 (18.2)	116 (27.3)
	Catz et al. [75]	Hebrew English Italian Danish	425	46.9 (18.2)	116 (27.3)
	Itzkovich et al. [76]	Hebrew Danish English German Italian	425	46.9 (18.2)	116 (27.3)
	Glass et al. [81]	English Italian Hebrew	425	46.9 (18.2)	116 (27.3)
	Ackerman et al. [79]	English	114	(12–64)	22 (19)
	Anderson et al. [80]	English	390	45.3 (17.9)	96 (24.6)
	Bluvshtein et al. [77]	Hebrew Danish English German Italian	261	40.1 (17.1)	n.a.
	Invernizzi et al. [83]	Italian	103	50.33 (15.35)	19 (18.33)
	Riberto et al. [85]	Portuguese (Brazil)	83	36.1 (15.4)	26 (31.3)
	Zarco-Periñán et al. [86]	Spanish	64	44.79 (20.5)	21 (32.8)
	Athanasiou et al. [87]	Greek	2	37	2 (100)
	Unalan et al. [88]	Turkish	204	39.7 (13.7)	60 (29.4)
	Wannapakhe et al. [89]	Thai	31	46 (17, 20–79)	11 (35.5)
	de Almeida et al. [84]	Portuguese (Brazil)	30	41.5 (14.7)	20 (66.7)
	Itzkovich et al. [78]	Hebrew	35	62 (15)	16 (46)
	Saberi et al. [90]	Persian	279	33.7 (10.13)	70 (25.1)
	Cho et al. [91]	Korean	42	47.32 (14.27)	8 (20)
SCIM-SR	Fekete et al. [92]	German	99	48 (35–64)	26 (26.3)
	Anguilar-Rodriguez et al. (2015)	Spanish	100	55.4 (15.2)	32 (32)
	Michailidou et al. [95]	English	174	47 (12)	63 (36)
	Michailidou et al. [95]	Greek	45	61 (17)	22 (48.8)
	Bonavita et al. [96]	Italian	116	45.5 (17.7)	36 (31)
	Prodinger et al. [93]	German French Italian	1530	52.33 (14.63)	437 (28.5)
	Wilartratsami et al. [97]	Thai	32	44.97 (20.31, 20–80)	4 (12.5)

n number of participants of the study, *n.a.* not available

Table 22 Evaluation of quality and risk of bias

Authors	Item of COSMIN checklist									
	1	2	3	4	5	6	7	8	9	10
Catz et al. [67]	+	+	−	−	−	+	−	+	+	−
Catz et al. [68]	?	?	−	−	+	−	−	−	−	−
Scivoletto et al. [69]	?	+	−	−	+	+	+	−	−	−
Catz et al. [70]	+	+	−	−	−	+	−	+	+	−
Itzkovich et al. [72]	?	?	+	−	+	−	−	−	−	−
Itzkovich et al. [71]	?	+	−	−	−	+	−	+	+	−
Van Hedel et al. [73]	?	?	−	−	+	−	+	+	+	+
Catz et al. [74]	n.a.	n.a.	n.a.	n.a.	n.a.	n.a.	n.a.	n.a.	n.a.	n.a.
Catz et al. [75]	+	+	−	−	−	−	−	−	−	−
Catz et al. [75]	?	?	−	+	−	+	−	+	+	−
Itzkovich et al. [76]	?	?	+	−	−	−	−	−	−	−
Glass et al. [81]	?	?	+	+	+	+	−	+	+	−
Ackerman et al. [79]	?	+	−	−	+	−	−	−	−	+
Anderson et al. [80]	?	?	−	+	−	+	+	+	+	−
Bluvshtein et al. [77]	?	?	−	−	+	+	−	+	+	−
Invernizzi et al. [83]	?	+	−	+	−	+	−	+	+	−
Riberto et al. [85]	?	+	−	−	−	+	−	+	+	−
Zarco-Periñán et al. [86]	?	+	−	+	+	+	−	+	+	+
Athanasiou et al. [87]	?	+	−	−	−	−	−	−	−	−
Unalan et al. [88]	?	+	−		I	+	−	+	+	−
Wannapakhe et al. [89]	?	+	−	+	+	+	−	−	−	−
de Almeida et al. [84]	?	+	−	−	−	−	−	+	+	−
Itzkovich et al. [78]	?	?	−	−	−	+	−	−	−	−
Saberi et al. [90]	?	+	−	+	+	+	−	+	+	−
Cho et al. [91]	?	+	−	−	−	+	−	+	+	−
Fekete et al. [92]	?	+	−	−	+	+	−	+	+	−
Anguilar-Rodriguez et al. (2015)	?	+	−	−	−	+	−	+	+	−
Michailidou et al. [95]	?	+	−	+	−	−	−	+	+	−
Michailidou et al. [95]	?	+	−	+	−	−	−	+	+	−
Bonavita et al. [96]	?	+	+	−	+	+	−	+	+	−
Prodinger et al. [93]	?	+	−	−	+	−	−	−	−	−
Wilartratsami et al. [97]	?	+	−	+	+	+	−	+	+	−

Item 1 PROM development, *Item 2* content validity, *Item 3* structural validity, *Item 4* internal consistency, *Item 5* cross-cultural validity/measurement invariance, *Item 6* reliability, *Item 7* measurement error, *Item 8* criterion validity, *Item 9* hypothesis testing for construct validity, *Item 10* responsiveness, + sufficient, − insufficient, ? indeterminate

Table 23 Characteristics of the studies validating IPA

Authors	Language	n	Age mean (SD, range) year	Gender % Female
Sibley et al. [98]	English	213	(20-75)	n.a.
Larsson Lund et al. [99]	Swedish	161	52 (18.2, 17–48)	31 (23)
Noonan et al. [41]	English	145	48.7 (17.4, 21–86)	66 (45.5)
Suttiwong et al. [100]	Thai	139	34.2 (8.4, 18–55)	29 (20.9)
Noonan et al. [42]	English	n.a.	n.a.	n.a.

n number of participants of the study, *n.a.* not available

Table 24 Evaluation of quality and risk of bias

| Authors | Item of COSMIN checklist | | | | | | | | | |
	1	2	3	4	5	6	7	8	9	10
Sibley et al. [98]	+	+	+	+	+	+	−	+	+	−
Larsson Lund et al. [99]	?	+	+	−	+	−	−	−	−	−
Noonan et al. [41]	?	+	−	+	+	+	+	+	+	−
Suttiwong et al. [100]	?	+	+	+	−	+	−	+	+	−
Noonan et al. [42]	n.a.	n.a.	n.a.	n.a.	n.a.	n.a.	n.a.	n.a.	n.a.	n.a.

Item 1 PROM development, *Item 2* content validity, *Item 3* structural validity, *Item 4* internal consistency, *Item 5* cross-cultural validity/measurement invariance, *Item 6* reliability, *Item 7* measurement error, *Item 8* criterion validity, *Item 9* hypothesis testing for construct validity, *Item 10* responsiveness, + sufficient, − insufficient, ? indeterminate

Table 25 Characteristics of the studies validating LTPA

Authors	Language	n	Age mean (SD, range) year	Gender % Female
Cummings et al. [101]	French (Canada)	7	n.a.	n.a.
Ginis et al. [2]	English	103	48.1 (12.7)	25 (25)

n number of participants of the study, *n.a.* not available

Table 26 Evaluation of quality and risk of bias

| Authors | Item of COSMIN Check List | | | | | | | | | |
	1	2	3	4	5	6	7	8	9	10
Cummings et al. [101]	?	+	−	−	+	+	−	−	−	+
Ginis et al. [2]	?	?	−	−	+	+	−	+	+	−

Item 1 PROM development, *Item 2* content validity, *Item 3* structural validity, *Item 4* internal consistency, *Item 5* cross-cultural validity/measurement invariance, *Item 6* reliability, *Item 7* measurement error, *Item 8* criterion validity, *Item 9* hypothesis testing for construct validity, *Item 10* responsiveness, + sufficient, − insufficient, ? indeterminate

Table 27 Characteristics of the studies validating MSES

Authors	Language	n	Age mean (SD, range) year	Gender % Female
Middleton et al. [102]	English	108	45.26 (15.99)	28 (25.9)
Rajati et al. [106]	Persian	204	40.84 (9.22)	72 (33.6)
Middleton et al. [103]	English	161	48.5 (15.1)	43 (26.7)
Miller [105]	English	162	45.8 (13.4)	51 (31.5)
Brooks et al. [104]	English	274	46.82 (13.46)	89 (32.5)

n number of participants of the study, *n.a.* not available

3.14 Moorong Self-Efficacy Scale (MSES)

Was developed by Middleton in 2003 [102] to measure self-efficacy in persons with SCI. The authors generated 20 original scale items during development, which were refined to the final 16-item version. It was validated in English [102–105], and Persian [106]. It is an SCI-specific measure of self-efficacy that assesses confidence in performing daily activities. It comprises 16 items and two subscales: (a) Daily Activities and (b) Social Functioning. Each item is rated on a 7-point Likert-type scale ranging from 1 (very uncertain) to 7 (very certain). The MSES is found to be related to depression and anxiety, functional limitations, and participation. Table 27 summarizes the papers' authors and languages and Table 28 shows the quality of the studies.

Table 28 Evaluation of quality and risk of bias

Authors	Item of COSMIN checklist									
	1	2	3	4	5	6	7	8	9	10
Middleton et al. [102]	+	+	+	+	+	+	−	+	+	+
Rajati et al. [106]	?	+	+	+	+	+	−	+	+	−
Middleton et al. [103]	?	−	+	−	−	−	−	+	+	−
Miller [105]	?	?	+	−	−	−	−	+	+	−
Brooks et al. [104]	?	+	+	−	+	−	−	−	−	−

Item 1 PROM development, *Item 2* content validity, *Item 3* structural validity, *Item 4* internal consistency, *Item 5* cross-cultural validity/measurement invariance, *Item 6* reliability, *Item 7* measurement error, *Item 8* criterion validity, *Item 9* hypothesis testing for construct validity, *Item 10* responsiveness, + sufficient, − insufficient, ? indeterminate

Table 29 Characteristics of the studies validating ESES

Authors	Language	n	Age mean (SD, range) year	Gender % Female
Kroll et al. [107]	English	368	n.a.	147 (40)
Nooijen et al. [109]	Dutch	53	51.5 (12.3)	9 (17)
Pisconti et al. [108]	Portuguese (Brazil)	76	n.a.	10 (13.2)

n number of participants of the study, *n.a.* not available

Table 30 Evaluation of quality and risk of bias

Authors	Item of COSMIN checklist									
	1	2	3	4	5	6	7	8	9	10
Kroll et al. [107]	+	+	+	+	−	+	−	+	+	−
Nooijen et al. [109]	?	+	−	+	−	−	−	+	+	−
Pisconti et al. [108]	?	+	−	+	−	+	−	+	+	−

Item 1 PROM development, *Item 2* content validity, *Item 3* structural validity, *Item 4* internal consistency, *Item 5* cross-cultural validity/measurement invariance, *Item 6* reliability, *Item 7* measurement error, *Item 8* criterion validity, *Item 9* hypothesis testing for construct validity, *Item 10* responsiveness, + sufficient, − insufficient, ? indeterminate

3.15 Exercise Self-Efficacy Scale (ESES)

The ESES was translated into English [107], Portuguese (Brazil) [108], and Dutch [109]. It is an SCI-specific scale developed to measure perceived exercise self-efficacy for various types of physical activities. Consisting of 10 items, level of self-confidence regarding performing regular physical activities and exercise, a sample item is: "I am confident that I can overcome barriers and challenges concerning physical activity and exercise if I try hard enough." Respondents answer using a 4-point scale: not at all true, rarely true, sometimes true, and always true. The minimum score is 10, and the maximum score 40. A higher score indicates higher exercise self-efficacy. Table 29 summarizes the papers' authors and languages and Table 30 shows the quality of the studies.

3.16 Nottwil Environmental Factors Inventory Short Form (NEFI)

The NEFI is an interviewer-administered assessment of perceived environmental barriers and facilitators. It was validated by Juvalta et al. in English [110] and Swiss [110] and by Ballert et al. in German [111], French [111], and Italian [111]. It is based on outcomes of the International Classification of Functioning, Disability, and Health's Core Sets for SCI project and is composed of 56 items covering 13 environmental factors as perceived barriers and perceived facilitators for different participation domains (productive life vs. social/community life), including items on overcoming and avoidance of barriers. The short form of NEFI focuses on the perceived impact of environmental barriers on participation in general, while refraining from assessing facilitators and overcoming and avoiding barriers. The NEFI short form consists of 14 items with three response options: 0 (no influence/not applicable), 1 (made my life a little harder), and 2 (made my life a lot harder). Table 31 summarizes the papers' authors and languages and Table 32 shows the quality of the studies.

3.17 Participation Measure–Post-Acute Care (PM-PAC)

The PM-PAC was designed to assess participation in the community. It contains 51 questions, with 42 questions used to create scores for the domains Communication; Mobility; Domestic Life; Interpersonal Relationships; Role Functioning; Work and Employment; Education; Economic Life; and Community, Social, and Civic Life. A higher score indicates better participation [41, 42, 112]. Table 33 summarizes the papers' authors and languages and Table 34 shows the quality of the studies.

Table 31 Characteristics of the studies validating NEFI

Authors	Language	n	Age mean (SD, range) year	Gender % Female
Ballert et al. [111]	German French Italian	1549	55.36	441 (28.5)
Juvalta et al. [110]	English/Swiss	37	45.5 (12.6, 25-65)	13 (35)

n number of participants of the study, *n.a.* not available

Table 32 Evaluation of quality and risk of bias

Authors	Item of COSMIN checklist									
	1	2	3	4	5	6	7	8	9	10
Ballert et al. [111]	?	?	+	+	+	–	–	–	–	–
Juvalta et al. [110]	+	+	–	–	–	–	–	–	–	–

Item 1 PROM development, *Item 2* content validity, *Item 3* structural validity, *Item 4* internal consistency, *Item 5* cross-cultural validity/measurement invariance, *Item 6* reliability, *Item 7* measurement error, *Item 8* criterion validity, *Item 9* hypothesis testing for construct validity, *Item 10* responsiveness, + sufficient, – insufficient, ? indeterminate

Table 33 Characteristics of the studies validating PM-PAC

Authors	Language	n	Age mean (SD, range) year	Gender % Female
Noonan et al. [41]	English	n.a.	n.a.	n.a.
Noonan et al. [42]	English	145	48.7 (17.4, 21–86)	66 (45.5)
Chang et al. [112]	English	520	45.1 (13.6)	124 (24)

n number of participants of the study, *n.a.* not available

Table 34 Evaluation of quality and risk of bias

Authors	Item of COSMIN checklist									
	1	2	3	4	5	6	7	8	9	10
Noonan et al. [41]	n.a.	n.a.	n.a.	n.a.	n.a.	n.a.	n.a.	n.a.	n.a.	n.a.
Noonan et al. [42]	?	+	–	+	+	+	+	+	+	–
Chang et al. [112]	+	+	+	–	–	–	–	–	–	–

Item 1 PROM development, *Item 2* content validity, *Item 3* structural validity, *Item 4* internal consistency, *Item 5* cross-cultural validity/measurement invariance, *Item 6* reliability, *Item 7* measurement error, *Item 8* criterion validity, *Item 9* hypothesis testing for construct validity, *Item 10* responsiveness, + sufficient, – insufficient, ? indeterminate

3.18 Participation Objective and Participation Subjective (POPS)

The POPS assesses the participation in 26 life activities from an objective (frequency) and subjective (importance and level of satisfaction) perspective. The developer's scoring algorithm was used to calculate objective and subjective overall scores and domain scores (Domestic Life; Major Life Areas; Transportation; Interpersonal Interactions and Relationships; and Community, Recreational and Civic Life) [41]. Table 35 summarizes the authors and languages of the papers and Table 36 shows the quality of the studies.

3.19 Canadian Occupational Performance Measure (COPM)

The COPM is an individualized, client-centered outcome measure. In a semi-structured interview, individuals identify up to five occupational activities considered a problem for themselves. This step is the basis for identifying treatment goals. The individuals are then asked to use a 10-point scale to assess their current performance and satisfaction with each of the selected issues. The therapist evaluates the COPM performance and satisfaction score dividing the sum of the assigned score by the number of problems identified. After the treatment, the individuals are asked again to self-rate their level of performance and satisfaction for the same problems. The scores are used by the therapist to calculate change scores. It was validated in the Italian for the SCI Population [10]. Table 35 summarizes the papers' authors and languages and Table 36 shows the quality of the studies.

3.20 Quadriplegia Index of Function (QIF)

The QIF was developed in 1980 to provide a sensitive functional scale for measuring gains in individuals with tetraplegia during rehabilitation. The QIF evaluates ten self-care areas and mobility: transfers, grooming, bathing, feeding, dressing, wheelchair mobility, bed activities, bladder

program, bowel program, and understanding for personal care. In 1999, Marino RJ et al. developed the short form [113]. Table 35 summarizes the papers' authors and languages and Table 36 shows the quality of the studies.

3.21 Life Space Assessment (LSA)

For the LSA, participants were asked to consider within the prior 4 weeks how frequently they traveled out of the room in which they slept (life-space level 1 [LS 1]), outside of their home to places such as the porch or garage (LS 2), into their neighborhood (LS 3), into town (LS 4), and outside of town (LS 5). Possible responses were never (scored as 0 for that LS level), less than once a week (scored as a 1), 1–3 times per week [2], 4–6 times per week [3], and daily [4]. For each LS level, participants reported if personal assistance (the assistance of another, scored as a 1) or equipment (scored as 1.5) was needed. It was validated in SCI population in 2016 in English [114]. Table 35 summarizes the papers' authors and languages and Table 36 shows the quality of the studies.

3.22 Access to Information and Technology (AIT)

A new AIT instrument addressed a gap in measuring environmental barriers for people with SCI, stroke, or TBI. This instrument includes items on devices and technology to transmit and receive information such as phones, computers, and internet services, as well as items that address the usability and understandability of information. It was validated in English [115]. Table 35 summarizes the papers' authors and languages and Table 36 shows the quality of the studies.

3.23 Physical Activity Instrument-SCI (PAI-SCI)

The PAI-SCI is a 7-day recall, 14-item questionnaire that focuses on activities engaged in by individuals with SCI/D. Relevant activities for

Table 35 Characteristics of the studies of scale, test, or questionnaire with less than two validations

Scale, test, or questionnaire	Authors	Language	n	Age mean (SD, range) year	Gender % Female
FAM	Hadian et al. [120]	Persian	200	35.7 (7.2)	76 (62)
FAI	Hsieh et al. [121]	Chinese (Taiwan)	233	41.1 (12.6)	40 (17.2)
LORS-III	Velozo et al. [122]	English	201	n.a.	n.a.
SIF	Johansson et al. [123]	Swedish	29	42	4 (13.8)
OPHI	Lynch and Bridle [124]	English	143	n.a.	31 (21.7)
COVS	Barker et al. [125]	English	41		n.a.
SCIA&P Basic Data set	Post et al. [126]	Dutch	n.a.	n.a.	n.a.
BPAQ-MI]	Vasudevan et al. [127]	English	10	n.a.	n.a.
RNL	Hitzig et al. [128]	English	618	n.a.	117 (18.9)
IMPACT-S	Post et al. [129]	Dutch	275	40.4 (15.8)	94 (34.1)
PAR-PRO	Ostir et al. [130]	English	594	74	364 (61.4)
InSCI	Fekete et al. [131]	English	n.a.	n.a.	n.a.
ACIRF	Laleh et al. [132]	Persian	100	n.a.	25 (25)
KAP	Noonan et al. [41]	English	145	48.7 (17.4, 21–86)	66 (45.5)
POPS	Noonan et al. [42]	English	145	48.7 (17.4, 21–86)	66 (45.5)
COPM	Berardi et al. [10]	Italian	39	53 (15)	12 (29)
QIF	Marino and Goin [113]	English	95	31.2 (13.2, 16–68)	10 (10.5)
LSA	Lanzino et al. [114]	English	50	n.a.	n.a.
AIT	Hahn et al. [115]	English	209	46 (14)	45 (22)
PAI-SCI	Butler et al. [116]	English	45	54.2 (16.6)	n.a.
Life-H 3.1	Goh et al. [117]	Malaysian	29	n.a.	n.a.
Sunnaas ADL index	Bathen and Vardeberg [118]	Norwegian	16	n.a.	n.a.
RIPSCI	Neufeld and Lysack [119]	English	139	39.9 (12.2)	45 (32.4)
HEI	Norin et al. [133]	Swedish	122	63 (9)	35 (29)

n number of participants of the study, *n.a.* not available

Table 36 Evaluation of quality and risk of bias

Authors	Item of COSMIN Check List									
	1	2	3	4	5	6	7	8	9	10
Hadian et al. [120]	?	+	−	+	−	+	−	+	+	−
Hsieh et al. [121]	?	−	+	−	−	−	−	−	−	−
Velozo et al. [122]	+	+	+	−	−	−	−	−	−	−
Johansson et al. [123]	?	?	−	−	−	−	−	+	+	−
Lynch and Bridle [124]	+	+		−	−	−	−	+	+	−
Barker et al. [125]	?	?	−	−	+	+	−	+	+	−
Post et al. [126]	+	+	−	−	−	−	−	−	−	−
Vasudevan et al. [127]	+	+	−	+	+	+	−	+	+	−
Hitzig et al. [128]	?	?	+	+	+	−	−	−	−	−
Post et al. [129]	+	+	−	+	+	+	−	+	+	+
Ostir et al. [130]	+	+	+	+	+	−	−	−	−	−
Fekete et al. [131]	+	+	−	−	−	−	−	−	−	−
Laleh et al. [132]	+	+	−	−	+	+	−	−	+	−
Noonan et al. [41]	?	+	−	+	+	+	+	+	+	−
Noonan et al. [42]	?	+	−	+	+	+	+	+	+	−
Berardi et al. [10]	?	+	−	+	−	+	−	+	+	+
Marino and Goin [113]	+	+	+	−	+	−	−	+	+	−
Lanzino et al. [114]	?	+	−	+	+	+	+	−	−	−
Hahn et al. [115]	+	+	+	−	+	−	−	−	−	−
Butler et al. [116]	?	?	−	+	−	+	−	−	−	−
Goh et al. [117]	?	+	−	−	+	+	+	+	+	+
Bathen and Vardeberg [118]	+	+	−	−	−	+	−	−	−	−
Neufeld and Lysack [119]	+	+	+	+	+	−	−	+	+	−
Norin et al. [133]	?	+	−	−	+	−	−	+	+	−

Item 1 PROM development, Item 2 content validity, Item 3 structural validity, Item 4 internal consistency, Item 5 cross-cultural validity/measurement invariance, Item 6 reliability, Item 7 measurement error, Item 8 criterion validity, Item 9 hypothesis testing for construct validity, Item 10 responsiveness, + sufficient, − insufficient, ? indeterminate

persons without SCI were substituted for activities performed by people with SCI. For example, "how often did you walk outside your home not specifically for exercise?" was changed to "how often did you wheel outside of your home not specifically for exercise?" The scale was validated in 2008 for the SCI population [116]. Table 35 summarizes the papers' authors and languages and Table 36 shows the quality of the studies.

3.24 LIFE Habits Assessment 3.1 (LIFE-H 3.1)

The short form of LIFE-H 3.1 consists of 77 items covering 12 life habit domains—nutrition, fitness, personal care, communication, housing, mobility, interpersonal relationships, responsibilities, community life, education, employment, and recreation. It was validated in the Malaysian language [117]. Table 35 summarizes the papers' authors and languages and Table 36 shows the quality of the studies.

3.25 Sunnaas ADL Index

The Sunnaas ADL Index contains ratings on 12 daily activities. These are believed to be the most important activities necessary for adults to live independently in the community. They include both PADL (personal activities of daily living) and I-ADL activities (instrumental activities of daily living) [118]. Table 35 summarizes the papers' authors and languages and Table 36 shows the quality of the studies.

3.26 Risk Inventory for Persons with Spinal Cord Injury (RISCI)

Modeled after the 27-item Physical Risk Assessment Inventory (PRAI), the final RISCI scale consisted of 12 items which (after statistical analysis toward the end of the study) we labeled "physical risk" (4 items), "SCI-specific mobility risk" (4 items), and "social risk" (4 items). The

RISCI scale instructions to participants were: "I will read out an activity to you, and then I want you to say how risky this activity is for the average person with an SCI. Your choices are 0¼ not risky at all, 1 = low risk, 2 = medium risk, 3 = high risk, 4 = extremely risky. I can show you the list of activities as I read them if it will be easier for you." It was validated in the English language in 2010 [119]. Table 35 summarizes the papers' authors and languages and Table 36 shows the quality of the studies.

3.27 Function Assessment Measure (FAM)

The FAM initially evaluated the disability and functional performance in brain-injured patients. In 2012, Reza Hadian et al. validated and translated the Persian version of the FAM among a sample of SCI patients [120]. The FAM has been translated into several languages, including Portuguese and German. The FAM has 12 items, which include five main domains: self-care, mobility, communication, psychosocial, and cognition. The FAM is not a self-report measure and it is administered by raters. Each response scores between 1 (total dependence) and 7 (normal independence). Table 35 summarizes the papers' authors and languages and Table 36 shows the quality of the studies.

3.28 Frenchay Activities Index (FAI)

The FAI consists of domestic chores, work/leisure activities, and outdoor activities. It was validated in Taiwan in 2007 for a person with SCI [121]. The FAI is designed to assess the patient's frequency of doing IADL over the recent past, which corresponds to the "participation" of International Classification of Functioning, Disability, and Health but not to assess whether he/she can perform IADL. The FAI has been used with the elderly, persons with stroke, amputations, tremors, or leg ulcers. The FAI is composed of 15 items. Response categories of the items measure the frequency of engaging in activity from 0 (never or none) to 3 (daily or weekly). Some items were changed. For example, the item "walking outside" of the FAI is not appropriate for SCI patients because most SCI patients cannot walk and they usually depend on a wheelchair for mobility. Thus, we modified this item as "going outside (with or without wheelchair)" in this study. This study demonstrated that the revised 13-item FAI assesses a single, unidimensional IADL for SCI patients living in the community. The revised FAI shows the potential for assessment of IADL in SCI patients. Table 35 summarizes the papers' authors and languages and Table 36 shows the quality of the studies.

3.29 Level of Rehabilitation Scale-III (LORS-III)

The LORS scale was created in 1977 to evaluate and compare inpatient rehabilitation programs' effectiveness on an ongoing basis. Since then, the scale revised into LORS-III [122]. In 1995, more than 40 inpatient rehabilitation facilities in the United States used the LORS-III. The LORS-III focuses on functional independence with a scale consisting of 17 measurements representing abilities in ADL, mobility, communication, cognition, and memory. All items, except for the memory items, score admission, discharge, and 3-month follow-up data on a 5-point scale, ranging from 0 (complete dependence) to 4 (independent or normal function). Memory items are scored only at admission on a 2-point scale: 0 (impaired) and 1 (nonimpaired). Table 35 summarizes the papers' authors and languages and Table 36 shows the quality of the studies.

3.30 Spinal Cord Index of Function (SIF)

In 2009, Johansson et al. evaluated the validity and responsiveness of the SIF [123], an instrument on the activity level, measuring the ability to perform various transfers in non-walking patients with a spinal cord lesion in Gothenburg,

Sweden. SIF is an instrument developed by the authors and physiotherapists with substantial experience in SCI rehabilitation at the Sahlgrenska University Hospital, Gothenburg, and consists of nine parameters: [1] moving legs up in bed; [2] turning to the side; [3] getting into a sitting position; [4] transferring from bed to wheelchair; [5] transferring from wheelchair to bed with a difference in the level; [6] transferring from wheelchair to shower chair; [7] transferring from wheelchair to toilet; [8] transferring from floor to wheelchair; and [9] wheelchair maneuvering. The scores for each item range from 1 to 6. Score 1 means that the patient cannot perform the activity without maximum help. Score 6 means that the patient can perform the activity independently, without supervision, and in a safe manner, within a reasonable time. The maximum score is 54 points. Table 35 summarizes the papers' authors and languages and Table 36 shows the quality of the studies.

3.31 Occupational Performance History Interview (OPHI)

The OPHI was developed to gather reliable, valid data about individuals' past and present occupational performances. It is a structured interview instrument intended to provide a holistic picture of an individual's adaptation process amid everyday occupational performance. Developed within the framework of the Model of Human Occupation, the OPHI assesses five content areas likely to be of common concern to occupational therapists, regardless of their particular areas of practice: organization of daily living routines; life roles; interests, values, and goals; perceptions of control and ability; and environmental influences. The OPHI was designed to collect accurate and clinically useful information about individuals' past and present performances in work, play, and self-care, as well as their motivations and routines. In 1993, Lynch and Bridle validated OPHI in persons with SCI [124]. Table 35 summarizes the papers' authors and languages and Table 36 shows the quality of the studies.

3.32 Clinical Outcome Variables Scale (COVS)

COVS is a clinician-rated, composite measure of mobility used routinely across the continuum of care provided by Queensland Spinal Cord Injuries Service (QSCIS). It was validated in Australia [125]. It consists of 13 items, which comprise rolling (2 items), lying to sitting (1 item), sitting balance (1 item), transfers (2 items), ambulation (4 items), wheelchair mobility (1 item), and arm function (2 items). According to detailed guidelines, all 13 items are rated by a clinician through observation and assessment of task performance. Each COVS item is scored on a 7-point scale ranging from 1 (fully dependent mobility) to 7 (normal independent mobility). COVS scores are generally reported as a single composite score ranging from 13 to 91. Table 35 summarizes the papers' authors and languages and Table 36 shows the quality of the studies.

3.33 International Spinal Cord Injury Activities and Participation (SCIA&P) Basic Data Set

Data collection on living with SCI should be in the form of a common international data set to facilitate comparisons regarding injuries, treatments, and outcomes between individuals with SCI, treatment centers, and countries. The International SCI Data Set project was started in Vancouver in 2002 to select elements to be included in the International SCI Data Set. Basic data sets consist of a minimum amount of data that clinicians might want to collect on most or on all individuals with SCI whom they serve.

In 2015, Post et al. developed an International SCIA&P Basic Data Set [126]. They worked with an international working group of experts in SCI participation and quality of life research, together with the Executive Committee of the International SCI Standards and Data Sets. The working group selected items for the A&P data set that cover categories in the ICF Chaps. 4

(Mobility), 5 (Self-care), 6 (Domestic life), 7 (Interpersonal interactions and relationships), 8 (Major life areas), and 9 (Community, social and civic life). The A&P Basic Data Set thus consists of 8 items relating to Chaps. 4 and 5 of the ICF and 16 items relating to Chaps. 6–9. The SCIA&P Basic Data Set uses a 3-point verbal rating scale of 0 = not satisfied, 1 = somewhat satisfied, and 2 = very satisfied. Table 35 summarizes the papers' authors and languages and Table 36 shows the quality of the studies.

3.34 Barriers to Physical Activity Questionnaire for People with Mobility Impairments (BPAQ-MI)

In 2005, Vasudevan et al. developed the Barriers to Physical Activity Questionnaire for people with Mobility Impairments (BPAQ-MI) in English [127]. The BPAQ-MI measures barriers to physical activities across the intrapersonal, interpersonal, organizational, and community domains. The BPAQ-MI contains 63 items and includes eight subscales or factors: health; beliefs and attitudes; family; friends; fitness center built environment; staff and policy community built environment; and safety. Table 35 summarizes the papers' authors and languages and Table 36 shows the quality of the studies.

3.35 Reintegration to Normal Living (RNL)

The RNEL was validated for people with SCI in 2012, in Canada [128]. The RNL Index covers such areas of involvement in recreational and social activities, perceived ability to move within their communities, and the degree of comfort people have with their roles in the family and other relationships. The RNL Index is an 11-item measure of community reintegration covering participation in recreational and social activities, movement within the community, and degree of comfort the individual has in his/her role in the family and with other relationships [25]. The RNL Index has three alternate scoring systems: (1) visual analog scale (VAS), (2) 3-point scoring system, and (3) 4-point scoring system. Higher scores representing their levels of participation. Table 35 summarizes the papers' authors and languages and Table 36 shows the quality of the studies.

3.36 ICF Measure of Participation an ACTivities Questionnaire (IMPACT-S)

IMPACT-S is an ICF-based questionnaire that measures activities and participation. It was validated by Post et al. in 2007 in the Netherlands [129]. IMPACTS consists of 33 items in 9 scales, reflecting the nine activities and participation chapters of the International Classification of Functioning, Disability, and Health (ICF). The activity chapters are Learning and applying knowledge; General tasks and demands; Communication; Mobility; Self-care. Participation chapters are Domestic life; Interpersonal interactions and relationships; Major life areas; community, social, and civic life. IMPACT-S scores are summarized into nine scale scores, two subtotal scores for Activities and Participation, and one IMPACT-S total score. All summary scores are averaged item scores, converted into 0–100 scales. IMPACT-S is a reliable and valid generic measure of activity limitations and participation restrictions that fits the ICF. Table 35 summarizes the papers' authors and languages and Table 36 shows the quality of the studies.

3.37 New Measure of Participation (PAR-PRO)

PAR-PRO was developed by Ostir et al. in the United States in 2006 [130]. The PAR-PRO participation instrument was designed to measure the frequency a life situation occurs within a defined time. It is a measure of participation in domestic activities and the community and

includes 20 elements to which people can respond with: "0 = Never participated"; "1 = Monthly participation"; "2 = Biweekly participation"; "3 = Participation weekly "; and" 4 = Daily/almost daily participation. Table 35 summarizes the papers' authors and languages and Table 36 shows the quality of the studies.

3.38 International Spinal Cord Injury Community Survey (InSCI)

The InSCI questionnaire includes 125 questions, of which $n = 70$ (56.0%) assess functioning ($n = 28$, body functions and structures; $n = 42$, activities and participation); $n = 45$ (36.0%) contextual factors ($n = 26$, environmental factors; $n = 19$, personal factors); $n = 2$ (1.6%) lesion characteristics, and $n = 8$ (6.4%) appraisal of health and well-being. It was validated in English language [131]. Table 35 summarizes the papers' authors and languages and Table 36 shows the quality of the studies.

3.39 Attention to Clothing and Impact of Its Restrictive Factors in Iranian Patients with Traumatic Spinal Cord Injury (ACIRF-SCI)

The ACIRF-SCI is a 19-item questionnaire that includes five domains related to aspects of clothing: functional, medical, attitude, aesthetic, and emotional. It was validated in 2015 in the Persian language [132]. Table 35 summarizes the papers' authors and languages and Table 36 shows the quality of the studies.

3.40 Keele Assessment of Participation (KAP)

The KAP contains 11 questions asking about autonomy in conducting life activities in the subdomains: Mobility; Self-Care; Domestic Life; Interpersonal Interactions and Relationships;

Major Life Areas; and Community, Social, and Civic Life. The mean score for each question in the KAP was compared to similar domains within the participation instruments. A lower score on a question in the KAP indicates better perceived participation. It was validated in the English language [41]. Table 35 summarizes the papers' authors and languages and Table 36 shows the quality of the studies.

3.41   Housing Enabler

The Housing Enabler consists of two parts: (1) the individual component, including a dichotomous assessment of functional limitations and dependence on mobility devices (walking aids or wheelchair) present or not (resulting in a functional profile), assessed through interview and observation; and (2) the environmental component, comprising the section's exterior surroundings (28 items), entrances (46 items) and indoor environment (87 items), containing 161 items in all. The environmental barriers in the environmental component are dichotomously assessed as present or not. It was validated in Swedish in 2019 [133]. Table 35 summarizes the papers' authors and languages and Table 36 shows the quality of the studies.

4   Conclusions

This chapter reports all assessment tools described in the literature to assess people's neurological status with an SCI. Among the 48 tools included in this chapter, most scales evaluate the aspect of independence, participation, and environmental factors. The most common assessment tools are the functional independence measure (FIM) which is a multidimensional instrument that evaluates the performance in the motor and cognitive/social domains, and the Spinal Cord Independence Measure III (SCIM-III) which is designed for patients with an SCI to make the functional assessments, including self-care, respiration, sphincter management, and mvobility.

References

1. Barbetta DC, Cassemiro LC, Assis MR. The experience of using the scale of functional Independence measure in individuals undergoing spinal cord injury rehabilitation in Brazil. Spinal Cord. 2014. https://doi.org/10.1038/sc.2013.179.
2. Ginis KAM, Phang SH, Latimer AE, Arbour-Nicitopoulos KP. Reliability and validity tests of the leisure time physical activity questionnaire for people with spinal cord injury. Arch Phys Med Rehabil. 2012. https://doi.org/10.1016/j.apmr.2011.11.005.
3. Castelnuovo G, Giusti EM, Manzoni GM, et al. What is the role of the placebo effect for pain relief in neurorehabilitation? Clinical implications from the Italian consensus conference on pain in neurorehabilitation. Front Neurol. 2018. https://doi.org/10.3389/fneur.2018.00310.
4. Marquez MA, De Santis R, Ammendola V, et al. Cross-cultural adaptation and validation of the "spinal cord injury-falls concern scale" in the Italian population. Spinal Cord. 2018;56(7):712–8. https://doi.org/10.1038/s41393-018-0070-6.
5. Berardi A, De Santis R, Tofani M, et al. The Wheelchair Use Confidence Scale: Italian translation, adaptation, and validation of the short form. Disabil Rehabil Assist Technol. 2018;13(4):i. https://doi.org/10.1080/17483107.2017.1357053.
6. Anna B, Giovanni G, Marco T, et al. The validity of rasterstereography as a technological tool for the objectification of postural assessment in the clinical and educational fields: pilot study. In: Advances in intelligent systems and computing. 2020. https://doi.org/10.1007/978-3-030-23884-1_8.
7. Panuccio F, Berardi A, Marquez MA, et al. Development of the pregnancy and motherhood evaluation questionnaire (PMEQ) for evaluating and measuring the impact of physical disability on pregnancy and the management of motherhood: a pilot study. Disabil Rehabil. 2020;2020:1–7. https://doi.org/10.1080/09638288.2020.1802520.
8. Amedoro A, Berardi A, Conte A, et al. The effect of aquatic physical therapy on patients with multiple sclerosis: a systematic review and meta-analysis. Mult Scler Relat Disord. 2020. https://doi.org/10.1016/j.msard.2020.102022.
9. Dattoli S, Colucci M, Soave MG, et al. Evaluation of pelvis postural systems in spinal cord injury patients: outcome research. J Spinal Cord Med. 2018;43:185–92.
10. Berardi A, Galeoto G, Guarino D, et al. Construct validity, test-retest reliability, and the ability to detect change of the Canadian occupational performance measure in a spinal cord injury population. Spinal Cord Ser Cases. 2019. https://doi.org/10.1038/s41394-019-0196-6.
11. Ponti A, Berardi A, Galeoto G, Marchegiani L, Spandonaro C, Marquez MA. Quality of life, concern of falling and satisfaction of the sit-ski aid in

sit-skiers with spinal cord injury: observational study. Spinal Cord Ser Cases. 2020. https://doi.org/10.1038/s41394-020-0257-x.

12. Panuccio F, Galeoto G, Marquez MA, et al. General sleep disturbance scale (GSDS-IT) in people with spinal cord injury: a psychometric study. Spinal Cord. 2020. https://doi.org/10.1038/s41393-020-0500-0.

13. Monti M, Marquez MA, Berardi A, Tofani M, Valente D, Galeoto G. The multiple sclerosis intimacy and sexuality questionnaire (MSISQ-15): validation of the Italian version for individuals with spinal cord injury. Spinal Cord. 2020. https://doi.org/10.1038/s41393-020-0469-8.

14. Galeoto G, Colucci M, Guarino D, et al. Exploring validity, reliability, and factor analysis of the Quebec user evaluation of satisfaction with assistive technology in an Italian population: a cross-sectional study. Occup Ther Heal Care. 2018. https://doi.org/10.1080/07380577.2018.1522682.

15. Colucci M, Tofani M, Trioschi D, Guarino D, Berardi A, Galeoto G. Reliability and validity of the Italian version of Quebec user evaluation of satisfaction with assistive technology 2.0 (QUEST-IT 2.0) with users of mobility assistive device. Disabil Rehabil Assist Technol. 2019. https://doi.org/10.1080/17483107.2019.1668975.

16. Berardi A, Galeoto G, Lucibello L, Panuccio F, Valente D, Tofani M. Athletes with disability' satisfaction with sport wheelchairs: an Italian cross sectional study. Disabil Rehabil Assist Technol. 2020. https://doi.org/10.1080/17483107.2020.1800114.

17. Moher D, Shamseer L, Clarke M, et al. Preferred reporting items for systematic review and meta-analysis protocols (PRISMA-P) 2015 statement. Rev Esp Nutr Human Diet. 2016. https://doi.org/10.1186/2046-4053-4-1

18. Mokkink LB, Terwee CB, Patrick DL, et al. The COSMIN study reached international consensus on taxonomy, terminology, and definitions of measurement properties for health-related patient-reported outcomes. J Clin Epidemiol. 2010. https://doi.org/10.1016/j.jclinepi.2010.02.006.

19. Terwee CB, Prinsen CAC, Chiarotto A, et al. COSMIN methodology for evaluating the content validity of patient-reported outcome measures: a Delphi study. Qual Life Res. 2018. https://doi.org/10.1007/s11136-018-1829-0.

20. Mokkink LB, de Vet HCW, Prinsen CAC, et al. COSMIN risk of bias checklist for systematic reviews of patient-reported outcome measures. Qual Life Res. 2018. https://doi.org/10.1007/s11136-017-1765-4.

21. Latimer AE, Ginis KAM, Craven BC, Hicks AL. The physical activity recall assessment for people with spinal cord injury: validity. Med Sci Sports Exerc. 2006. https://doi.org/10.1249/01.mss.0000183851.94261.d2.

22. Ginis KAM, Latimer AE, Hicks AL, Craven BC. Development and evaluation of an activity measure for people with spinal cord injury. Med Sci Sports Exerc. 2005. https://doi.org/10.1249/01.mss.0000170127.54394.eb.

23. McClure LA, Boninger ML, Ozawa H, Koontz A. Reliability and validity analysis of the transfer assessment instrument. Arch Phys Med Rehabil. 2011. https://doi.org/10.1016/j.apmr.2010.07.231.

24. Tsai CY, Rice LA, Hoelmer C, Boninger ML, Koontz AM. Basic psychometric properties of the transfer assessment instrument (version 3.0). Arch Phys Med Rehabil. 2013. https://doi.org/10.1016/j.apmr.2013.05.001.

25. Lynn A Worobey, Christina K Zigler, Randall Huzinec, Stephanie K Rigot, JongHun Sung, Laura A Rice. Reliability and validity of the revised transfer assessment instrument. Top Spinal Cord Inj Rehabil. 2018. https://doi.org/10.1310/sci2403-217LK.

26. Baghel P, Walia S, Noohu MM. Reliability and validity of transfer assessment instrument version 3.0 in individuals with acute spinal cord injury in early rehabilitation phase. Hong Kong Physiother J. 2018. https://doi.org/10.1142/S1013702518500099.

27. Grey N, Kennedy P. The functional independence measure: a comparative study of clinician and self ratings. Paraplegia. 1993. https://doi.org/10.1038/sc.1993.74.

28. Dodds TA, Martin DP, Stolov WC, Deyo RA. A validation of the functional Independence measurement and its performance among rehabilitation inpatients. Arch Phys Med Rehabil. 1993. https://doi.org/10.1016/0003-9993(93)90119-U.

29. Hall KM, Cohen ME, Wright J, Call M, Werner P. Characteristics of the functional independence measure in traumatic spinal cord injury. Arch Phys Med Rehabil. 1999. https://doi.org/10.1016/S0003-9993(99)90260-5.

30. Küçükdeveci AA, Yavuzer G, Elhan AH, Sonel B, Tennant A. Adaptation of the functional independence measure for use in Turkey. Clin Rehabil. 2001. https://doi.org/10.1191/026921501676877265.

31. Lawton G, Lundgren-Nilsson Å, Biering-Sørensen F, et al. Cross-cultural validity of FIM in spinal cord injury. Spinal Cord. 2006. https://doi.org/10.1038/sj.sc.3101895.

32. da Silva GA, Schoeller SD, Gelbcke FL, de Carvalho ZMF, da Silva EM. Functional assessment of people with spinal cord injury: use of the functional independence measure - FIM. Texto e Context Enferm. 2012. https://doi.org/10.1590/S0104-07072012000400025.

33. Saltychev M, Lähdesmäki J, Jokinen P, Laimi K. Pre- and Postintervention factor structure of functional Independence measure in patients with spinal cord injury. Rehabil Res Pract. 2017. https://doi.org/10.1155/2017/6938718.

34. Ravaud MD, Alain Yelnik J-F. Construct validity of the functional independence measure (FIM): questioning the Unidimensionality of the scale and the "value" of FIM scores. Scand J Rehabil Med. 1999;31(1):31–41. https://doi.org/10.1080/003655099444704.

35. Lundgren-Nilsson Å, Tennant A, Grimby G, Sunnerhagen KS. Cross-diagnostic validity in a generic instrument: an example from the functional Independence measure in Scandinavia. Health Qual Life Outcomes. 2006. https://doi.org/10.1186/1477-7525-4-55.

36. Masedo AI, Hanley M, Jensen MP, Ehde D, Cardenas DD. Reliability and validity of a self-report FIM™ (FIM-SR) in persons with amputation or spinal cord injury and chronic pain. Am J Phys Med Rehabil. 2005. https://doi.org/10.1097/01.PHM.0000154898.25609.4A.

37. Hoenig H, Branch LG. McIntyre L, Hoff J, Horner RD. The validity in persons with spinal cord injury of a self-reported functional measure derived from the functional independence measure. Spine (Phila Pa 1976). 1999;24(6):539–43, discussion 543–4. https://doi.org/10.1097/00007632-199903150-00007. PMID: 10101817.

38. Middleton JW, Harvey LA, Batty J, Cameron I, Quirk R, Winstanley J. Five additional mobility and locomotor items to improve responsiveness of the FIM in wheelchair-dependent individuals with spinal cord injury. Spinal Cord. 2006. https://doi.org/10.1038/sj.sc.3101872.

39. Steinerte V, Vetra A. The World Health Organisation disability assessment scale (WHODAS II): links between self-rated health and objectively defined and clinical parameters in the population of spinal cord injury. SHS Web Conf. 2016. https://doi.org/10.1051/shsconf/20163000042.

40. De Wolf AC, Tate RL, Lannin NA, Middleton J, Lane-Brown A, Cameron ID. The world health or ganizati on disability assessment scale, WHODAS II: reliabil ity and validity in the measurement of activity and par ticipati on in a spinal cord injury population. J Rehabil Med. 2012. https://doi.org/10.2340/16501977-1016.

41. Noonan VK, Kopec JA, Noreau L, Singer J, Masse LC, Dvorak MF. Comparing the reliability of five participation instruments in persons with spinal conditions. J Rehabil Med. 2010. https://doi.org/10.2340/16501977-0583.

42. Noonan VK, Kopec JA, Noreau L, et al. Measuring participation among persons with spinal cord injury: comparison of three instruments. Top Spinal Cord Inj Rehabil. 2010. https://doi.org/10.1310/sci1504-49.

43. Chiu TY, Finger ME, Fellinghauer CS, et al. Validation of the World Health Organization disability assessment schedule 2.0 in adults with spinal cord injury in Taiwan: a psychometric study. Spinal Cord. 2019. https://doi.org/10.1038/s41393-018-0231-7.

44. Jette AM, Tulsky DS, Ni P, et al. Development and initial evaluation of the spinal cord injury-functional index. Arch Phys Med Rehabil. 2012. https://doi.org/10.1016/j.apmr.2012.05.008.

45. Tulsky DS, Jette AM, Kisala PA, et al. Spinal cord injury-functional index: item banks to measure physical functioning in individuals with spinal cord injury. Arch Phys Med Rehabil. 2012. https://doi.org/10.1016/j.apmr.2012.05.007.

46. Sinha R, Slavin MD, Kisala PA, Ni P, Tulsky DS, Jette AM. Functional ability level development and validation: providing clinical meaning for spinal cord injury functional index scores. Arch Phys Med Rehabil. 2015. https://doi.org/10.1016/j.apmr.2014.11.008.

47. Heinemann AW, Dijkers MP, Ni P, Tulsky DS, Jette A. Measurement properties of the spinal cord injury-functional index (SCI-FI) short forms. Arch Phys Med Rehabil. 2014. https://doi.org/10.1016/j.apmr.2014.01.031.

48. Slavin MD, Ni P, Tulsky DS, et al. Spinal cord injury–functional index/assistive technology short forms. Arch Phys Med Rehabil. 2016;97(10):1745–1752.e7. https://doi.org/10.1016/j.apmr.2016.03.029.

49. Whiteneck GG, Charlifue SW, Gerhart KA, Overholser JD, Richardson GN. Quantifying handicap: a new measure of long-term rehabilitation outcomes. Arch Phys Med Rehabil. 1992. https://doi.org/10.5555/uri:pii:000399939290185Y.

50. Tozato F, Tobimatsu Y, Wang CW, Iwaya T, Kumamoto K, Ushiyama T. Reliability and validity of the Craig handicap assessment and reporting technique for Japanese individuals with spinal cord injury. Tohoku J Exp Med. 2005. https://doi.org/10.1620/tjem.205.357.

51. Walker N, Mellick D, Brooks CA, Whiteneck GG. Measuring participation across impairment groups using the Craig handicap assessment reporting technique. Am J Phys Med Rehabil. 2003. https://doi.org/10.1097/01.PHM.0000098041.42394.9A.

52. Golhasani-Keshtan F, Ebrahimzadeh MH, Fattahi AS, Soltani-Moghaddas SH, Omidi-Kashani F. Validation and cross-cultural adaptation of the Persian version of Craig handicap assessment and reporting technique (CHART) short form. Disabil Rehabil. 2013. https://doi.org/10.3109/09638288.2013.768710.

53. Whiteneck GG, Harrison-Felix CL, Mellick DC, Brooks CA, Charlifue SB, Gerhart KA. Quantifying environmental factors: a measure of physical, attitudinal, service, productivity, and policy barriers. Arch Phys Med Rehabil. 2004. https://doi.org/10.1016/j.apmr.2003.09.027.

54. Soni S, Walia S, Noohu MM. Hindi translation and evaluation of psychometric properties of Craig Hospital inventory of environmental factors instrument in spinal cord injury subjects. J Neurosci Rural Pract. 2016. https://doi.org/10.4103/0976-3147.172170.

55. Van De Velde D, Bracke P, Van Hove G, et al. Measuring participation when combining subjective and objective variables: the development of the Ghent participation scale (GPS). Eur J Phys Rehabil Med. 2016;52:527–40.

56. Van De Velde D, Coorevits P, Sabbe L, et al. Measuring participation as defined by the World Health Organization in the international classification of functioning, disability and health. Psychometric properties of the Ghent partici-

pation scale. Clin Rehabil. 2017. https://doi.org/10.1177/0269215516644310.

57. Kirchberger I, Cieza A, Biering-Sørensen F, et al. ICF Core sets for individuals with spinal cord injury in the early post-acute context. Spinal Cord. 2010. https://doi.org/10.1038/sc.2009.128.

58. Herrmann KH, Kirchberger I, Stucki G, Cieza A. The comprehensive ICF core sets for spinal cord injury from the perspective of occupational therapists: a worldwide validation study using the Delphi technique. Spinal Cord. 2011. https://doi.org/10.1038/sc.2010.168.

59. Henao Lema CP, Pérez Parra JE. Appearance and concurrent validity of an instrument to assess disability in people with chronic spinal cord injury based on the icf core set. Rev Ciencias la Salud. 2013.

60. Tatlı HU, Köseoğlu BF, Özcan DS, Akselim SK, Doğan A. Validation and application of the international classification of functioning core set for spinal cord injury in the Turkish patients. Turkish J Phys Med Rehabil. 2019. https://doi.org/10.5606/tftrd.2019.3045.

61. Ballert CS, Stucki G, Biering-Sørensen F, Cieza A. Towards the development of clinical measures for spinal cord injury based on the international classification of functioning, disability and health with Rasch analyses. Arch Phys Med Rehabil. 2014. https://doi.org/10.1016/j.apmr.2014.05.006.

62. Chen HC, Yen TH, Chang KH, Lin YN, Wang YH, Liou TH. Developing an ICF core set for sub-acute stages of spinal cord injury in Taiwan: a preliminary study. Disabil Rehabil. 2015. https://doi.org/10.3109/09638288.2014.895871.

63. Washburn RA, Zhu W, McAuley E, Frogley M, Figoni SF. The physical activity scale for individuals with physical disabilities: development and evaluation. Arch Phys Med Rehabil. 2002. https://doi.org/10.1053/apmr.2002.27467.

64. Covotta A, Gagliardi M, Berardi A, et al. Physical activity scale for the elderly: translation, cultural adaptation, and validation of the Italian version. Curr Gerontol Geriatr Res. 2018. https://doi.org/10.1155/2018/8294568.

65. Mat Rosly M, Halaki M, Mat Rosly H, Davis GM, Hasnan N, Husain R. Malaysian adaptation of the physical activity scale for individuals with physical disabilities in individuals with spinal cord injury. Disabil Rehabil. 2020. https://doi.org/10.1080/09638288.2018.1544294.

66. Van Den Berg-Emons RJ, L'Ortye AA, Buffart LM, et al. Validation of the physical activity scale for individuals with physical disabilities. Arch Phys Med Rehabil. 2011. https://doi.org/10.1016/j.apmr.2010.12.006.

67. Catz A, Itzkovich M, Agranov E, Ring H, Tamir A. SCIM - spinal cord independence measure: a new disability scale for patients with spinal cord lesions. Spinal Cord. 1997. https://doi.org/10.1038/sj.sc.3100504.

68. Catz A, Itzkovich M, Agranov E, Ring H, Tamir A. The spinal cord independence measure (SCIM): sensitivity to functional changes in subgroups of spinal cord lesion patients. Spinal Cord. 2001. https://doi.org/10.1038/sj.sc.3101118.

69. Scivoletto G, Tamburella F, Laurenza L, Molinari M. The spinal cord independence measure: how much change is clinically significant for spinal cord injury subjects. Disabil Rehabil. 2013. https://doi.org/10.3109/09638288.2012.756942.

70. Catz A, Itzkovich M, Steinberg F, et al. The Catz-Itzkovich SCIM: a revised version of the spinal cord independence measure. Disabil Rehabil. 2001. https://doi.org/10.1080/096382801750110919.

71. Itzkovich M, Tamir A, Philo O, et al. Reliability of the Catz-Itzkovich spinal cord independence measure assessment by interview and comparison with observation. Am J Phys Med Rehabil. 2003. https://doi.org/10.1097/01.PHM.0000057226.22271.44.

72. Itzkovich M, Tripolski M, Zeilig G, et al. Rasch analysis of the Catz-Itzkovich spinal cord independence measure. Spinal Cord. 2002. https://doi.org/10.1038/sj.sc.3101315.

73. Van Hedel HJA, Dietz V, Meiners T, et al. Walking during daily life can be validly and responsively assessed in subjects with a spinal cord injury. Neurorehabil Neural Repair. 2009. https://doi.org/10.1177/1545968308320640.

74. Catz A, Itzkovich M, Tamir A, et al. [SCIM--spinal cord independence measure (version II): sensitivity to functional changes]. Harefuah. 2002;141(12):1025–1031, 1091.

75. Catz A, Itzkovich M, Tesio L, et al. A multicenter international study on the spinal cord independence measure, version III: Rasch psychometric validation. Spinal Cord. 2007. https://doi.org/10.1038/sj.sc.3101960.

76. Itzkovich M, Gelernter I, Biering-Sorensen F, et al. The spinal cord Independence measure (SCIM) version III: reliability and validity in a multi-center international study. Disabil Rehabil. 2007. https://doi.org/10.1080/09638280601046302.

77. Bluvshtein V, Front L, Itzkovich M, et al. SCIM III is reliable and valid in a separate analysis for traumatic spinal cord lesions. Spinal Cord. 2011. https://doi.org/10.1038/sc.2010.111.

78. Itzkovich M, Shefler H, Front L, et al. SCIM III (spinal cord independence measure version III): reliability of assessment by interview and comparison with assessment by observation. Spinal Cord. 2018. https://doi.org/10.1038/sc.2017.97.

79. Ackerman P, Morrison SA, McDowell S, Vazquez L. Using the spinal cord Independence measure III to measure functional recovery in a post-acute spinal cord injury program. Spinal Cord. 2010. https://doi.org/10.1038/sc.2009.140.

80. Anderson KD, Acuff ME, Arp BG, et al. United States (US) multi-center study to assess the validity and reliability of the spinal cord Independence

measure (SCIM III). Spinal Cord. 2011. https://doi.org/10.1038/sc.2011.20.

81. Glass CA, Tesio L, Itzkovich M, et al. Spinal cord independence measure, version III: applicability to the UK spinal cord injured population. J Rehabil Med. 2009. https://doi.org/10.2340/16501977-0398.

82. Catz A, Itzkovich M. Spinal cord Independence measure: comprehensive ability rating scale for the spinal cord lesion patient. J Rehabil Res Dev. 2007. https://doi.org/10.1682/JRRD.2005.07.0123.

83. Invernizzi M, Carda S, Milani P, et al. Development and validation of the Italian version of the spinal cord Independence measure III. Disabil Rehabil. 2010. https://doi.org/10.3109/09638280903437246.

84. de Almeida C, Coelho JN, Riberto M. Applicability, validation and reproducibility of the spinal cord Independence measure version III (SCIM III) in patients with non-traumatic spinal cord lesions. Disabil Rehabil. 2016. https://doi.org/10.3109/09638288.2015.1129454.

85. Riberto M, Tavares DA, Rimoli JRJ, et al. Validation of the Brazilian version of the spinal cord Independence measure III. Arq Neuropsiquiatr. 2014. https://doi.org/10.1590/0004-282x20140066.

86. Zarco-Periñan MJ, Barrera-Chacón MJ, García-Obrero I, Mendez-Ferrer JB, Alarcon LE, Echevarria-Ruiz De Vargas C Development of the Spanish version of the Spinal Cord Independence Measure version III: cross-cultural adaptation and reliability and validity study. Disabil Rehabil. 2014. https://doi.org/10.3109/09638288.2013.864713.

87. Athanasiou A, Alexandrou A, Paraskevopoulos E, Foroglou N, Prassas Bamidis PD. Towards a Greek adaptation of the spinal cord Independence measure (SCIM). In: Proceedings of the 15th European congress of neurosurgery (EANS 14); 2015. p. 181–4. https://doi.org/10.13140/RG.2.1.1669.0087.

88. Unalan H, Misirlioglu TO, Erhan B, et al. Validity and reliability study of the Turkish version of spinal cord Independence measure-III. Spinal Cord. 2015. https://doi.org/10.1038/sc.2014.249.

89. Wannapakhe J, Saensook W, Keawjoho C, Amatachaya S. Reliability and discriminative ability of the spinal cord independence measure III (Thai version). Spinal Cord. 2016. https://doi.org/10.1038/sc.2015.114.

90. Saberi H, Vosoughi F, Derakhshanrad N, et al. Development of Persian version of the spinal cord Independence measure III assessed by interview: a psychometric study. Spinal Cord. 2018. https://doi.org/10.1038/s41393-018-0160-5.

91. Cho DY, Shin H-I, Kim H-R, et al. Reliability and validity of the Korean version of the spinal cord Independence measure III. Am J Phys Med Rehabil. 2020;99(4):305–9. https://doi.org/10.1097/PHM.0000000000001327.

92. Fekete C, Eriks-Hoogland I, Baumberger M, et al. Development and validation of a self-report version of the spinal cord Independence measure (SCIM III). Spinal Cord. 2013. https://doi.org/10.1038/sc.2012.87.

93. Prodinger B, Ballert CS, Brinkhof MWG, Tennant A, Post MWM. Metric properties of the spinal cord independence measure – self report in a community survey. J Rehabil Med. 2016. https://doi.org/10.2340/16501977-2059.

94. Aguilar-Rodríguez M, Peña-Pachés L, Grao-Castellote C, Torralba-Collados F, Hervás-Marín D, Giner-Pascual M. Adaptation and validation of the Spanish self-report version of the spinal cord Independence measure (SCIM III). Spinal Cord. 2015. https://doi.org/10.1038/sc.2014.225.

95. Michailidou C, Marston L, De Souza LH. Translation into Greek and initial validity and reliability testing of a modified version of the SCIM III, in both English and Greek, for self-use. Disabil Rehabil. 2016. https://doi.org/10.3109/09638288.2015.1035454.

96. Bonavita J, Torre M, China S, Bressi F, Bonatti E, Capirossi R. Validation of the Italian version of the spinal cord Independence measure (SCIM III) self-report. Spinal Cord. 2016;54:553–60.

97. Wilartratsami S, Luksanapruksa P, Santipas B, et al. Cross-cultural adaptation and psychometric testing of the Thai version of the spinal cord Independence measure III—self report. Spinal Cord. 2020. https://doi.org/10.1038/s41393-020-00556-7.

98. Sibley A, Kersten P, Ward CD, White B, Mehta R, George S. Measuring autonomy in disabled people: validation of a new scale in a UK population. Clin Rehabil. 2006. https://doi.org/10.1177/0269215506070808.

99. Lund ML, Fisher AG, Lexell J, Bernspång B. Impact on participation and autonomy questionnaire: internal scale validity of the Swedish version for use in people with spinal cord injury. J Rehabil Med. 2007. https://doi.org/10.2340/16501977-0031.

100. Suttiwong J, Vongsirinavarat M, Vachalathiti R, Chaiyawat P. Impact on participation and autonomy questionnaire: psychometric properties of the Thai version. J Phys Ther Sci. 2013. https://doi.org/10.1589/jpts.25.769.

101. Cummings I, Lamontagne ME, Sweet SN, Spivock M, Batcho CS. Canadian-French adaptation and test-retest reliability of the leisure time physical activity questionnaire for people with disabilities. Ann Phys Rehabil Med. 2019. https://doi.org/10.1016/j.rehab.2018.12.002.

102. Middleton JW, Tate RL, Geraghty TJ. Self-efficacy and spinal cord injury: psychometric properties of a new scale. Rehabil Psychol. 2003;48(4):281–8.

103. Middleton JW, Tran Y, Lo C, Craig A. Reexamining the validity and dimensionality of the Moorong self-efficacy scale: improving its clinical utility. Arch Phys Med Rehabil. 2016. https://doi.org/10.1016/j.apmr.2016.05.027.

104. Brooks J, Smedema SM, Tu WM, Eagle D, Catalano D, Chan F. Psychometric validation of the Moorong self-efficacy scale in people with spinal cord injury:

a brief report. Rehabil Couns Bull. 2014. https://doi.org/10.1177/0034355214523506.

105. Miller SM. The measurement of self-efficacy in persons with spinal cord injury: psychometric validation of the Moorong self-efficacy scale. Disabil Rehabil. 2009. https://doi.org/10.1080/09638280802378025.

106. Rajati F, Ghanbari M, Hasandokht T, Hosseini SY, Akbarzadeh R, Ashtarian H. Persian version of the Moorong self-efficacy scale: psychometric study among subjects with physical disability. Disabil Rehabil. 2017. https://doi.org/10.1080/09638288.2016.1226404.

107. Kroll T, Kehn M, Ho PS, Groah S. The SCI exercise self-efficacy scale (ESES): development and psychometric properties. Int J Behav Nutr Phys Act. 2007. https://doi.org/10.1186/1479-5868-4-34.

108. Pisconti F, Santos SMS, Lopes J, Cardoso JR, Lavado EL. Cross-cultural and psychometric properties assessment of the exercise self-efficacy scale in individuals with spinal cord injury. Acta Medica Port. 2017. https://doi.org/10.20344/amp.8884.

109. Nooijen CFJ, Post MWM, Spijkerman DCM, Bergen MP, Stam HJ, Van Den Berg-Emons RJG. Exercise self-efficacy in persons with spinal cord injury: psychometric properties of the Dutch translation of the exercise self-efficacy scale. J Rehabil Med 2013. https://doi.org/10.2340/16501977-1112.

110. Juvalta S, Post MWM, Charlifue S, et al. Development and cognitive testing of the Nottwil environmental factors inventory in Canada, Switzerland and the USA. J Rehabil Med. 2015. https://doi.org/10.2340/16501977-1982.

111. Ballert CS, Post MW, Brinkhof MW, Reinhardt JD. Psychometric properties of the Nottwil environmental factors inventory short form. Arch Phys Med Rehabil. 2015. https://doi.org/10.1016/j.apmr.2014.09.004.

112. Chang FH, Ni P, Coster WJ, Whiteneck GG, Jette AM. Measurement properties of a modified measure of participation for persons with spinal cord injury. J Spinal Cord Med. 2016. https://doi.org/10.1080/10790268.2016.1157956.

113. Marino RJ, Goin JE. Development of a short-form quadriplegia index of function scale. Spinal Cord. 1999; https://doi.org/10.1038/sj.sc.3100772.

114. Lanzino D, Sander E, Mansch B, Jones A, Gill M, Hollman J. Life space assessment in spinal cord injury. Top Spinal Cord Inj Rehabil. 2016;22(3):173–82. https://doi.org/10.1310/sci2203-173.

115. Hahn EA, Garcia SF, Lai JS, et al. Measuring access to information and technology: environmental factors affecting persons with neurologic disorders. Arch Phys Med Rehabil. 2016. https://doi.org/10.1016/j.apmr.2016.01.027.

116. Butler JA, Miller T, O'Connell S, Jelinek C, Collins EG. Physical activity inventory for patients with spinal cord injury. SCI Nurs. 2008;25(3):20–8.

117. Goh HT, Ramachandram K, Ahmad-Fauzi A, Subamanian P. Test-retest reliability and validity of the Malay version LIFE habits assessment (LIFE-H

3.1) to measure social participation in adults with physical disabilities. J Geriatr Phys Ther. 2016. https://doi.org/10.1519/JPT.0000000000000064.

118. Bathen T, Vardeberg K. Test-retest reliability of sunnaas ADL index. Scand J Occup Ther. 2001. https://doi.org/10.1080/110381201750464494.

119. Neufeld S, Lysack C. The "risk inventory for persons with spinal cord injury": development and preliminary validation of a risk assessment tool for spinal cord injury. Disabil Rehabil. 2010. https://doi.org/10.3109/09638280903095957.

120. Hadian MR, Yekaninejad MS, Salehin F, et al. Cross-cultural adaptation and reliability evaluation of Iranian version of functional assessment measure in spinal cord injury patients. Neurol Neurochir Pol. 2012. https://doi.org/10.5114/ninp.2012.30268.

121. Hsieh CL, Jang Y, Yu TY, Wang WC, Sheu CF, Wang YH. A Rasch analysis of the Frenchay Activities Index in patients with spinal cord injury. Spine (Phila Pa 1976). 2007. https://doi.org/10.1097/01.brs.0000255095.08523.39.

122. Velozo CA, Magalhaes LC, Pan AW, Leiter P. Functional scale discrimination at admission and discharge: Rasch analysis of the level of rehabilitation scale-III. Arch Phys Med Rehabil. 1995. https://doi.org/10.1016/S0003-9993(95)80523-0.

123. Johansson C, Bodin P, Kreuter M. Validity and responsiveness of the spinal cord index of function: an instrument on activity level. Spinal Cord. 2009. https://doi.org/10.1038/sc.2009.57.

124. Lynch KB, Bridle MJ. Construct validity of the occupational performance history interview. Occup Ther J Res. 1993. https://doi.org/10.1177/153944929301300402.

125. Barker RN, Amsters DI, Kendall MD, Pershouse KJ, Haines TP. Reliability of the clinical outcome variables scale when administered via telephone to assess mobility in people with spinal cord injury. Arch Phys Med Rehabil. 2007. https://doi.org/10.1016/j.apmr.2007.02.032.

126. Post MW, Charlifue S, Biering-Sørensen F, et al. Development of the international spinal cord injury activities and participation basic data set. Spinal Cord. 2016. https://doi.org/10.1038/sc.2015.188.

127. Vasudevan V, Rimmer JH, Kviz F. Development of the barriers to physical activity questionnaire for people with mobility impairments. Disabil Health J. 2015. https://doi.org/10.1016/j.dhjo.2015.04.007.

128. Hitzig SL, Romero Escobar EM, Noreau L, Craven BC. Validation of the reintegration to normal living index for community-dwelling persons with chronic spinal cord injury. Arch Phys Med Rehabil. 2012. https://doi.org/10.1016/j.apmr.2011.07.200.

129. Post MWM, de Witte LP, Reichrath E, Verdonschot MM, Wijlhuizen GJ, Perenboom RJM. Development and validation of impact-s, an ICF-based questionnaire to measure activities and participation. J Rehabil Med. 2008. https://doi.org/10.2340/16501977-0223.

130. Ostir GV, Granger CV, Black T, et al. Preliminary results for the PAR-PRO: a measure of home and

community participation. Arch Phys Med Rehabil. 2006. https://doi.org/10.1016/j.apmr.2006.04.024.

131. Fekete C, Post MWM, Bickenbach J, et al. A structured approach to capture the lived experience of spinal cord injury: data model and questionnaire of the international spinal cord injury community survey. Am J Phys Med Rehabil. 2017. https://doi.org/10.1097/PHM.0000000000000622.

132. Laleh L, Latifi S, Koushki D, Matin M, Javidan AN, Yekaninejad MS. Assessment of attention to cloth-ing and impact of its restrictive factors in Iranian patients with traumatic spinal cord injury (ACIRF-SCI): Introduction of a new questionnaire. Top Spinal Cord Inj Rehabil. 2015;21(3):257–65. https://doi.org/10.1310/sci2103-257.

133. Norin L, Iwarsson S, Haak M, Slaug B. The housing enabler instrument: assessing threats to reliability and validity. Br J Occup Ther. 2019. https://doi.org/10.1177/0308022618782329.

Measuring Upper Limb Function in Spinal Cord Injury

Francescaroberta Panuccio, Marina D'Angelo, Giulia Grieco, and Marco Tofani

1 Introduction

Tetraplegia results in varying degrees of functional losses in the neck, trunk, and upper and lower limbs, depending on the severity and injury level. The impairment of arm and hand function is one of the most devastating aspects of a spinal cord injury (SCI) at the cervical level because greatly impacts independence and quality of life [1]. For persons with tetraplegia after cervical spinal cord injury (SCI), the loss of hand function poses a significant functional deficit [2]. In fact, impaired motor and sensory functions in arms and hands are among the most debilitating results of the cervical spinal cord injury (SCI).

However, restoration of hand and arm function during rehabilitation is crucial considering their key role in activities of daily living (ADL) and the level of independence [3]. Full recovery from a complete SCI is exceedingly rare, and the majority of injured people are disabled during the most productive periods of their lives. Previous studies show that arm and hand function restoration is a high priority for individuals with tetraplegia. They are judged to be most desirable to regain before

bowel, bladder, sexual function, or walking ability. Moreover, most persons with tetraplegia expected enhanced quality of life if their hand function could be improved [4]. Quantitative assessment of hand function in people with tetraplegia is important not only for day-to-day clinical practice but also for evaluating emerging therapies. Evaluation of the efficacy of rehabilitation and experimental interventions can be achieved by standardized tests that assess upper extremity function validly.

This chapter aims to describe and evaluate assessment tools on upper limb function in people with SCI through a systematic review.

2 Materials and Methods

This study was conducted by a research group composed of medical doctors and health professionals from the "Sapienza" University of Rome and the "Rehabilitation & Outcome Measure Assessment" (R.O.M.A.) association. In the last few years, the R.O.M.A. association has worked with several studies and validations of outcome measures in Italy for the Spinal Cord Injury population [5, 6, 7–18].

This chapter describes all assessment tools regarding upper limb function resulting from a systematic review conducted on PubMed, Scopus, and Web of Science. For specific details on methodology, see chapter "Methodological Approach to Identifying Outcome Measures in Spinal Cord

F. Panuccio · M. D'Angelo · G. Grieco
R.O.M.A. Rehabilitation Outcome Measures
Assessment, Non-Profit Organization, Rome, Italy

M. Tofani (✉)
Department of Neurorehabilitation and Robotics,
Bambino Gesù Paediatric Hospital, Rome, Italy
e-mail: marco.tofani@uniroma1.it

© The Author(s), under exclusive license to Springer Nature Switzerland AG 2021
G. Galeoto et al. (eds.), *Measuring Spinal Cord Injury*,
https://doi.org/10.1007/978-3-030-68382-5_8

Injury." Eligibility criteria for considering studies for this chapter were validation studies and cross-cultural adaptation studies, studies about the upper limb function, studies about tests, questionnaires, and self-reported and performance-based outcome measures, studies with a population of people of SCI and population ≥18 years old. Study selection: the selection of studies was conducted in accordance with the 27-item PRISM Statement for Reporting Systematic Reviews [19]. For the data collection, the authors followed recommendations from the COnsensus-based Standards for the selection of health Measurement Instruments (COSMIN) initiative [20]. Study quality and risk of bias were assessed using COSMIN Check List [21, 22].

3   Results

For this chapter, 33 papers were considered. The authors found 17 assessment tools that evaluate upper limb function in persons with SCI. In Fig. 1, a flow chart of included studies is reported [21, 22]. The assessment tools are described subsequently.

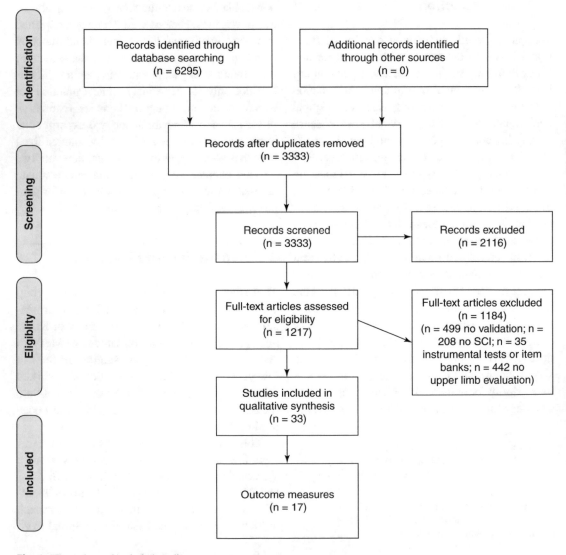

Fig. 1 Flow chart of included studies

3.1 Van Lieshout Test (VLT)

The VLT is an instrument to assess the quality of arm–hand skilled performance (AHSP) in persons with a cervical spinal cord injury (C-SCI). The VLT was developed in 2004 by Van Lieshout and colleagues as a specific tool to assess hand function in CSCI. The VLT was validated in the Dutch [23–25] and Italian language [1]. However, English and German versions are available from the author. The VLT is composed of 19 tasks, and it makes a distinction between basic and complex activities. The possible ways of performing each task are described in six hierarchical levels, resulting in a score from 0 to 5. This tool is responsive to changes in arm/hand skilled performance during rehabilitation in people with C-SCI. In 2006, Post et al. developed a short version of the VLT (VLT-SV) to have a more useful instrument for research purposes [26, 27]. In 2018, the short version of VLT was validated in Italian [28]. The VLT-SV includes 10 of the 19 tasks of the original VLT, and the level of perfor-

mance of each task is scored within a range from 0 (worst arm/hand function) to 5 (best arm/hand function). The administration time is 25–35 min. Table 1 summarizes the papers' authors and languages and Table 2 shows the quality of the studies.

3.2 Motor Capacities Scale (MCS)

The MCS is specifically designed for people with tetraplegia who undergo a functional surgery of upper limbs. In 2004, Fattal validated MCS in France [29, 30]. The purpose of the MCS is to focus on the elementary motor abilities required to achieve ADL. MCS contains 60 items. The resulting MCS includes six functional categories, each with a different number of tasks: transfers, repositioning on Bobath's couch, repositioning on wheelchair seat, locomotion in a manual wheelchair and an electric wheelchair, motor capacities of spatial exploration, and motor capacities for grasping and gripping. Functional categories were

Table 1 Characteristics of the studies validating VLT

Authors	Language	n	Age mean (SD, range) year	Gender % Female
Berardi et al. [28]	Italian	61	47 (14.76)	12 (20)
Galeoto et al. [12]	Italian	50	48 (18)	22 (44)
Post et al. [26]	Dutch	55	42.1 (13.5)	9 (16.4)
Spooren et al. [23]	Dutch	60	38.9	14 (23.3)
Spooren et al. [24]	Dutch	61	41 (15)	12 (19.7)
Spooren et al. [25]	Dutch	73	40 (15.5)	20 (27.4)
Franke et al. [27]	Dutch	55	38 (12.93, 18–64)	15 (27)

n number of participants of the study, n.a. not available

Table 2 Evaluation of quality and risk of bias

Authors	Item of COSMIN checklist									
	1	2	3	4	5	6	7	8	9	10
Berardi et al. [28]	?	+	–	+	–	+	–	+	+	–
Galeoto et al. [12]	?	+	–	+	–	+	–	+	+	+
Post et al. [26]	+	+	–	+	–	+	–	+	+	–
Spooren et al. [23]	+	+	–	–	+	–	–	+	+	–
Spooren et al. [24]	?	–	+	–	–	–	–	–	–	–
Spooren et al. [25]	?	–	+	–	–	–	–	–	–	–
Franke et al. [27]	?	?	+	–	–	–	–	–	–	+

Item 1 PROM development, *Item 2,* content validity, *Item 3* structural validity, *Item 4* internal consistency, *Item 5* cross-cultural validity/measurement invariance, *Item 6* reliability, *Item 7* measurement error, *Item 8* criterion validity, *Item 9* hypothesis testing for construct validity, *Item 10*: responsiveness, + sufficient, – insufficient, ? indeterminate

Table 3 Characteristics of the studies validating MCS

Authors	Language	n	Age mean (SD, range) year	Gender % Female
Fattal [29]	French	52	11 (21.59)	n.a.
Fattal et al. [30]	French	27	n.a.	6 (22)

N number of participants of the study, *n.a.* not available

Table 4 Evaluation of quality and risk of bias

Authors	Item of COSMIN checklist									
	1	2	3	4	5	6	7	8	9	10
Fattal [29]	+	+	−	+	+	+	−	+	+	−
Fattal et al. [30]	?	?	−	−	+	−	−	−	−	+

Item 1 PROM development, *Item 2* content validity, *Item 3* structural validity, *Item 4* internal consistency, *Item 5* cross-cultural validity/measurement invariance, *Item 6* reliability, *Item 7* measurement error, *Item 8* criterion validity, *Item 9* hypothesis testing for construct validity, *Item 10,* responsiveness, + sufficient, − insufficient, *?* indeterminate

Table 5 Characteristics of the studies validating CUE-T

Authors	Language	n	Age mean (SD, range) year	Gender % Female
Marino et al. [32]	English	30	44.8	7 (23.3)
Marino et al. [31]	English	154	36.7 (11.1)	9 (5.8)
Oleson and Marino [33]	English	46	44 (21)	4 (8.7)
Marino et al. [35]	English	50	48.1 (18.2, 17–81)	14 (28)
Marino et al. [34]	English	85	41.9 (18.1, 15–79)	27 (16)

n number of participants of the study; *n.a.* not available

Table 6 Evaluation of quality and risk of bias

Authors	Item of COSMIN checklist									
	1	2	3	4	5	6	7	8	9	10
Marino et al. [32]	+	+	−	−	+	−	−	−	−	−
Marino et al. [31]	+	+	+	+	+	+	−	+	+	−
Oleson and Marino [33]	?	?	+	−	+	−	−	+	+	−
Marino et al. [35]	?	?	+	−	−	−	−	+	+	−
Marino et al. [34]	?	+	−	−	+	−	+	+	+	+

Item 1 PROM development, *Item 2* content validity, *Item 3* structural validity, *Item 4* internal consistency, *Item 5* cross-cultural validity/measurement invariance, *Item 6* reliability, *Item 7* measurement error, *Item 8* criterion validity, *Item 9* hypothesis testing for construct validity, *Item 10* responsiveness, + sufficient, − insufficient, *?* indeterminate

defined at the request of both experts. Table 3 summarizes the papers' authors and languages and Table 4 shows the quality of the studies.

3.3 Capabilities of Upper Extremity Test (CUE-T)

The CUE was developed by Marino et al. in 1998 in the United States [31]. The test has as its model a questionnaire of the same name: CUE-Q. The CUE-Q was validated in the United States by Ralph J. Marino et al. [32–35]. So CUE-Q 32 items formed the basis of the test items on the CUE-T. The Capabilities of Upper Extremity-Questionnaire (CUE-Q) was developed to fill a gap in upper extremity assessment in patients with spinal cord injury. Table 5 summarizes the papers' authors and languages and Table 6 shows the quality of the studies.

3.4 Graded Redefined Assessment of Strength, Sensibility and Prehension (GRASSP)

The GRASSP was developed by Sukhvinder Kalsi-Ryan, in Switzerland and Toronto in 2012. It was validated in English and Swiss [34, 36–40]. The GRASSP consists of five subtests performed separately and yields five subtest scores for both right and left. The scores are interpreted separately rather than as one global score because each score provides specific information about the upper limb, and all subtests do not share internal consistency. In 2018, Vestra et al. validated the second version of GRASSP in the Swiss language [41]. Table 7 summarizes the papers' authors and languages and Table 8 shows the quality of the studies.

3.5 Neuromuscular Recovery Scale (NRS) to the Upper Extremities

The initial version of the NRS (Behrman et al. 2012) consisted of 11 motor tasks evaluated in the overground and body weight-supported treadmill environments, with each task focusing on the trunk and lower extremity function. The NRS has since been extended in three ways. The first change to the NRS was the inclusion of three upper extremity items to assess the recovery of upper extremity function in individuals with tetraplegia. These three upper extremity items are the (1) forward reach and grasp, (2) door open and pull, and (3) overhead press. It was validated in English language [42, 43]. Table 9 summarizes the papers' authors and languages and Table 10 shows the quality of the studies.

Table 7 Characteristics of the studies validating GRASSP and GRASSP second version

	Authors	Language	n	Age mean (SD, range) year	Gender % Female
GRASSP	Kalsi-Ryan et al. [40]	English	n.a.	n.a.	n.a.
	Kalsi-Ryan et al. [36]	English	72	39.7 (10.7)	n.a.
	Kalsi-Ryan et al. [36]	English	n.a.	n.a.	n.a.
	Velstra et al. [39]	Swiss	74	49 (18, 18–87)	23 (21.1)
	Kalsi-Ryan et al. [38]	Swedish English	53	49.6 (15.6, 18–83)	5 (13)
	Marino et al. [34]	English	85	41.9 (18.1, 15–79)	27 (16)
GRASSP II	Velstra et al. [41]	Swiss	77	50.61 (20.24)	25 (32.4)

n number of participants of the study, *n.a.* not available

Table 8 Evaluation of quality and risk of bias

Authors	Item of COSMIN checklist									
	1	2	3	4	5	6	7	8	9	10
Kalsi-Ryan et al. [40]	+	+	–	–	–	–	–	–	–	–
Kalsi-Ryan et al. [36]	?	?	+	–	+	+	–	+	+	–
Kalsi-Ryan et al. [36]	+	+	–	–	–	–	–	–	–	–
Velstra et al. [39]	?	?	–	–	–	–	–	+	+	+
Kalsi-Ryan et al. [38]	?	?	+	+	+	–	+	+	+	+
Marino et al. [34]	?	+	–	–	+	–	+	+	+	+
Velstra et al. [41]	+	+	+	–	–	–	–	–	–	–

Item 1 PROM development, *Item 2* content validity, *Item 3* structural validity, *Item 4* internal consistency, *Item 5* cross-cultural validity/measurement invariance, *Item 6* reliability, *Item 7* measurement error, *Item 8* criterion validity, *Item 9* hypothesis testing for construct validity, *Item 10* responsiveness, + sufficient, – insufficient, ? indeterminate

Table 9 Characteristics of the studies validating NRS

Authors	Language	n	Age mean (SD, range) year	Gender % Female
Harkema et al. [42]	English	152	36 (15)	29 (19)
Tester et al. [43]	English	72	36 (15)	15 (21)

n number of participants of the study, *n.a.* not available

Table 10 Evaluation of quality and risk of bias

| Authors | Item of COSMIN checklist | | | | | | | | | |
	1	2	3	4	5	6	7	8	9	10
Harkema et al. [42]	+	+	+	−	+	−	−	−	−	−
Tester et al. [43]	?	?	+	−	−	−	−	−	−	+

Item1 PROM development, *Item 2* content validity, *Item 3* structural validity, *Item 4* internal consistency, *Item 5* cross-cultural validity/measurement invariance, *Item 6* reliability, *Item 7* measurement error, *Item 8* criterion validity, *Item 9* hypothesis testing for construct validity, *Item 10* responsiveness, + sufficient, − insufficient, ? indeterminate

Table 11 Characteristics of the studies of scale, test, or questionnaire with less than two validations

	Authors	Language	n	Age mean (SD, range) year	Gender % Female
AuSpinal	Coates et al. [2]	English	8	n.a.	n.a.
Handheld myometer	Larson et al. [44]	English	24	53.3	1 (4.2)
DHI	Misirlioglu et al. [3]	Turkish	40	8 (20)	25.6 (10.1)
WAnT	Jacobs et al. [45]	English	43	10 (23.3)	34.4 (10.3)
TRI-HFT	Kapadia et al. [46]	English	21	n.a.	n.a.
Swedish tetraplegia surgery satisfaction questionnaire	Bunketorp-Käll et al.[4]	Swedish	58	47 (23–78)	15 (25.9)
RAHFT	Kowalczewski et al. [47]	English	13	(24–56)	n.a.
K-B scale	Dahlgren et al. [48]	Swedish	55	39 (18–72)	12 (22)
IMPA	Shin et al. [49]	Korean	n.a.	n.a.	n.a.
Automated tools to quantify hand and wrist motor function	Grasse et al. [50]	English	13	32.15 (13.92)	4 (30.8)
FST	Triolo et al. [51]	English	10	25	8 (80)

n number of participants of the study, *n.a.* not available

3.6   AuSpinal

SK Coates et al. developed AuSpinal in Australia in 2011 [2] to quantify unilateral hand function in people with tetraplegia. Seven tasks were selected from an array of existing hand assessments and modified to ensure appropriateness for this population and sensitivity to change in people with poor hand function. The final version of AuSpinal consisted of seven tasks. Four tasks were based on the Sollerman Hand Function Test elements and involved manipulating a key, coin, telephone, and metal nut. Two tasks were modified from the Rehabilitation Engineering Laboratory Hand Function Test for Functional Electrical Stimulation Assisted–Grasping, and included manipulating a can of soft drink and a credit card. The last task was modified from the Upper Extremity Function Test, but instead of manipulating small ball bearings, it involved

manipulating a small, chocolate-covered candy mimicking a pill. Administration of the AuSpinal takes approximately 15 min per hand. The scores for each task were summed with a maximum possible score of 86. Table 11 summarizes the papers' authors and languages and Table 12 shows the quality of the studies.

3.7   Handheld Myometer

In 2010, the Handheld Myometer was validated for people with SCI [44]. It is a test that involves the use of a portable myometer. This test evaluates the strength of the "SECOND-DIGIT" adductors, the "FIFTH-DIGIT" adductors, and the opposites of the thumb able participants and in subjects with weakness. Table 11 summarizes the papers' authors and languages and Table 12 shows the quality of the studies.

Table 12 Evaluation of quality and risk of bias

Authors	Item of COSMIN checklist									
	1	2	3	4	5	6	7	8	9	10
Coates et al. [2]	+	+	−	+	−	+	−	−	−	−
Larson et al. [44]	+	+	−	−	+	+	−	−	−	−
Misirlioglu et al. [3]	?	−	+	+	+	−	−	+	+	
Jacobs et al. [45]	?	−	−	−	+	+	−	−	−	−
Kapadia et al. [46]	+	+	+	−	+	+	−	+	+	−
Bunketorp-Käll et al. [4]	+	+	−	+	−	+	−	−	−	−
Kowalczewski et al. [47]	+	+	+	−	−	−	−	−	−	−
Dahlgren et al. [48]	+	+	+	−	−	−	−	+	+	
Shin et al. [49]	+	+	−	−	−	−	−	−	−	−
Grasse et al. [50]	+	+	−	−	−	+	+	+	+	−
Triolo et al. [51]	?	+	−	−	+	+	−	−	−	−

Item1 PROM development, *Item 2* content validity, *Item 3* structural validity, *Item 4* internal consistency, *Item 5* cross-cultural validity/measurement invariance, *Item 6* reliability, *Item 7* measurement error, *Item 8* criterion validity, *Item 9* hypothesis testing for construct validity, *Item 10* responsiveness, + sufficient, − insufficient, *?* indeterminate

3.8   Duruöz Hand Index (DHI)

The DHI is a self-report questionnaire developed primarily to assess hand-related activity limitations in patients with rheumatoid arthritis (RA). It was validated in Turkey for people with SCI [3]. As an inexpensive, easy to administer tool that requires no special equipment or training, the DHI shows promise as an outcome measure of hand-related activity It contains 18 items related to the ability of the hand during performing kitchen tasks (8 items), dressing (2 items), maintaining personal hygiene (2 items), performing office tasks (2 items), and other general items (4 items). Patients rate their ability from "0" (no difficulty) to "5" (impossible to do), and these six levels of answers allow a highly sensitive grading of hand-related activity limitation. The total score of the questionnaire, ranging from 0 to 90, indicates greater impairment or more difficulty with higher scores, whereas less impairment or difficulty with lower scores. No training is required before administration and it takes less than 3 min to administer the whole questionnaire. Table 11 summarizes the papers' authors and languages and Table 12 shows the quality of the studies.

3.9   Wingate Anaerobic Testing (WAnT)

The WAnt is a muscular power assessment commonly used in research and sports training, involves 30 s of maximal efforts printing on an arm or leg cycle ergometer. In 2002, Jacobs et al. examined test–retest reliability of arm WAnT performance in persons with complete SCI and paraplegia in Miami, Florida, USA [45]. The WAnt has been validated in the general population compared to several tasks that are considered generally to be measures of anaerobic fitness involving both the lower and upper limbs. Table 11 summarizes the papers' authors and languages and Table 12 shows the quality of the studies.

3.10   Toronto Rehabilitation Institute–Hand Function Test (TRI-HFT)

It was validated in people with SCI by N. Kapadia et al. in Toronto, Ontario, Canada in 2012 [46]. TRI-HFT is a test to measure palmar grasp, lateral pinch, and pulp pinch, as these are the most frequently used hand postures in ADLs. The TRI-HFT consists of two parts. The first part of the test assesses the individuals' ability to manipulate objects that they may encounter in their daily lives (Items 1–11). To manipulate these objects, they must use one of the following: a lateral pinch, a pulp pinch, or a palmar grasp. The second part of the test measures the strength of their lateral pinch or pulp pinch and palmar grasp (Items 12–14). The two parts of the TRI-HFT should be administered sequentially, and each test component should be presented to the individual in the order shown on the scoring form. The individual may take as much time as required and is scored when he/she completes the task or when he/she stops trying to accomplish the task. There is no time limit within which the task must be performed. The results of the test are entered on a paper record. The TRIHFT should preferably be administered by a hand or upper extremity specialist (physiotherapist or occupational therapist). The entire valuation for both hands can be completed in less than 30 min. When the assessment is to be recorded on videotape, the camera should be positioned at a 45° angle opposite the involved upper extremity at 1 m height. The score range is 0–7 for each item. Table 11 summarizes the papers' authors and languages and Table 12 shows the quality of the studies.

3.11 Swedish Tetraplegia Surgery Satisfaction Questionnaire

In 2017, Bunketorp-Käll et al. validated the Swedish version to evaluate reconstructive surgery satisfaction [4]. Similar to the original version of the questionnaire, participants are asked to respond to statements on a 5-point Likert-type scale ranging from 1 to 5 (i.e., strongly disagree, disagree, neutral, agree, and strongly agree). The first section of the questionnaire was divided into the following categories: (1) satisfaction, (2) activities, and (3) occupation/schooling. The second section consists of one question about the appearance and

cosmesis of the hand after the surgery, together with two questions about changes in the functional ability of participants after triceps- and hand/wrist surgery, respectively. The third section contains questions where participants are asked to list activities in which function was improved after surgery. Similarly, a question was added where individuals are asked to report whether the surgery has complicated certain tasks. In two final questions, participants were asked to mention any other disadvantages with the surgery and to give general comments, if any. Table 11 summarizes the papers' authors and languages and Table 12 shows the quality of the studies.

3.12 ReJoyce Automated Hand Function Test (RAHFT)

In 2011, Kowalczewski et al. validated RAHFT for people with SCI in Alberta, Canada [47]. This test is connected to the ReJoyce (Rehabilitation Joystick for Computer Exercise) on which subjects perform various movement tasks while playing computer games. The ReJoyce provides the requisite signals. It is a passive workstation comprising a segmented arm that presents the user with a variety of spring-loaded manipulanda. Each manipulandum is instrumented with one or more sensors, whose signals are fed to a computer. The signals are analyzed with custom software to control computer games and to run the "ReJoyce Automated Hand Function Test" (RAHFT). Kowalczewski et al. compared and validated the RAHFT against two widely used clinical tests, the Action Research Arm Test (ARAT), and the Fugl–Meyer Assessment (FMA). The RAHFT consists of three parts: a functional range of motion (fROM), grasp, key grip, pronation–supination tasks, and placement tasks. The users (subjects or therapists) initiated the RAHFT software program by clicking on a desktop icon. It ran automatically, taking its cues from signals from the ReJoyce device or inputs from the subject's computer keyboard. As the test component of the test with a three-dimensional animation. The user was then allowed up to 60 s to perform the task. If the task was completed within this time, the user or therapist could advance to the next task by depressing the keyboard spacebar. Table 11 summarizes the papers' authors and languages and Table 12 shows the quality of the studies.

3.13 Klein–Bell Adl Scale (K-BSCALE)

Validated in Sweden [48], the scale measures the patient's level of independence in the basic ADL with 170 items divided into six dimensions: dressing, bladder management, mobility, baths and hygiene, use of the telephone, and nutrition. Table 11 summarizes the papers' authors and languages and Table 12 shows the quality of the studies.

3.14 Intentional Movement Performance Ability (IMPA)

In 2013, Sung Yul Shin et al. worked to develop IMPA in Korea, a new assessment method for evaluating the motor function of patients who are suffering from physical weakness after a stroke, incomplete spinal cord injury (iSCI), or other diseases [49]. IMPA is a scale that measures how well the patient can perform his/her intended movement. They used a robotic device to obtain the information of interaction between the patient and the robot and used it to assess the patients. The IMPA is defined by the root mean square of the interactive torque, while the subject performs given periodic movement with the robot. IMPA is proposed to determine the level of the subject's impaired motor function quantitatively. The method is indirectly tested by asking the healthy subjects to lift a barbell to disturb their motor function. The IMPA has the potential to provide proper information on the subject's motor function level. Table 11 summarizes the papers' authors and languages, and Table 12 shows the quality of the studies.

3.15 Automated Tools to Quantify Hand and Wrist Motor Function

The system consisted of seven devices that were each designed to measure either the force or range of motion (ROM) of simple hand and wrist movements. It was validated in the English language [50]. Table 11 summarizes the papers' authors and languages and Table 12 shows the quality of the studies.

3.16 Functional Standing Test (FST)

The 18 subtests included in the original FST are listed below in increasing order of assumed difficulty. Manipulation of light objects on the countertop or low shelves (test items 1 through 6) was assumed to be a mild challenge to postural control mechanisms while moving heavier objects to and from higher locations or across the midline (items 13 through 18) was assumed to be more demanding. Items common to both the FST and Jebsen Test of Hand Function are designated by asterisks. It was validated in 1994 [51]. Table 11 summarizes the papers' authors and languages and Table 12 shows the quality of the studies.

4 Conclusions

This chapter reports on all assessment tools described in the literature to evaluate upper limb functioning in SCI people. Among the 33 papers included in this chapter, 17 tools resulted in evaluating the arm–hand skilled performance and sensorimotor and prehension functions. The most common assessment tools are the Van Lieshout Test (VLT), which is an instrument to assess the quality of arm–hand skilled performance, and the Graded Redefined Assessment Of Strength, Sensibility And Prehension (GRASSP), a clinical impairment measure of sensorimotor and prehension function through three domains (strength, sensation, and prehension).

References

1. Galeoto G, Berardi A, De Santis R, et al. Validation and cross-cultural adaptation of the Van Lieshout test in an Italian population with cervical spinal cord injury: a psychometric study. Spinal Cord Ser Cases. 2018;15(4):49. https://doi.org/10.1038/s41394-018-0083-6.
2. Coates SK, Harvey LA, Dunlop SA, Allison GT. The AuSpinal: a test of hand function for people with tetraplegia. Spinal Cord. 2011. https://doi.org/10.1038/sc.2010.86.
3. Misirlioglu TO, Unalan H, Karamehmetoglu SS. Validation of Duruöz hand index in patients with tetraplegia. J Hand Ther. 2016. https://doi.org/10.1016/j.jht.2015.10.001.
4. Bunketorp-Käll L, Wangdell J, Reinholdt C, Fridén J. Satisfaction with upper limb reconstructive surgery in individuals with tetraplegia: the development and reliability of a Swedish self-reported satisfaction questionnaire. Spinal Cord. 2017. https://doi.org/10.1038/sc.2017.12.
5. Castelnuovo G, Giusti EM, Manzoni GM, et al. What is the role of the placebo effect for pain relief in neurorehabilitation? Clinical implications from the Italian consensus conference on pain in neurorehabilitation. Front Neurol. 2018. https://doi.org/10.3389/fneur.2018.00310.
6. Marquez MA, De Santis R, Ammendola V, et al. Cross-cultural adaptation and validation of the "spinal cord injury-falls concern scale" in the Italian population. Spinal Cord. 2018;56(7):712–8. https://doi.org/10.1038/s41393-018-0070-6.
7. Dattoli S, Colucci M, Soave MG, et al. Evaluation of pelvis postural systems in spinal cord injury patients: outcome research. J Spinal Cord Med. 2018;43:185–92.
8. Berardi A, Galeoto G, Guarino D, et al. Construct validity, test-retest reliability, and the ability to detect change of the Canadian occupational performance measure in a spinal cord injury population. Spinal Cord Ser Cases. 2019. https://doi.org/10.1038/s41394-019-0196-6.
9. Ponti A, Berardi A, Galeoto G, Marchegiani L, Spandonaro C, Marquez MA. Quality of life, concern of falling and satisfaction of the sit-ski aid in sit-skiers with spinal cord injury: observational study. Spinal Cord Ser Cases. 2020. https://doi.org/10.1038/s41394-020-0257-x.
10. Panuccio F, Galeoto G, Marquez MA, et al. General sleep disturbance scale (GSDS-IT) in people with spinal cord injury: a psychometric study. Spinal Cord. 2020. https://doi.org/10.1038/s41393-020-0500-0.
11. Monti M, Marquez MA, Berardi A, Tofani M, Valente D, Galeoto G. The multiple sclerosis intimacy and sexuality questionnaire (MSISQ-15): validation of the Italian version for individuals with spinal cord injury. Spinal Cord. 2020. https://doi.org/10.1038/s41393-020-0469-8.
12. Galeoto G, Colucci M, Guarino D, et al. Exploring validity, reliability, and factor analysis of the Quebec user evaluation of satisfaction with assistive Technology in an Italian Population: a cross-sectional study. Occup Ther Heal Care. 2018. https://doi.org/10.1080/07380577.2018.1522682.
13. Colucci M, Tofani M, Trioschi D, Guarino D, Berardi A, Galeoto G. Reliability and validity of the Italian version of Quebec user evaluation of satisfaction with assistive technology 2.0 (QUEST-IT 2.0) with users of mobility assistive device. Disabil Rehabil Assist Technol. 2019. https://doi.org/10.1080/17483107.2019.1668975.
14. Berardi A, Galeoto G, Lucibello L, Panuccio F, Valente D, Tofani M. Athletes with disability' satisfaction with sport wheelchairs: an Italian cross sectional study. Disabil Rehabil Assist Technol. 2020. https://doi.org/10.1080/17483107.2020.1800114.
15. Berardi A, De Santis R, Tofani M, et al. The Wheelchair Use Confidence Scale: Italian translation, adaptation, and validation of the short form. Disabil Rehabil Assist Technol. 2018;13(4):i. https://doi.org/10.1080/17483107.2017.1357053.
16. Anna B, Giovanni G, Marco T, et al. The Validity of Rasterstereography as a Technological Tool for the Objectification of Postural Assessment in the Clinical and Educational Fields: Pilot Study. In: Advances in intelligent systems and computing; 2020. https://doi.org/10.1007/978-3-030-23884-1_8.
17. Panuccio F, Berardi A, Marquez MA, et al. Development of the pregnancy and motherhood evaluation questionnaire (PMEQ) for evaluating and measuring the impact of physical disability on pregnancy and the management of motherhood: a pilot study. Disabil Rehabil. 2020;2020:1–7. https://doi.org/10.1080/09638288.2020.1802520.
18. Amedoro A, Berardi A, Conte A, et al. The effect of aquatic physical therapy on patients with multiple sclerosis: a systematic review and meta-analysis. In: Mult Scler Relat Disord; 2020. https://doi.org/10.1016/j.msard.2020.102022.
19. Moher D, Shamseer L, Clarke M, et al. Preferred reporting items for systematic review and meta-analysis protocols (PRISMA-P) 2015 statement. Rev Esp Nutr Human Diet. 2016. https://doi.org/10.1186/2046-4053-4-1
20. Mokkink LB, Terwee CB, Patrick DL, et al. The COSMIN study reached international consensus on taxonomy, terminology, and definitions of measurement properties for health-related patient-reported outcomes. J Clin Epidemiol. 2010. https://doi.org/10.1016/j.jclinepi.2010.02.006.
21. Terwee CB, Prinsen CAC, Chiarotto A, et al. COSMIN methodology for evaluating the content validity of patient-reported outcome measures: a Delphi study. Qual Life Res. 2018; https://doi.org/10.1007/s11136-018-1829-0.
22. Mokkink LB, de Vet HCW, Prinsen CAC, et al. COSMIN risk of bias checklist for systematic reviews

of patient-reported outcome measures. Qual Life Res. 2018. https://doi.org/10.1007/s11136-017-1765-4.

23. Spooren AIF, Janssen-Potten YJM, Post MWM, Kerckhofs E, Nene A, Seelen HAM. Measuring change in arm hand skilled performance in persons with a cervical spinal cord injury: responsiveness of the Van Lieshout test. Spinal Cord. 2006. https://doi.org/10.1038/sj.sc.3101957.

24. Spooren AIF, Arnould C, Smeets RJEM, Snoek G, Seelen HAM. Reference values for the transformed Van Lieshout hand function test for tetraplegia. Spinal Cord. 2013. https://doi.org/10.1038/sc.2013.73.

25. Spooren AIF, Arnould C, Smeets RJEM, Bongers HMH, Seelen HAM. Improvement of the Van Lieshout hand function test for tetraplegia using a Rasch analysis. Spinal Cord. 2013. https://doi.org/10.1038/sc.2013.54.

26. Post MWM, Van Lieshout G, Seelen HAM, Snoek GJ, Ijzerman MJ, Pons C. Measurement properties of the short version of the Van Lieshout test for arm/hand function of persons with tetraplegia after spinal cord injury. Spinal Cord. 2006. https://doi.org/10.1038/sj.sc.3101937.

27. Franke AC, Snoek GJ, De Groot S, Nene AV, Spooren AIF, Post MWM. Arm hand skilled performance in persons with a cervical spinal cord injury – long-term follow-up. Spinal Cord. 2013. https://doi.org/10.1038/sc.2012.95.

28. Berardi A, Biondillo A, Màrquez MA, et al. Validation of the short version of the Van Lieshout test in an Italian population with cervical spinal cord injuries: a cross-sectional study. Spinal Cord. 2018;57:339–45.

29. Fattal C. Motor capacities of upper limbs in tetraplegics: a new scale for the assessment of the results of functional surgery on upper limbs. Spinal Cord. 2004. https://doi.org/10.1038/sj.sc.3101551.

30. Fattal C, Enjalbert M, Teissier J, Coulet B, Fachin-Martins E. Responsiveness of the motor capacities scale to upper limb reconstructive surgery in persons with tetraplegia due to cervical spinal cord injury. Spinal Cord. 2020. https://doi.org/10.1038/s41393-020-0456-0.

31. Marino RJ, Shea JA, Stineman MG. The capabilities of upper extremity instrument: reliability and validity of a measure of functional limitation in tetraplegia. Arch Phys Med Rehabil. 1998. https://doi.org/10.1016/S0003-9993(98)90412-9.

32. Marino RJ, Patrick M, Albright W, et al. Development of an objective test of upper-limb function in tetraplegia: the capabilities of upper extremity test. Am J Phys Med Rehabil. 2012. https://doi.org/10.1097/PHM.0b013e31824fa6cc.

33. Oleson CV, Marino RJ. Responsiveness and concurrent validity of the revised capabilities of upper extremity-questionnaire (CUE-Q) in patients with acute tetraplegia. Spinal Cord. 2014. https://doi.org/10.1038/sc.2014.77.

34. Marino RJ, Sinko R, Bryden A, et al. Comparison of responsiveness and minimal clinically impor-

tant difference of the capabilities of upper extremity test (CUE-T) and the graded redefined assessment of strength, sensibility and prehension (GRASSP). Top Spinal Cord Inj Rehabil. 2018. https://doi.org/10.1310/sci2403-227.

35. Marino RJ, Kern SB, Leiby B, Schmidt-Read M, Mulcahey MJ. Reliability and validity of the capabilities of upper extremity test (CUE-T) in subjects with chronic spinal cord injury. J Spinal Cord Med. 2015. https://doi.org/10.1179/2045772314Y.0000000272.

36. Kalsi-Ryan S, Curt A, Verrier MC, Fehlings MG. Development of the graded redefined assessment of strength, sensibility and Prehension (GRASSP): reviewing measurement specific to the upper limb in tetraplegia. J Neurosurg Spine. 2012. https://doi.org/10.3171/2012.6.aospine1258.

37. Kalsi-Ryan S, Beaton D, Curt A, et al. The graded redefined assessment of strength sensibility and prehension: reliability and validity. J Neurotrauma. 2012. https://doi.org/10.1089/neu.2010.1504.

38. Kalsi-Ryan S, Beaton D, Ahn H, et al. Responsiveness, sensitivity, and minimally detectable difference of the graded and redefined assessment of strength, sensibility, and Prehension, version 1.0. J Neurotrauma. 2016. https://doi.org/10.1089/neu.2015.4217.

39. Velstra IM, Curt A, Frotzler A, et al. Changes in strength, sensation, and Prehension in acute cervical spinal cord injury: European Multicenter responsiveness study of the GRASSP. Neurorehabil Neural Repair. 2015. https://doi.org/10.1177/1545968314565466.

40. Kalsi-Ryan S, Curt A, Fehlings M, Verrier M. Assessment of the hand in tetraplegia using the graded redefined assessment of strength, sensibility and Prehension (GRASSP). Top Spinal Cord Inj Rehabil. 2009;14(4):34–46. https://doi.org/10.1310/sci1404-34.

41. Velstra IM, Fellinghauer C, Abel R, Kalsi-Ryan S, Rupp R, Curt A. The graded and redefined assessment of strength, sensibility, and Prehension version 2 provides interval measure properties. J Neurotrauma. 2018. https://doi.org/10.1089/neu.2017.5195.

42. Harkema SJ, Shogren C, Ardolino E, Lorenz DJ. Assessment of functional improvement without compensation for human spinal cord injury: extending the neuromuscular recovery scale to the upper extremities. J Neurotrauma. 2016. https://doi.org/10.1089/neu.2015.4213.

43. Tester NJ, Lorenz DJ, Suter SP, et al. Responsiveness of the neuromuscular recovery scale during outpatient activity-dependent rehabilitation for spinal cord injury. Neurorehabil Neural Repair. 2016. https://doi.org/10.1177/1545968315605181.

44. Larson CA, Tezak WD, Malley MS, Thornton W. Assessment of postural muscle strength in sitting: reliability of measures obtained with hand-held dynamometry in individuals with spinal cord injury. J Neurol Phys Ther. 2010. https://doi.org/10.1097/NPT.0b013e3181cf5c49.

45. Jacobs PL, Mahoney ET, Johnson B. Reliability of arm Wingate anaerobic testing in persons with com-

plete paraplegia. J Spinal Cord Med. 2003. https://doi.org/10.1080/10790268.2003.11753674.

46. Kapadia N, Zivanovic V, Verrier M, Popovic M. Toronto rehabilitation institute-hand function test: assessment of gross motor function in individuals with spinal cord injury. Topics Spinal Cord Injury Rehabil. 2012. https://doi.org/10.1310/sci1802-167.

47. Kowalczewski J, Ravid E, Prochazka A. Fully-automated test of upper-extremity function. Proc Ann Int Conf IEEE Eng Med Biol Soc. 2011. https://doi.org/10.1109/IEMBS.2011.6091710.

48. Dahlgren A, Karlsson AK, Lundgren-Nilsson Å, Fridén J, Claesson L. Activity performance and upper extremity function in cervical spinal cord injury patients according to the Klein-Bell ADL scale. Spinal Cord. 2007. https://doi.org/10.1038/sj.sc.3101993.

49. Shin SY, Kim JY, Lee S, Lee J, Kim SJ, Kim C. Intentional movement performance ability (IMPA): a method for robot-aided quantitative assessment of motor function. IEEE Int Conf Rehabil Robotics. 2013. https://doi.org/10.1109/ICORR.2013.6650498.

50. Grasse KM, Hays SA, Rahebi KC, et al. A suite of automated tools to quantify hand and wrist motor function after cervical spinal cord injury. J Neuroeng Rehabil. 2019. https://doi.org/10.1186/s12984-019-0518-8.

51. Triolo RJ, Bevelheimer T, Eisenhower G, Wormser D. Inter-rater reliability of a clinical test of standing function. J Spinal Cord Med. 1995. https://doi.org/10.1080/10790268.1995.11719375.

Measuring Urological Aspects in Spinal Cord Injury

Giulia Grieco, Francescaroberta Panuccio,
Marina D'Angelo, and Maria Auxiliadora Marquez

1 Introduction

Spinal cord injury presents a grave event in a patient's life, with consequences that can be very long-term and far-reaching. The level of the injury along the spine determines the degree of disability experienced by the patient. One aspect of the patient's life that may be affected by SCI is bladder function, as coordinated lower urinary tract function depends on an intact neural axis. Bladder contractility and the occurrence of reflex contractions depend on an intact sacral spinal cord and its afferent and efferent connections. Generally, SCI results in absent sensation below the level of the lesion. Patients with upper motor neuron lesions can have a local reflex of bladder contraction, but this is often countered by high sphincter pressure caused by smooth and striated sphincter dyssynergia. Other complications include detrusor hyperreflexia or areflexia, or insufficiency, urinary incontinence following bladder overactivity, or dysuria, and chronic retention due to an areflexic bladder [1].

People with SCI show limited participation across many major life domains such as decreased employment, limited social role, family role, and limited access to recreational and leisure activities. One important factor responsible for this limitation is urinary incontinence [2]. For this reason, people with SCI have to learn and acquire the technique of catheterization. The clean intermittent self-catheterization (CISC) has become a commonly recommended procedure for patients with incomplete voiding, especially in the neurogenic population, thereby decreasing the incidence of urinary tract infections, high vesicle pressure, reflux, and renal failure. CISC has thus contributed to a decrease in the morbidity and mortality of these patients and improved their quality of life.

Clinicians have to know the most common tests and questionnaires about urological aspects in people with SCI to assess their problems and limits and the best incontinence management technique to guarantee their independence and acceptance over their condition.

The objective of this study is to describe and evaluate the assessment tools on urological aspects in people with SCI through a systematic review of cross-sectional studies.

G. Grieco · F. Panuccio (✉) · M. D'Angelo
R.O.M.A. Rehabilitation Outcome Measures
Assessment, Non-Profit Organization, Rome, Italy

M. Auxiliadora Marquez
Universidad Fernando Pessoa-Canarias,
Las Palmas, Spain

2 Materials and Methods

This study was conducted by a research group composed of medical doctors and health professionals from the "Sapienza" University of Rome and the "Rehabilitation & Outcome

Measure Assessment" (R.O.M.A.) association. In the last few years, the R.O.M.A. association has worked with several studies and validated several outcome measures in Italy for the SPI population [3–16].

This chapter describes all assessment tools on urological aspects resulted from a systematic review conducted on PubMed, Scopus, and Web of science. For specific methodology details, see chapter "Methodological Approach to Identifying Outcome Measures in Spinal Cord Injury." Eligibility criteria for considering studies for this chapter were validation studies and cross-cultural adaptation studies, studies about the urological aspects, studies about tests, questionnaires, and self-reported and performance-based outcome measures, studies with a population of people of SCI and population ≥18 years old. Study selection: The selection of studies was conducted in accordance with the 27-item PRISM Statement for Reporting Systematic Reviews [17]. For the data collection, the authors followed the recommendations from the COnsensus-based Standards to select the health Measurement Instruments (COSMIN) initiative [18]. The study quality and risk of bias were assessed using COSMIN Check List [19, 20].

3 Results

For this chapter, 36 papers were considered. The authors found 20 assessment tools that evaluate the urological area in persons with SCI. See Fig. 1 for a flow chart of the included reported studies.

3.1 Qualiveen

The Qualiveen is an extensive questionnaire specifically developed for urinary dysfunction due to neurological dysfunctions/diseases. It comprises 30 questions that assess the general and urinary quality of life in patients with neurological disabilities [1]. Costa et al. developed the Qualiveen questionnaire in 2000 for French-speaking SCI patients [1]. It was quickly translated and vali-

dated for the SCI population into Portuguese [21], German [22], Italian [23], Persian [24], and Polish [25]. Because of the similarity of urinary problems in patients with SCI and multiple sclerosis (MS), the Qualiveen questionnaire was validated and used for patients with MS. It has 30 articles focusing on four aspects of patients' lives: worrying about the frequency, frequency of operations, fears, and feelings. Each article is assigned a score from 1 to 4, which defines the degree of severity. There is also a Short-Form version, the SF–Qualiveen, validated in Dutch [26] and Polish [25]. Table 1 summarizes the papers' authors and languages and Table 2 shows the quality of the studies.

3.2 Intermittent Catheterization Difficulty Questionnaire (ICDQ)

In 2016, Guinet-Lacoste et al. constructed and validated ICDQ in France. ICDQ evaluates and quantifies patients' difficulties during CISC. ICDQ has 13 items that concern ease of catheter insertion and withdrawal, the presence of pain, limb spasticity, urethral sphincter spasms, and local urethral bleeding during catheterization. ICDQ also evaluates the frequency and intensity of these difficulties. The response options are arranged on a 4-point Likert type scale, with 0 indicating "none" and 3 indicating "very difficult" in terms of the use of the catheter. The ICDQ is a valid test for evaluating catheter use and of patients' difficulties during CISC [27]. It was validated in 2020 in Arabic (Tunisia) language [28]. Table 3 summarizes the papers' authors and languages and Table 4 shows the quality of the studies.

3.3 Intermittent Self Catheterization Questionnaire (ISC-Q)

Pinder et al. developed in France ISC-Q in 2012. ISC-Q evaluates aspects of quality of life specific to the needs of individuals performing

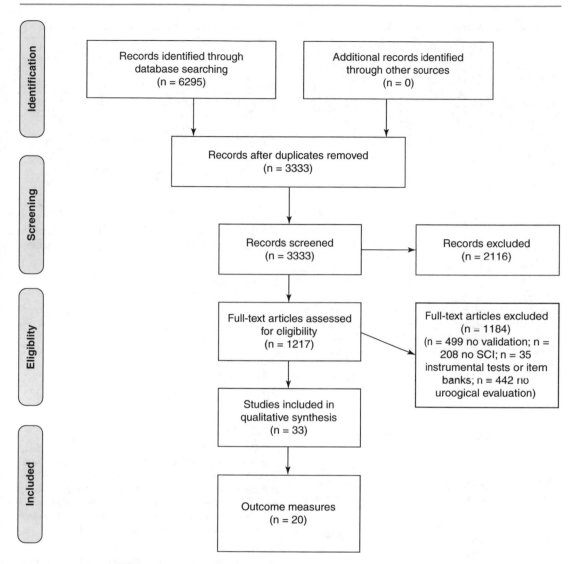

Fig. 1 Flow chart of included studies

Table 1 Characteristics of the studies validating Qualivee

	Authors	Language	n	Age mean (SD, range) year	Gender % Female
Qualivee	Costa, P. (2000)	English	20	35.8 (11.81)	4 (20)
	Pannek, J. (2007)	French	29	n.a.	n.a.
	D'Ancona, C.A.L. (2008)	French	281	41 (17–87)	59 (21)
	Bonniaud, V. (2011)	German	439	43.5	94 (21.4)
	Nikfallah, A. (2014)	Portuguese (Portugal)	33	n.a.	n.a.
	Przydacz, M. (2020)	Italian	128	43.5 ± 15.9	30 (23.4)
SF-Qualivee	Reuvers, S.H.M. (2017)	Dutch	57	53.2 (14.6)	20 (35.1)
	Przydacz, M. (2020)	Polish	126	n.a.	39 (31)

n number of participants of the study, *n.a.* not available

Table 2 Evaluation of quality and risk of bias

Authors	Items of the COSMIN Checklist									
	1	2	3	4	5	6	7	8	9	10
Costa, P. (2000)	+	+	+	−	−	+	−	−	−	−
Pannek, J.	?	+	−	+	+	+	−	−	−	−
D'Ancona, C.A.L. (2008)	?	+	−	+	−	+	−	+	+	−
Bonniaud, V. (2011)	?	+	−	+	+	+	+	+	+	+
Nikfallah, A. (2014)	?	+	−	+	+	+	−	+	+	−
Przydacz, M. (2020)	?	+	−	+	+	+	−	+	+	−
Reuvers, S.H.M. (2017)	?	+	−	+	+	+	−	+	+	−
Przydacz, M. (2020)	?	+	−	+	+	+	−	+	+	−

Item 1: PROM development, *Item 2* content validity, *Item 3*: structural validity, *Item 4*: internal consistency, *Item 5* cross-cultural validity/measurement invariance, *Item 6* reliability, *Item 7* measurement error, *Item 8* criterion validity, *Item 9* hypothesis testing for construct validity, *Item 10* responsiveness, + sufficient, − insufficient, ? indeterminate

Table 3 Characteristics of the studies validating ICDQ

Authors	Language	n	Age mean (SD, range) year	Gender % Female
Guinet-Lacoste, A. (2016)	French	6	49.5 (13)	3 (50)
Ghroubi, S. (2020)	Arabic (Tunisia)	30	40.6 (15.3)	7 (23.3)

n number of participants of the study, *n.a.* not available

Table 4 Evaluation of quality and risk of bias

Authors	Items of the COSMIN Checklist									
	1	2	3	4	5	6	7	8	9	10
Guinet-Lacoste, A. (2016)	+	+	−	+	−	+	−	−	−	−
Ghroubi, S. (2020)	?	+	−	+	−	+	−	−	−	−

Item 1 PROM development, *Item 2* content validity, *Item 3* structural validity, *Item 4* internal consistency, *Item 5* cross-cultural validity/measurement invariance, *Item 6* reliability, *Item 7* measurement error, *Item 8* criterion validity, *Item 9* hypothesis testing for construct validity, *Item 10* responsiveness, + sufficient, − insufficient, ? indeterminate

Table 5 Characteristics of the studies validating ISC-Q

Authors	Language	n	Age mean (SD, range) year	Gender % Female
Pinder, B. (2012)	English French German	306	46.1 (12.4)	104 (34.0)
Scivoletto, G. (2017)	Italian	217	43 (10.1)	75 (34.4)
Campos Ximenes, R.R. (2018)	Portuguese (Brazil)	30	35 (11.9)	11 (36.7)
Yesil, H. (2020)	Turkish	60	30.07 (12.6)	20 (33.3)

n number of participants of the study, *n.a.* not available

Table 6 Evaluation of quality and risk of bias

Authors	Item of COSMIN checklist									
	1	2	3	4	5	6	7	8	9	10
Pinder, B. (2012)	+	+	+	+	−	+	+	+	+	−
Scivoletto, G. (2017)	?	+	−	+	−	+	+	+	+	−
Campos Ximenes, R.R. (2018)	?	+	−	−	+	−	−	−	−	−
Yesil, H. (2020)	?	+	−	+	−	+	−	+	+	−

Item 1: PROM development, *Item 2* content validity, *Item 3* structural validity, *Item 4* internal consistency, *Item 5* cross-cultural validity/measurement invariance, *Item 6* reliability, *Item 7* measurement error, *Item 8* criterion validity, *Item 9* hypothesis testing for construct validity, *Item 10* responsiveness, + sufficient, − insufficient, ? indeterminate

Intermittent Self-Catheterization (ISC). ISC-Q is a self-reported outcome measure. The questionnaire contains four domains: ease of use, convenience, discreetness, and psychological well-being. The total 24 items are rated on a 5-point Likert-type scale (ranging from strongly agree to strongly disagree). The ISC-Q is psychometrically robust, with excellent internal consistency, adequate test-retest reliability, and good validity [29]. It was validated into Portuguese (Brazil) in 2018 [30], Italian in 2017 [31], and Turkish in 2020 [32]. Table 5 summarizes the papers' authors and languages and Table 6 shows the quality of the studies.

3.4 Neurogenic Bladder Symptom Score (NBSS)

Welk et al. developed the NBSS to assess lower urinary tract symptoms in patients with neurogenic lower urinary tract dysfunction (NLUTD). It was validated in English in 2013 [33, 34], Polish [35], and Portuguese (Brazil) in 2019. The NBSS is a comprehensive questionnaire for the assessment of lower urinary tract symptoms and evaluation of consequences of NLUTD. It can be applied both in men and women with congenital or acquired NLUTD. The scale evaluates three domains that best represent the spectrum of neurogenic bladder dysfunction: (1) Incontinence (eight questions), (2) storage and voiding (seven questions), and (3) consequences (seven questions). Two additional questions (first and last) are directed respectively to the method of bladder emptying and the impact of NLUTD on QoL and complete the 24 NBSS items. The NBSS has a possible score of 0–74, where the higher the score, the greater the severity of the symptoms. According to clinical utility, the authors validated each of the domains as an independent subscale, so that they can be used in combination or separately. The questionnaire can be self-administered [36]. In 2020, Welk et al. validated the short form [37]. Table 7 summarizes the papers' authors and languages and Table 8 shows the quality of the studies.

3.5 Multiple Sclerosis Intimacy and Sexuality Questionnaire (MSISQ)

The original version of MSISQ was in English and consisted of 19 items that have been translated and validated into Persian and Portuguese.

In 2018, Noordhoff et al. validated the Dutch version of MSISQ-15 for patients with SCI in 2018 [38]. The Italian version was also validated in an SCI population [13]. It evaluated symptoms of sexual dysfunction (SD) in MS patients, divided into three dimensions. Categorized as primary SD are symptoms resulting from neurologic changes that directly influence sexual function, such as impaired genital sensation, erectile dysfunction, orgasm dysfunction, decreased vaginal lubrication, and loss or reduction of libido. Secondary SD includes symptoms that arise from MS and indirectly influence sexual function, such as muscle tightness, spasticity, bladder and bowel function, pain, or discomfort in the body's nongenital areas. Tertiary SD refers to the psychological, emotional, social, and cultural aspects of MS that impact sexual function. Table 9 summarizes the papers' authors and languages and Table 10 shows the quality of the studies.

Table 8 Evaluation of quality and risk of bias

Authors	Item of COSMIN Check List									
	1	2	3	4	5	6	7	8	9	10
Costa, P. (2000)	+	+	−	−	−	−	−	−	−	−
Pannek, J. (2007)	?	+	+	−	−	−	−	+	+	−
D'Ancona, C.A.L. (2008)	?	+	−	+	+	+	−	+	+	−
Bonniaud, V. (2011)	?	+	−	+	−	−	−	+	+	−
Nikfallah, A. (2014)	+	+	−	−	−	−	−	−	−	−

Item 1 PROM development, *Item 2* content validity, *Item 3* structural validity, *Item 4* internal consistency, *Item 5* cross-cultural validity/measurement invariance, *Item 6* reliability, *Item 7* measurement error, *Item 8* criterion validity, *Item 9* hypothesis testing for construct validity, *Item 10* responsiveness, + sufficient, − insufficient, ? indeterminate

Table 7 Characteristics of the studies validating NBSS

	Authors	Language	n	Age mean (SD, range) year	Gender % Female
NBSS	Welk, B. (2013)	English	11	(30–70)	n.a.
	Welk, B. (2014)	English	80	(39–43)	n.a.
	Liidtke Cintra, L.K. (2019)	Portuguese (Brazil)	66	n.a.	n.a.
	Przydacz, M. (2020)	Polish	274	46.8	80 (73)
NBSS-SF	Welk, B. (2020)	English	1479	n.a.	592 (40)

n number of participants of the study, *n.a.* not available

Table 9 Characteristics of the studies validating MSISQ-15

Authors	Language	n	Age mean (SD, range) year	Gender % Female
Noordhoff, T. (2018)	Dutch	48	41.3 (11.9)	8 (16.3)
Monti, M. (2020)	Italian	65	40.4 (11.9)	18 (27.7)

n number of participants of the study, *n.a.* not available

Table 10 Evaluation of quality and risk of bias

Authors	Item of COSMIN Check List									
	1	2	3	4	5	6	7	8	9	10
Noordhoff, T. (2018)	?	+	−	+	+	+	−	+	+	−
Monti, M. (2020)	?	+	−	+	−	+	−	+	+	−

Item 1 PROM development, *Item 2* content validity, *Item 3,* structural validity, *Item 4* internal consistency, *Item 5* cross-cultural validity/measurement invariance, *Item 6* reliability, *Item 7* measurement error, *Item 8* criterion validity, *Item 9* hypothesis testing for construct validity, *Item 10* responsiveness, + sufficient,− insufficient, ? indeterminate

3.6 King's Health Questionnaire (KHQ)

The KHQ is designed to sensitively measure the effects of the symptoms of urinary incontinence on the quality of life, and it can be used to grade the improvement after treatment. It was validated for the SCI population in the Turkish language [39]. Table 11 summarizes the papers' authors and languages and Table 12 shows the quality of the studies.

3.7 Monitoring Efficacy of Neurogenic Bowel Dysfunction Treatment on Response (MENTOR)

MENTOR is a tool in three dimensions, the components of each are: (1) bowel/defecation symptoms through the NBD score; (2) special attention symptoms (SAS), which are the elements of comorbidity that may link to poor bowel man-

Table 11 Characteristics of the studies of scale, test, or questionnaire with less than two validations

	Authors	Language	n	Age mean (SD, range) year	Gender % Female
I-APS	Walia, P. (2016)	English	20	35.8 (11.81)	4 (20)
I-CAT	Guinet-Lacoste, A. (2016)	French	29	n.a.	n.a.
I-QOL	Schurch, B. (2007)	Fench	43	n.a.	n.a.
InCaSaQ	Guinet-Lacoste, A. (2014)	French	16	53 (14.4)	6 (37.5)
USQNB-IC	Tractenberg, R.E. (2018)	English	336	46.7 (13.64, 18−75)	101 (30.1)
Self-report questionnaire assessing the bodily and physiological sensations of orgasm	Dubray, S. (2016)	French (Canadian)	227	36.55 (18−73)	115 (50.7)
SAQ	Merghati-Khoei, E. (2015)	Persian	200	n.a.	54 (27)
PSDS-H	Paneri, V. (2014)	Hindi	30	n.a.	2 (6.7)
KHQ	Karapolat, K. (2018)	Turkish	50	34.4 (10.92)	26 (74.3)
MENTOR	Emmanuel, A. (2019)	English	241	49 (15, 20−86)	102 (42)
SAIQ	Brockway, J.A. (1980)	English	11	28.6 (22−64)	3 (27.3)
KCAASS	Kendall, M. (2003)	English	n.a.	n.a.	n.a.

n number of participants of the study, *n.a.* not available

Table 12 Evaluation of quality and risk of bias

Authors	Item of COSMIN Check List									
	1	2	3	4	5	6	7	8	9	10
Walia, P. (2016)	+	+	−	+	−	−	−	−	−	−
Guinet-Lacoste, A. (2016)	+	+	+	+	−	+	−	−	−	−
Schurch, B. (2007)	?	?	−	+	−	−	+	+	+	+
Guinet-Lacoste, A. (2014)	+	+	−	+	+	+	−	−	−	−
Tractenberg, R.E. (2018)	+	+	+	+	+	+	+	−	−	−
Dubray, S. (2016)	+	+	+	+	+	+	−	+	+	−
Merghati-Khoei, E. (2015)	?	+	+	+	+	+	−	−	−	−
Paneri, V. (2014)	+	+	−	+	−	+	−	−	−	−
Karapolat, K. (2018)	?	+	−	+	−	+	−	+	+	−
Emmanuel, A. (2019)	+	+	−	−	+	−	−	−	−	−
Brockway, J.A. (1980)	+	+	−	−	−	+	−	+	+	−
Kendall, M. (2003)	+	+	+	−	−	−	−	−	−	−

Item 1 PROM development, *Item 2* content validity, *Item 3* structural validity, *Item 4* internal consistency, *Item 5* cross-cultural validity/measurement invariance, *Item 6* reliability, *Item 7* measurement error, *Item 8* criterion validity, *Item 9* hypothesis testing for construct validity, *Item 10* responsiveness, + sufficient, − insufficient, ? indeterminate

agement; and (3) patient perception of satisfaction with their bowel function. It was validated in the English language [40]. Table 11 summarizes the papers' authors and languages and Table 12 shows the quality of the studies.

3.8 The Sexual Attitude and Information Questionnaire (SAIQ)

The revised SAIQ is comprised of four scales: (1) Sexual Information, (2) Sexual Behavior Acceptability, (3) Sexual Concerns, and (4) Nonsexual Concerns. In addition, there is a rating of overall concern about one's ability to have a satisfying sexual relationship. It was validated in 1980 in English [41]. Table 11 summarizes the papers' authors and languages and Table 12 shows the quality of the studies.

3.9 Incontinence–Activity Participation Scale (I-APS)

Walia et al., in 2016, developed I-APS in India for the English-speaking population. I-APS is specifically addressing the issues of activity limitation and participation restriction in SCI subjects with bladder problems. The I-PAS contains 16 items with 12 items in ADL and 4 items in occupation/education. The maximum score is 80, which indicates the maximum limitation during the activity. A score ≤16 indicates "No limitation." The I-APS is a valid comprehensive instrument that measures the activity limitation and participation restrictions due to SCI's bladder problems. Table 11 summarizes the papers' authors and languages and Table 12 shows the quality of the studies.

3.10 Intermittent Catheterization Acceptance Test (I-CAT)

In 2016, Guinet-Lacoste et al. constructed and validated I-CAT. Thanks to the nine neuro-rehabilitation and urology departments in French university hospitals, I-CAT was developed and validated primarily in French and English. I-CAT evaluates the psychological acceptance of Clean Intermittent Self Catheterization (CISC) in neurological and non-neurological populations. I-CAT contains 13 items and one global question. The first 5 items concern multiple fears about self-catheterization, the other 8 items concern self-esteem. The global ICAT score and dimension scores compute as the sum of the responses given for each item: (0 = strongly disagree, 1 = disagree, 2 = neither agree nor disagree, 3 = agree, 4 = strongly agree). The I-CAT is an acceptable, comprehensive, and reliable questionnaire for evaluating a patient's CISC acceptance [42]. Table 11 summarizes the papers' authors and languages and Table 12 shows the quality of the studies.

3.11 Lower Urinary Tract Symptoms Treatment Constraints Assessment (LUTS-TCA)

LUTS TCA, composed of 22 independent items, evaluates a broad sample of constraints due to urinary treatment. Thus social, psychological, environmental, and financial constraints, but also beliefs', doubts', and patients' feeling (with the proposed treatment) are necessary to be taken into account in the discussion of the proposition, the pursuit, and obviously, in the evaluation of the treatment. It was validated in French in 2018 [43]. Table 11 summarizes the papers' authors and languages and Table 12 shows the quality of the studies.

3.12 Incontinence Quality of Life (I-QOL)

Schurch et al., in 2007, worked in Zurich, Switzerland, and Paris, France, to assess the reliability, validity, responsiveness, and minimally important difference (MID) of I-QOL. I-QOL evaluates the quality of life for patients with urinary incontinence due to neurogenic detrusor overactivity. The I-QOL consists of 22 items evaluating concerns relating to incontinence. Subjects assign a value on a 5-point scale from 1 (extremely) to 5 (not at all) for each item. For all items, higher scores indicate better incontinence related QOL. The 22 items are divided into three subscales: avoidance and limiting behavior, psychosocial impact, and social embarrassment. I-QOL is a reliable, valid, and responsive measuring tool for incontinence-related QOL in neurogenic patients [44]. Table 11 summarizes the paper's authors and languages and Table 12 shows the quality of the studies.

3.13 Intermittent Catheterization Satisfaction Questionnaire (InCaSaQ)

In 2014, Guinet-Lacoste et al. worked in France to construct and validate a specific tool to evaluate patient satisfaction with intermittent self-catheterization in France. The InCaSaQ contains eight questions in four categories: (1) packaging (discretion and bulk of the package, hygiene and robustness, opening, and possible fixation of the catheter); (2) lubrification: means used for lubrification (spontaneous, gel, water); (3) the catheter itself: (holding, pushing and into the urinary meatus, ease of progression and insertion comfort, ease with which you could void); (4) after catheterization: the ease with which the catheter could be disposed of. Response options are ranked on a 4-point Likert-type scale, with 0 indicating "not at all satisfied" and 3 indicating "extreme satisfaction" with using a catheter [45]. Table 11 summarizes the papers' authors and languages and Table 12 shows the quality of the studies.

3.14 Knowledge, Comfort, Approach, and Attitudes toward Sexuality Scale (KCAASS)

This scale is composed of three subscales. The Knowledge subscale asked participants to indicate their current level of knowledge related to 14 topics on a scale from 1 to 4, where 1 was no knowledge, and 4 was excellent. The Comfort subscale followed the format used by Dunn et al. and asked participants to rate their comfort level on a scale from 1 to 4, where 1 was nil discomfort, and 4 was high discomfort in dealing with 26 different scenarios. The Attitude subscale provided participants with seven statements on SCI and sexuality. Participants were asked to indicate whether they agreed or disagreed with the statement on a scale from 1 to 4 where 1 was disagreed strongly, and 4 was agreed strongly. The participants are also asked to identify in a yes or no response format whether these statements would have elicited different responses if related to people who did not have an SCI [46]. Table 11 summarizes the papers' authors and languages and Table 12 shows the quality of the studies.

3.15 Self-Report Questionnaire Assessing the Bodily and Physiological Sensations of Orgasm

In 2016, Dubray et al. developed and validated a brief self-report measurement of orgasm by assessing bodily and physiologic sensations perceived during climax by able-bodied individuals in Montreal, Canada. Two versions of the questionnaire were created, with 3 items differing according to sex-specific responses (e.g., clitoral pulsation vs. penile contraction). Using a 5-point Likert-type scale of 0–4 (0¼ not at all, 1¼ somewhat, 2¼ moderately, 3¼ a lot, 4¼ extremely), participants are asked to rate the extent to which they experienced each of these sensations during ejaculation or orgasm. The questionnaire includes 28 bodily and physiologic sensations associated with orgasm and organized into four categories: cardiovascular, muscular, autonomic, and dysreflexic sensations [47]. Table 11 summarizes the papers' authors and languages and Table 12 shows the quality of the studies.

3.16 Sexual Adjustment Questionnaire (SAQ)

This instrument was developed by Merghati-Khoei et al. in 2013 to assess the spinal cord injured population's sexual health holistically, and it is validated in Iran. SAQ contains 11 items that assess the sexual adjustment in SCI. Each item was rated on a 5-point response (completely agree to completely disagree). Developed measures included social life, sexual adjustment, sexual activity, sexual fantasies, partnership satisfaction, and sexual performance [48]. Table 11 summarizes the papers' authors and languages and Table 12 shows the quality of the studies.

3.17 Perceived Sexual Distress Scale (PSDS)

The PSDS was developed in 2014 by Paneri et al. into Hindi for persons with spinal cord injury (SCI) [35]. PSDS-H is a behavior instrument, a 38-item questionnaire. The scale is of ordinal kind (5-point, frequency type, self- and interviewer-rated). Respondents have to answer each statement regarding how often the problem bothered them over the last 4 weeks. They are instructed to select one of five responses: "never, rarely, occasionally, frequently and always." Higher scores indicate a more frequently occurring behavior, whereas lower scores indicate that the behavior occurred less frequently. This tool is quite practical, taking 20–25 minutes to administer; and is applicable across a wide age range and for both genders. The measurable data gathered by the PSDS-H can help the rehabilitation team gain some insight regarding the effectiveness of interventions related to sexuality after SCI. The PSDS-H is a valid, self/interviewer-rated tool that can help inform the rehabilitation team about the level of an individual's perceived sexual distress post-SCI. It also provides an outcome measure to evaluate the efficacy of interventions related to sexuality post-injury. Table 11 summarizes the papers' authors and languages and Table 12 shows the quality of the studies.

3.18 Urinary Symptom Questionnaire for Individuals with Neuropathic Bladder Using Intermittent Catheterization (USQNB-IC)

Rochelle E. Tractenber validated the USQNB-IC in 2014. It is a Urinary Symptom Questionnaire (USQ) for individuals with neurogenic bladder (NB) in the United States. USQNB-IC focuses on upper and lower urinary tract signs and symptoms and contains 29 items. Each item is presented as a query about whether the respondent had experienced it during the past year (yes/no), with three additional required responses: average frequency (0–365); average severity (usually not at all severe; usually somewhat severe; usually severe; always very severe); and average impact on, or importance in, daily life (rarely affects my actions or decisions to go about my daily life; sometimes affects my actions or decisions to go about my daily life; usually affects my actions or decisions to go about my daily life; always affects my actions or decisions to go about my daily life) [36]. Table 11 summarizes the papers' authors and languages and Table 12 shows the quality of the studies.

4 Conclusions

This chapter reports all assessment tools described in the literature to assess urological aspects in people with SCI. This chapter's 20 tools found the resulting aspects: Intermittent Self-Catheterization, Neurogenic Bladder, and sexuality. The most common assessment tools include the Qualiveen which comprises 30 questions that assess the general and urinary quality of life; the Intermittent Self-Catheterization Questionnaire (ISC-Q) which is a self-reported outcome measure that contains domains such as ease of use, convenience, discreetness, and psychological well-being; the Neurogenic Bladder Symptom Score (NBSS) which assesses lower urinary tract symptoms in patients with neurogenic lower urinary tract dysfunction; and, the Multiple Sclerosis Intimacy and Sexuality Questionnaire (MSISQ) which evaluates symptoms of sexual dysfunction (SD) such as impaired genital sensation, reduction of libido, or symptoms indirectly influencing sexual function, such as spasticity, pain, or discomfort in nongenital areas of the body, or psychological, emotional, social, and cultural aspects that impact sexual function.

References

1. Costa P, Perrouin-Verbe B, Colvez A, et al. Quality of life in spinal cord injury patients with urinary difficulties: development and validation of Qualiveen. Eur Urol. 2001; https://doi.org/10.1159/000052421.
2. Walia P, Kaur J. Development and validation of Incontinence - Activity Participation Scale for spi-nal cord injury. Indian J Urol. 2017; https://doi.org/10.4103/0970-1591.203413.
3. Castelnuovo G, Giusti EM, Manzoni GM, et al. What is the role of the placebo effect for pain relief in neurorehabilitation? Clinical implications from the Italian consensus conference on pain in neurorehabilitation. Front Neurol. 2018; https://doi.org/10.3389/fneur.2018.00310.
4. Marquez MA, De Santis R, Ammendola V, et al. Cross-cultural adaptation and validation of the "spinal Cord Injury-Falls Concern Scale" in the Italian population. Spinal Cord. 2018;56(7):712–8. https://doi.org/10.1038/s41393-018-0070-6.
5. Dattoli S, Colucci M, Soave MG, et al. Evaluation of pelvis postural systems in spinal cord injury patients: Outcome research. J Spinal Cord Med. 2018;
6. Berardi A, Galeoto G, Guarino D, et al. Construct validity, test-retest reliability, and the ability to detect change of the Canadian Occupational Performance Measure in a spinal cord injury population. Spinal Cord Ser Cases. 2019; https://doi.org/10.1038/s41394-019-0196-6.
7. Ponti A, Berardi A, Galeoto G, Marchegiani L, Spandonaro C, Marquez MA. Quality of life, concern of falling and satisfaction of the sit-ski aid in sit-skiers with spinal cord injury: observational study. Spinal Cord Ser Cases. 2020; https://doi.org/10.1038/s41394-020-0257-x.
8. Panuccio F, Galeoto G, Marquez MA, et al. General Sleep Disturbance Scale (GSDS-IT) in people with spinal cord injury: a psychometric study. Spinal Cord. 2020; https://doi.org/10.1038/s41393-020-0500-0.
9. Monti M, Marquez MA, Berardi A, Tofani M, Valente D, Galeoto G. The Multiple Sclerosis Intimacy and Sexuality Questionnaire (MSISQ-15): validation of the Italian version for individuals with spinal cord injury. Spinal Cord. 2020; https://doi.org/10.1038/s41393-020-0469-8.
10. Galeoto G, Colucci M, Guarino D, et al. Exploring validity, reliability, and factor analysis of the Quebec user evaluation of satisfaction with assistive technology in an Italian population: a cross-sectional study. Occup Ther Heal Care. 2018; https://doi.org/10.1080/07380577.2018.1522682.
11. Colucci M, Tofani M, Trioschi D, Guarino D, Berardi A, Galeoto G. Reliability and validity of the Italian version of Quebec User Evaluation of Satisfaction with Assistive Technology 2.0 (QUEST-IT 2.0) with users of mobility assistive device. Disabil Rehabil Assist Technol. 2019; https://doi.org/10.1080/17483107.2019.1668975.
12. Berardi A, Galeoto G, Lucibello L, Panuccio F, Valente D, Tofani M. Athletes with disability' satisfaction with sport wheelchairs: an Italian cross sectional study. Disabil Rehabil Assist Technol. 2020; https://doi.org/10.1080/17483107.2020.1800114.
13. Berardi A, De Santis R, Tofani M, et al. The wheelchair use confidence scale: Italian translation, adaptation, and validation of the short form. Disabil Rehabil

Assist Technol. 2018;13(4):i. https://doi.org/10.1080/17483107.2017.1357053.

14. Anna B, Giovanni G, Marco T, et al. The validity of rasterstereography as a technological tool for the objectification of postural assessment in the clinical and educational fields: pilot study. In: Advances in Intelligent Systems and Computing; 2020. https://doi.org/10.1007/978-3-030-23884-1_8.

15. Panuccio F, Berardi A, Marquez MA, et al. Development of the Pregnancy and Motherhood Evaluation Questionnaire (PMEQ) for evaluating and measuring the impact of physical disability on pregnancy and the management of motherhood: a pilot study. Disabil Rehabil. 2020:1–7. https://doi.org/10.1080/09638288.2020.1802520.

16. Amedoro A, Berardi A, Conte A, et al. The effect of aquatic physical therapy on patients with multiple sclerosis: a systematic review and meta-analysis. Mult Scler Relat Disord. 2020; https://doi.org/10.1016/j.msard.2020.102022.

17. Moher D, Shamseer L, Clarke M, et al. Preferred reporting items for systematic review and meta-analysis protocols (PRISMA-P) 2015 statement. Rev Esp Nutr Hum Diet. 2016; https://doi.org/10.1186/2046-4053-4-1.

18. Mokkink LB, Terwee CB, Patrick DL, et al. The COSMIN study reached international consensus on taxonomy, terminology, and definitions of measurement properties for health-related patient-reported outcomes. J Clin Epidemiol. 2010; https://doi.org/10.1016/j.jclinepi.2010.02.006.

19. Terwee CB, Prinsen CAC, Chiarotto A, et al. COSMIN methodology for evaluating the content validity of patient-reported outcome measures: a Delphi study. Qual Life Res. 2018; https://doi.org/10.1007/s11136-018-1829-0.

20. Mokkink LB, de Vet HCW, Prinsen CAC, et al. COSMIN Risk of Bias checklist for systematic reviews of Patient-Reported Outcome Measures. Qual Life Res. 2018; https://doi.org/10.1007/s11136-017-1765-4.

21. D'Ancona CAL, Tamanini JT, Botega N, et al. Quality of life of neurogenic patients: Translation and validation of the Portuguese version of Qualiveen. Int Urol Nephrol. 2009; https://doi.org/10.1007/s11255-008-9402-3.

22. Pannek J, Märk R, Stöhrer M, Schurch B. Lebensqualität bei Deutschsprachigen patienten mit rückenmarkverletzungen und blasenfunktionsstörungen: Validierung der Deutschen adaption des Qualiveen®-fragebogens. Urol Ausgabe A. 2007; https://doi.org/10.1007/s00120-007-1425-3.

23. Bonniaud V, Bryant D, Pilati C, et al. Italian version of Qualiveen-30: Cultural adaptation of a neurogenic urinary disorder-specific instrument. Neurourol Urodyn. 2011; https://doi.org/10.1002/nau.20967.

24. Nikfallah A, Rezaali S, Mohammadi N, et al. Translation, cultural adaptation and validation of the qualiveen-30 questionnaire in persian for patients with spinal cord injury and multiple sclerosis. Low Urin Tract Symptoms. 2015;7(1):42–9.

25. Przydacz M, Kornelak P, Dudek P, Golabek T, Chlosta P. The urinary disorder-specific quality of life in patients after spinal cord injury: Polish translation, adaptation and validation of the Qualiveen and SF-Qualiveen. Spinal Cord. 2020; https://doi.org/10.1038/s41393-020-0499-2.

26. Reuvers SHM, Korfage IJ, Scheepe JR, T'Hoen LA, Sluis TAR, Blok BFM. The validation of the Dutch SF-Qualiveen, a questionnaire on urinary-specific quality of life, in spinal cord injury patients. BMC Urol. 2017; https://doi.org/10.1186/s12894-017-0280-9.

27. Guinet-Lacoste A, Jousse M, Tan E, Caillebot M, Le Breton F, Amarenco G. Intermittent catheterization difficulty questionnaire (ICDQ): a new tool for the evaluation of patient difficulties with clean intermittent self-catheterization. Neurourol Urodyn. 2016; https://doi.org/10.1002/nau.22686.

28. Ghroubi S, Chmak J, Borgi O, El Fani N, El Arem S, Elleuch MH. Translation and validation of the Intermittent Catheterisation Difficulty Questionnaire (ICDQ) in an Arabic population. Arab J Urol. 2020;18(1):22-26. https://doi.org/10.1080/2090598X.2019.1694762

29. Pinder B, Lloyd AJ, Elwick H, Denys P, Marley J, Bonniaud V. Development and psychometric validation of the intermittent self-catheterization questionnaire. Clin Ther. 2012; https://doi.org/10.1016/j.clinthera.2012.10.006.

30. Ximenes RRC, Carvalho ZM d F, Coutinho JFV, Braga DC d O, JMA C, RMB S. Cross-cultural adaptation and validation of the Intermittent SelfCatheterization Questionnaire. Rev da Rede Enferm do Nord. 2018; https://doi.org/10.15253/2175-6783.2018193315.

31. Scivoletto G, Musco S, De Nunzio C, et al. Minerva Urol e Nefrol. 2017; https://doi.org/10.23736/S0393-2249.16.02744-2.

32. Yeşil H, Akkoc Y, Yıldız N, et al. Reliability and validity of the Turkish version of the intermittent self-catheterization questionnaire in patients with spinal cord injury. Int Urol Nephrol. 2020;52(8):1437–42. https://doi.org/10.1007/s11255-020-02445-7.

33. Welk B, Morrow SA, Madarasz W, Potter P, Sequeira K. The conceptualization and development of a patient-reported neurogenic bladder symptom score. Res Reports Urol. 2013; https://doi.org/10.2147/RRU.S51020.

34. Welk B, Morrow S, Madarasz W, Baverstock R, Macnab J, Sequeira K. The Validity and reliability of the neurogenic bladder symptom score. J Urol. 2014; https://doi.org/10.1016/j.juro.2014.01.027.

35. Przydacz M, Dudek P, Golabek T, et al. Neurogenic bladder symptom score: Polish translation, adaptation and validation of urinary disorder-specific instrument for patients with neurogenic lower urinary tract dysfunction. Int J Clin Pract. 2020;74(10) https://doi.org/10.1111/ijcp.13582.

36. LKL C, JdeB J, Kawahara VI, et al. Cross-cultural adaptation and validation of the neurogenic bladder symptom score questionnaire for brazilian portu-

guese. Int Braz J Urol. 2019; https://doi.org/10.1590/S1677-5538.IBJU.2018.0335.

37. Welk B, Lenherr S, Elliott S, et al. The creation and validation of a short form of the Neurogenic Bladder Symptom Score. Neurourol Urodyn. 2020; https://doi.org/10.1002/nau.24336.

38. Noordhoff TC, Scheepe JR, 't Hoen LA, Sluis TAR, Blok BFM. The Multiple Sclerosis Intimacy and Sexuality Questionnaire (MSISQ-15): validation of the Dutch version in patients with multiple sclerosis and spinal cord injury. Neurourol Urodyn. 2018; https://doi.org/10.1002/nau.23804.

39. Karapolat H, Akkoç Y, Eyigör S, Tanıgör G. Bladder-related quality of life in people with neurological disorders: Reliability and validity of the Turkish version of the King's health questionnaire in people with spinal cord injury. Turkish J Urol. 2018; https://doi.org/10.5152/tud.2018.45556.

40. Emmanuel A, Krogh K, Kirshblum S, et al. Creation and validation of a new tool for the monitoring efficacy of neurogenic bowel dysfunction treatment on response: the MENTOR tool. Spinal Cord. 2020; https://doi.org/10.1038/s41393-020-0424-8.

41. Brockway JA, Steger JC. Sexual attitude and information questionnaire: reliability and validity in a spinal cord injured population. Sex Disabil. 1981; https://doi.org/10.1007/BF01102464.

42. Guinet-Lacoste A, Kerdraon J, Rousseau A, et al. Intermittent catheterization acceptance test (I-CAT): a tool to evaluate the global acceptance to practice clean intermittent self-catheterization. Neuerourol Urodyn. 2017; https://doi.org/10.1002/nau.23195.

43. Turmel N, Lévy P, Hentzen C, et al. Lower urinary tract symptoms treatment constraints assessment (LUTS-TCA): a new tool for a global evaluation of neurogenic bladder treatments. World J Urol. 2019;37(9):1917–25. https://doi.org/10.1007/s00345-018-2580-4.

44. Schurch B, Denys P, Kozma CM, Reese PR, Slaton T, Barron R. Reliability and validity of the incontinence quality of life questionnaire in patients with neurogenic urinary incontinence. Arch Phys Med Rehabil. 2007; https://doi.org/10.1016/j.apmr.2007.02.009.

45. Guinet-Lacoste A, Jousse M, Verollet D, et al. Validation of the InCaSaQ, a new tool for the evaluation of patient satisfaction with clean intermittent selfcatheterization. Ann Phys Rehabil Med. 2014; https://doi.org/10.1016/j.rehab.2014.02.007.

46. Kendall M, Booth S, Fronek P, Miller D, Geraghty T. The development of a scale to assess the training needs of professionals in providing sexuality rehabilitation following spinal cord injury. Sex Disabil. 2003; https://doi.org/10.1023/A:1023510925729.

47. Dubray S, Gérard M, Beaulieu-Prévost D, Courtois F. Validation of a self-report questionnaire assessing the bodily and physiological sensations of orgasm. J Sex Med. 2017; https://doi.org/10.1016/j.jsxm.2016.12.006.

48. Merghati-Khoei E, Maasoumi R, Rahdari F, et al. Psychometric properties of the Sexual Adjustment Questionnaire (SAQ) in the Iranian population with spinal cord injury. Spinal Cord. 2015; https://doi.org/10.1038/sc.2015.69.

Measuring Assistive Devices Management in Spinal Cord Injury

Anna Berardi, Giulia Grieco,
Francescaroberta Panuccio, Marina D'Angelo,
Maria Auxiliadora Marquez, and Marco Tofani

1   Introduction

An essential aspect of daily life for most persons with a spinal cord injury (SCI) is the dependence on a wheelchair [1]. For these persons, wheelchair use is conditional on achieving independent mobility. Independent mobility in the community for these patients requires proficient management of various wheelchair skills in order to deal with the varied and complex environmental barriers that an SCI patient experiences to participate in daily life activities [2].

Wheeled mobility is defined by the International Classification of Functioning, Disability, and Health (ICF) as "moving around using equipment: moving the whole body from place to place, on any surface or space, by using specific devices designed to facilitate moving or create other ways of moving around, such as moving down the street in a wheelchair or a walker." Participation is also an important rehabilitation outcome for persons with SCI. In the International Classification of Functioning, Disability, and Health, participation is defined as "involvement in life situations," including, for example, work and school, social relations, and community organizations. Participation restrictions are the problems that an individual may face in involvement in life situations [3].

Other problems that can limit an individual's independence include the frequent need for repairs, a high incidence of injuries because of tip-overs, and a high prevalence of upper limb overuse problems [4]. For these reasons, wheelchair training programs may help patients master the necessary skills for independence and mobility, allowing them to safely perform them [5].

It is important to search the most common tests that clinicians have to use to assess persons' mobility skills with SCI to guarantee independence during daily life. All rehabilitation clinicians must have access to measuring instruments that help them understand their client's difficulties when using a wheelchair. Therapists should have valid, reliable, and sensitive measuring tools at their disposal to objectively and systematically assess their patient's level of (Wheeled Mobility) WM performances, before, during, and after interventions [6]. Assessment tools of wheelchair user performance should make it possible to identify difficult environmental situations and the extent of the difficulties encountered by

A. Berardi (✉)
Department of Human Neurosciences, Sapienza University of Rome, Rome, Italy
e-mail: anna.berardi@uniroma1.it

G. Grieco · F. Panuccio · M. D'Angelo
R.O.M.A. Rehabilitation Outcome Measures Assessment, Non-Profit Organization, Rome, Italy

M. Auxiliadora Marquez
Universidad Fernando Pessoa-Canarias, Las Palmas, Spain

M. Tofani
Department of Neurorehabilitation and Robotics, Bambino Gesù Paediatric Hospital, Rome, Italy

wheelchair users. They should also guide interventions to improve users' performance so they can increase their autonomy and social participation. This study aims to describe and evaluate the assessment tools on assistive devices and wheelchairs in people with SCI through a systematic review of cross-sectional studies.

2   Materials and Methods

This study was conducted by a research group composed of medical doctors and health professionals from the "Sapienza" University of Rome and "Rehabilitation & Outcome Measure Assessment" (R.O.M.A.) association. R.O.M.A. association in the last few years has dealt with several studies and validation of many outcome measures in Italy for spinal cord injury population. This chapter describes all assessment tools regarding assistive devices and wheelchair resulting from a systematic review conducted on Pubmed, Scopus, and Web of science. For specific methodology details, see Chapter 3 "Methodological Approach to Identifying Outcome Measures in Spinal Cord Injury." Eligibility criteria for considering studies for this chapter were validation studies and cross-cultural adaptation studies, studies about the assistive devices and wheelchair, studies about tests, questionnaires, and self-reported and performance-based outcome measures with a population of people of SCI and population ≥ 18 years old. Study selection: the selection of studies was conducted in accordance with the 27-item PRISM Statement for Reporting Systematic Reviews [7]. For the data collection, the authors followed the recommendations from the COnsensus-based Standards for the selection of health Measurement Instruments (COSMIN) initiative [8]. Study quality and risk of bias were assessed using COSMIN Check List [9].

3   Results

For this chapter, 38 papers were considered. The authors found 22 assessment tools that evaluate the assistive devices management for persons with SCI. See Fig. 1 for a flow chart of included studies [9, 10].

3.1   Wheelchair Outcome Measure (WhOM)

Miller et al. developed the WhOM in English [11]. Three studies on French Canadian and English versions of WhOM have been conducted to investigate its measurement properties on various populations. In 2016, another WhOM version was developed in Farsi language for people with SCI [12]. The WhOM is the only tool to potentially measure participation across domains of the International Classification of Functioning, Disability, and Health (ICF). While many tools evaluate basic activities of daily living, the WhOM is specifically designed to capture the client's abilities in activities based on their needs. Asking questions such as "What activities in your home would you use your wheelchair to perform?" the WhOM measures the client's participation and engagement level. The WhOM is a client-centered wheelchair intervention measurement tool that allows clients to identify the activities they wish to complete when using their wheelchairs. It also provides clinicians with a tool to quantify outcomes of their interventions in a meaningful way to the client. The measure was designed through a mixed-method approach, including in-depth interviews of prescribers, individuals who use wheelchairs, and their associates. The WhOM has two parts, with the first part is designed to identify desired outcomes of participation in the home and community, and the second part

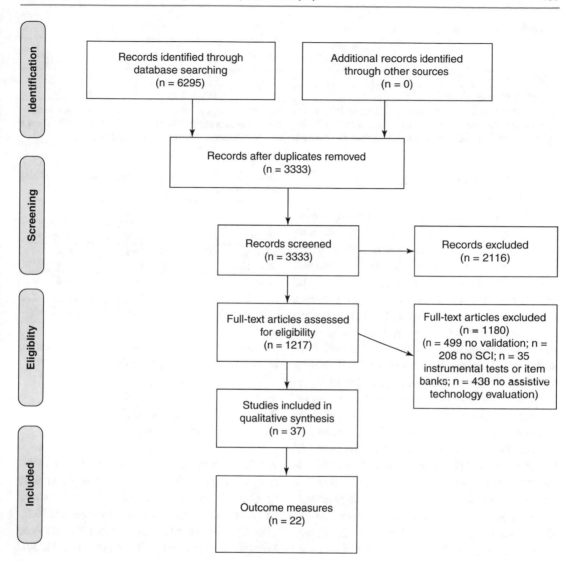

Fig. 1 Flow chart of included studies

Table 1 Characteristics of the studies validating WhoM

Authors	Language	n	Age mean (SD, range) year	Gender % Female
Miller et al. [11]	English	50	43.7 (10.7)	8 (16)
Alimohammad et al. [12]	Farsi	75	31.9 (9.5)	n.a.

n number of participants of the study, *n.a.* not available

is designed to address body structure and function. In the first part, clients rank the importance (Imp) of each identified goal on an 11-point scale that ranges 0–10 (0 5 no importance, 10 5 very important) and their level of satisfaction (Sat) with their performance (0 5 not satisfied at all, 10 5 extremely satisfied). The second part consists of three structured questions: the client's comfort while sitting in the wheelchair, satisfaction with body positioning in the wheelchair, and any experience of skin breakdown over the past month [12]. Table 1 summarizes the papers' authors and languages and Table 2 shows the quality of the studies.

Table 2 Evaluation of quality and risk of bias

Authors	Item of COSMIN checklist									
	1	2	3	4	5	6	7	8	9	10
Miller et al. [11]	?	+	−	−	−	+	+	+	+	−
Alimohammad et al. [12]	?	+	−	−	+	+	−	+	+	−

Item 1 PROM development, *Item 2* content validity, *Item 3* structural validity, *Item 4* internal consistency, *Item 5* cross-cultural validity/measurement invariance, *Item 6* reliability, *Item 7* measurement error, *Item 8* criterion validity, *Item 9* hypothesis testing for construct validity, *Item 10* responsiveness, + sufficient; − insufficient, ? indeterminate

3.2 Wheelchair Circuit

In 2002, Kilkens et al. [1, 13] assessed the validity and responsiveness of the Wheelchair Circuit, thanks to eight rehabilitation centers in the Netherlands. Wheelchair Circuit assesses manual wheelchair mobility in persons with SCI. The Wheelchair Circuit consists of eight different standardized items that are conditional on achieving independent wheelchair mobility. The items have a fixed sequence, on a hard and smooth floor surface or a motor-driven treadmill, all using a standard test wheelchair. During the circuit's performance, the ability to perform the test items, the performance time of the figure-of-eight shape and the 15-m sprint, and the peak heart rates during the 3% and 6% slope items on the treadmill were recorded. The main score of the Wheelchair Circuit is the ability score. All items that can be performed adequately and independently are assigned 1 point. There are 3 items that can also be scored as partially able (crossing a doorstep, mounting platform, transfer) and can then be assigned half a point. All points are summed to give an overall ability score. The ability score ranges from 0 to 8, is easy to calculate, and provides information about the subjects' ability to perform the various test items. There are two other scores that express subjects' performance on the Wheelchair Circuit: the performance time score and the physical strain score. The first is the sum of the performance times of the figure of-eight shape and the 15-m sprint. The second provides information on the physical strain induced by the performance of the 3% and 6% slope items. The two additional scores (performance time score, physical strain score) can provide more detailed information on wheelchair-related performance if desired [1]. Table 3 summarizes

Table 3 Characteristics of the studies validating Wheelchair Circuit

Authors	Language	n	Age mean (SD, range) year	Gender % Female
Kilkens et al. [13]	Dutch	27	n.a.	n.a.
Kilkens et al. [1]	Dutch	74	n.a.	n.a.

n number of participants of the study, *n.a.* not available

the papers' authors and languages and Table 4 shows the quality of the studies.

3.3 Adapted Manual Wheelchair Circuit (AMWC)

In 2011, Cowan et al. [14] worked to assess the test–retest reliability and discriminative validity of AMWC. The participants were individuals with SCI from centers in the United States and the Netherlands. This test was translated into Brazilian and Portuguese languages in 2018 [15]. The AMWC consists of 14 standard items considered essential to independent mobility in a manual wheelchair that must be performed in a fixed order with 2 min rests between each item: (1) a figure-eight shape; (2) a .012 m doorstep crossing; (3) a .04 m doorstep crossing; (4) a 10 m platform ascent; (5) a 15.0 m sprint; (6) a propelling over 4 m of artificial grass; (7) a 4 m 3% ramp ascent and descent; (8) a 4 m 6% ramp ascent and descent; (9) the opening and closing a door; (10) a 3 m 3% side slope; (11) holding a wheelie for 10 s; (12) propelling 3 m in a wheelie; (13) making a level transfer; (14) and, a 3-min overground wheeling test. All items performed correctly within the designated time are assigned 1 point, with half points available for each doorstep, platform, and transfer. The primary outcomes

Table 4 Evaluation of quality and risk of bias

Authors	Item of COSMIN checklist									
	1	2	3	4	5	6	7	8	9	10
Kilkens et al. [13]	−	−	−	−	−	+	−	−	−	−
Kilkens et al. [1]	+	+	−	−	+	−	−	+	+	+

Item 1 PROM development, *Item 2* content validity, *Item 3* structural validity, *Item 4* internal consistency, *Item 5* cross-cultural validity/measurement invariance, *Item 6* reliability, *Item 7* measurement error, *Item 8* criterion validity, *Item 9* hypothesis testing for construct validity, *Item 10* responsiveness, + sufficient, − insufficient, ? indeterminate

Table 5 Characteristics of the studies validating AMWC

Authors	Language	N	Age mean (SD, range) year	Gender % Female
Cowan et al. [14]	English Dutch	50	46 (13)	8 (16)
Ribeiro Neto et al. [15]	Portuguese (Brasil)	132	n.a.	132 (100)

N number of participants of the study, *n.a.* not available

Table 6 Evaluation of quality and risk of bias

Authors	Item of COSMIN checklist									
	1	2	3	4	5	6	7	8	9	10
Cowan et al. [14]	?	+	−	−	−	+	+	−	−	−
Ribeiro Neto et al. [15]	?	+	−	−	+	−	−	+	+	−

Item 1 PROM development, *Item 2* content validity, *Item 3* structural validity, *Item 4* internal consistency, *Item 5* cross-cultural validity/measurement invariance, *Item 6* reliability, *Item 7* measurement error, *Item 8* criterion validity, *Item 9* hypothesis testing for construct validity, *Item 10* responsiveness, + sufficient, − insufficient, ? indeterminate

are the sum ability score and the sum performance time. Secondary outcomes include individual task abilities and performances. Each item that is performed correctly and within the prescribed time is scored 1, with 0.5 values available for the doorstep, platform, and transfer items. The AMWC provides two results: (1) ability score, the sum of the scores of the 14 items; and (2) performance score, sum of time in seconds, of 3 items that should be performed in the shortest possible time [15]. Table 5 summarizes the papers' authors and languages and Table 6 shows the quality of the studies.

3.4 Self-Efficacy in Wheeled Mobility (SEWM)

Fliess-Douer et al. developed the new SEWM scale for perceived self-efficacy in manual wheeled mobility, based on the Generalized Perceived Self-efficacy Scale (GSE) and the spinal cord injury Exercise Self-Efficacy Scale (ESES). It was published in Belgium 2011. The SEWM scale was originally developed in English and translated into Dutch and Hebrew. In 2012, the perceived self-efficacy reliability and validity in the wheeled mobility scale were studied among elite athletes [16] with a spinal cord injury. Self-efficacy beliefs are defined as the confidence an individual has in performing a set of skills required to succeed in a specific task; perceiving self-efficacy is a major factor influencing behavior change, especially when complex skills need to be learned. Perceived self-efficacy influences, choice of activities, and motivational level and contributes to acquiring knowledge and refinement of new abilities. Perceived self-efficacy also influences individual judgments, effort, resilience, life choices, and perseverance in the face of difficulties. The initial item pool for the SEWM was based on the GSE and the ESES. The GSE consists of 10 items and assesses a general sense of perceived self-efficacy on a 4-point Likert-type scale (minimum score 0, maximum score 40). It aims to predict coping with daily difficulties and adaptation after experiencing all kinds of stressful life events. The ESES is a recently developed tool measuring SCI exercise self-efficacy in community-dwelling adults who participate in structured exercise programs and assess exercise self-efficacy beliefs in occasional and habitual exercisers with spinal cord injuries. Like the GSE, the ESES consists of 10 items assessed on a 4-point Likert-type scale (minimum score 0, maximum score 40). These scale items were reviewed and modified for presumed relevance to the SCI population and WM skills. Finally, 10 items were selected and constituted the 4-point Likert-type scale SEWM. The SEWM was reliable and valid in active spinal cord injury [17] and was validated in Hindi in 2015 [18]. Table 7 summarizes the authors and languages of the papers and Table 8 shows the quality of the studies.

3.5 Test of Wheeled Mobility (TOWM) and Wheelie Test

In 2012, Fliess-Douer et al. developed another two-wheeled mobility skill tests for manual wheelchair users with a spinal cord injury.

One is the TOWM, which is a comprehensive test based on daily wheeled mobility skills. The second is a short Wheelie test, aimed at fast and easy screening, developed following the realization that the ability to master a wheelie (balancing on the rear wheels), is perhaps the most important skill for the wheelchair user as wheelies permit access to areas and environments that would otherwise be inaccessible. TOWM consists of 30 standardized tasks that are conditional to mobility in persons with a spinal cord injury. The short wheelie test includes eight tasks related to the ability to perform a mature wheelie in challenging situations. The TOWM and the wheelie test tasks present different difficulty levels, hierarchically structured from the easiest to the most difficult. Including preparation and evaluation time, the estimated duration of the tests is 40 min. Both tests have the same four scoring methods: The ability score refers to all the tasks performed adequately and independently. Scores are assigned as 1 point if the participant completes the task successfully in the first trial; 0.5 points if they succeed on the second trial; 0 score for either a failure or avoiding trying. All scores are summed to give an overall ability score (TOWM min = 0, max = 30, wheelie test min = 0, max = 8). The ability score is easy to calculate and evaluate on the spot and provides information about the participant's ability to perform various test items. The TOWM and the wheelie tests are feasible and valid instruments for assessing manual wheelchair mobility in persons with spinal cord injury [19]. Table 9 summarizes the papers' authors and languages and Table 10 shows the quality of the studies.

Table 7 Characteristics of the studies validating SEWM

Authors	Language	n	Age mean (SD, range) year	Gender % Female
Fliess-Douer et al. [17]	English Dutch Hebrew French German	79	15.5 (6.63, 3–31)	30 (38)
Fliess-Douer et al. [17]	English Dutch Hebrew French German	47	38.2 (13.9, 18–75)	5 (11)
Swati et al. [18]	Hindi	n.a.	n.a.	n.a.

n number of participants of the study, *n.a.* not available

Table 8 Evaluation of quality and risk of bias

Authors	Item of COSMIN checklist									
	1	2	3	4	5	6	7	8	9	10
Fliess-Douer et al. [17]	?	+	−	+	+	−	−	+	+	−
Fliess-Douer et al. [17]	?	+	−	+	+	−	−	+	+	−
Swati et al. [18]	n.a.	n.a.	n.a.	n.a.	n.a.	n.a.	n.a.	n.a.	n.a.	n.a.

Item 1 PROM development, *Item 2* content validity, *Item 3* structural validity, *Item 4* internal consistency, *Item 5* cross-cultural validity/measurement invariance, *Item 6* reliability, *Item 7* measurement error, *Item 8* criterion validity, *Item 9* hypothesis testing for construct validity, *Item 10* responsiveness, + sufficient, − insufficient, ? indeterminate

3.6 Wheelchair Skills Test (WST)

Kirby et al. evaluated the practicality, safety, reliability, validity, and usefulness of a new WST in Halifax, Canada (2002) [20, 21]. Another version was published, until version 4.2, also in Spanish (2018) [2]. WST, version 1.0, consisted of 33 skills spanning the spectrum from skills as easy as applying the brakes to skills as difficult as performing a wheelie. Each skill is scored with a 3-point ordinal scale—0 for failure to complete the test criteria safely, 1 for partial completion (e.g., for the brake application skill, if the subject was successful on one side but not the other), and 2 for successful and safe completion [20]. Since its first publication, the WSP has evolved in different versions (e.g., 1.0, 2.4, 4.2). Version 4.2 offers the possibility of assessing manual and powered wheelchair users and scooter users as well. These modifications have been supported by clinical practice, research experience, feedback from users, and assessment of its measurement properties. The WST 4.2 for manual wheelchair users evaluates the subjects' capacity to perform specific skills in their specific wheelchairs and in a standardized way. This evaluation consists of 32 individual skills, in which the rater scores the success in accomplish-ing each skill in the following manner: "Pass" (score of 2), "Pass with difficulty" (score of 1), "Fail" (score of 0), "Not possible" (the wheelchair does not have the parts to allow this skill), and "Testing error" (testing of the skill was not sufficiently well observed to provide a score) [20]. Table 11 summarizes the papers' authors and languages and Table 12 shows the quality of the studies.

3.7 Quebec User Evaluation with Assistive Technology (Version 2.0) (QUEST 2.0)

The QUEST was developed to measure satisfaction on various types of assistive technology (AT) devices [22]. The instrument was designed based on the matching person and technology model. The first version of QUEST, QUEST 1.0, constituted 27 items that covered human, machine (or device) domains, and environment. Each item had a 5-point important scale and 5-point satisfaction scale [23]. The QUEST 2.0 has been established with the overall number of items reduced to 12, and the important scale removed [24]. QUEST's 12 items were divided into eight device and four services items with the same 5-point Likert-type

Table 9 Characteristics of the studies validating TOWM and Wheelie test

Authors	Language	n	Age Mean (SD, range) yr	Gender % Female
Fliess-Douer et al. [17]	Dutch	30	38.8 (8, 23–53)	n.a.
Fliess-Douer et al. [6]	Dutch	30	38.8 (8, 23–53)	n.a.

n number of participants of the study, *n.a.* not available

Table 11 Characteristics of the studies validating WST

Authors	Language	n	Age mean (SD, range) year	Gender % Female
Kirby et al. [20]	English	3	n.a.	n.a.
Kirby et al. [21]	English	117	n.a.	17 (24.5)
Passuni et al. [2]	Spanish	11	29.81 (12.18)	1 (9)

n number of participants of the study, *n.a.* not available

Table 10 Evaluation of quality and risk of bias

Authors	Item of COSMIN checklist									
	1	2	3	4	5	6	7	8	9	10
Fliess-Douer et al. [17]	+	+	−	−	+	+	+	−	−	−
Fliess-Douer et al. [6]	?	+	−	−	+	−	−	+	+	−

Item 1 PROM development, *Item 2* content validity, *Item 3* structural validity, *Item 4* internal consistency, *Item 5* crosscultural validity/measurement invariance, *Item 6* reliability, *Item 7* measurement error, *Item 8* criterion validity, *Item 9* hypothesis testing for construct validity, *Item 10* responsiveness, + sufficient, − insufficient, ? indeterminate

Table 12 Evaluation of quality and risk of bias

Authors	Item of COSMIN checklist									
	1	2	3	4	5	6	7	8	9	10
Kirby et al. [20]	+	+	−	−	+	+	−	−	−	−
Kirby et al. [21]	?	?	−	−	+	−	−	+	+	−
Passuni et al. [2]	?	+	−	−	+	+	−	−	−	−

Item 1 PROM development, *Item 2* content validity, *Item 3* structural validity, *Item 4* internal consistency, *Item 5* cross-cultural validity/measurement invariance, *Item 6* reliability, *Item 7* measurement error, *Item 8* criterion validity, *Item 9* hypothesis testing for construct validity, *Item 10* responsiveness, + sufficient, − insufficient, *?* indeterminate

Table 13 Characteristics of the studies validating QUEST 2.0

Authors	Language	n	Age mean (SD, range) year	Gender % Female
Chan and Chan [28]	Chinese	31	41.68 (11.17)	6 (19.4)
Hwang et al. [27]	Korean	70	40.9 (11.2)	15 (21.4)

n number of participants of the study, *n.a.* not available

scale (ranging from 1 = not satisfactory at all to 5 = very satisfactory). It was recommended to compute the scores by averaging the device, services, and total scores. Toward the end, the respondent was asked to select the three most important items from a 12-satisfaction item checklist. Both self-administration and interview formats were also suggested to be appropriate depending on the user's ability to complete a questionnaire [24]. To date, it is validated in several languages and for several populations of wheelchair users (Demers, Weiss-Lambrou, et al., 2002) [25, 26]. In 2006 the Chinese and in 2015 in Korean [27] language of QUEST 2.0 was validated for an SCI population [28] Table 13 summarizes the papers' authors and languages and Table 14 shows the quality of the studies.

3.8 Wheelchair Use Confidence Scale (WheelCon)

The Wheelchair Use Confidence Scale (WheelCon) [29] is a measurement scale that assesses self-efficacy with manual wheelchair use in six conceptual areas, including (1) the physical environment (34 items); (2) activi-

ties performed (11 items); (3) knowledge and problem-solving (8 items); (4) advocacy (4 items); (5) social situations (7 items); and (6) emotions (1 item). In 2015, Sakakibara BM et al. performed a rush analysis on the English version to create a short version [30]. In the same year, Rushton BW et al. translated and validated the French (Canada) version [31] and in 2018 Berardi A et al. validated the Italian version [5]. WheelCon-M-short form is a 21-item self-report questionnaire designed to measure wheelchair confidence in two areas: managing the physical environment (13 items) and managing the social environment (8 items). Each item is scored using a 10-point Likert-type scale ranging from "0" (not confident) to "10" (completely confident). Table 15 summarizes the papers' authors and languages and Table 16 shows the quality of the studies.

3.9 Assistive Technology Device Predisposition Assessment (ATD-PA)

The ATD-PA inquiry into subjective consumer satisfaction with current achievements various functional areas and asks the consumer to characterize aspects of their functioning, temperament, lifestyle, and views of a particular assistive device. It was validated in English [32, 33]. The ATD PA-Device Form is a 12-item self-assessment questionnaire, where respondents report their satisfaction from using the assistive device. The tool in question is patient-reported. It was validated in the Greek language [34]. Table 17 summarizes the paper's authors and languages and Table 18 shows the quality of the studies.

Table 14 Evaluation of quality and risk of bias

Authors	Item of COSMIN checklist									
	1	2	3	4	5	6	7	8	9	10
Chan and Chan [28]	?	+	+	−	+	−	−	+	+	−
Hwang et al. [27]	?	+	−	−	−	+	−	+	+	−

Item 1 PROM development, *Item 2* content validity, *Item 3* structural validity, *Item 4* internal consistency, *Item 5* cross-cultural validity/measurement invariance, *Item 6* reliability, *Item 7* measurement error, *Item 8* criterion validity, *Item 9* hypothesis testing for construct validity, *Item 10* responsiveness, + sufficient, − insufficient, ? indeterminate

Table 15 Characteristics of the studies validating WheelCon

Authors	Language	n	Age mean (SD, range) year	Gender % Female
Rushton et al.[31]	French (Canada)	18	n.a.	n.a.
Rushton et al. [29]	English	50	n.a.	n.a.
Berardi et al. [5]	Italian	21	n.a.	n.a.

n number of participants of the study, *n.a.* not available

Table 16 Evaluation of quality and risk of bias

Authors	Item of COSMIN checklist									
	1	2	3	4	5	6	7	8	9	10
Rushton et al. [31]	?	+	−	+	+	−	−	−	−	−
Rushton et al. [29]	+	+	−	+	+	+	+	+	+	+
Berardi et al. [5]	?	+	−	+	−	+	−	+	+	−

Item 1 PROM development, *Item 2* content validity, *Item 3* structural validity, *Item 4* internal consistency, *Item 5* cross-cultural validity/measurement invariance, *Item 6* reliability, *Item 7* measurement error, *Item 8* criterion validity, *Item 9* hypothesis testing for construct validity, *Item 10* responsiveness, + sufficient, − insufficient, ? indeterminate

Table 17 Characteristics of the studies validating FIM, FIM-SF, and FIM-5-AML

Scale, test, or questionnaire	Authors	Language	n	Age mean (SD, range) year	Gender % Female
ATD PA	Scherer and Cushman [32]	English	20	51.1 (16.4)	10 (50)
	Scherer and Cushman [33]	English	20	51.05 (16.44)	10 (50)
ATD PA device form	Koumpouros et al. [34]	Greek	115	62.45 (19.29)	64 (55.65)

n number of participants of the study, *n.a.* not available

Table 18 Evaluation of quality and risk of bias

Authors	Item of COSMIN checklist									
	1	2	3	4	5	6	7	8	9	10
Scherer and Cushman [32]	?	?	−	−	−	−	−	+	+	−
Scherer and Cushman [33]	?	?	−	+	−	−	−	+	+	−
Koumpouros et al. [34]	?	+	−	−	−	+	−	+	+	−

Item 1 PROM development, *Item 2* content validity, *Item 3* structural validity, *Item 4* internal consistency, *Item 5* cross-cultural validity/measurement invariance, *Item 6* reliability, *Item 7* measurement error, *Item 8* criterion validity, *Item 9* hypothesis testing for construct validity, *Item 10* responsiveness, + sufficient, − insufficient, ? indeterminate

3.10 Manual Wheelchair Slalom Test (MWST)

In 2011, Gagnon et al., in Montreal, Canada, developed a test to evaluate the mobility and rapidly changes directions when people wheel [35]. MWST was performed on an unobstructed indoor smooth and leveled concrete corridor, along which a slalom trajectory (linear length, 18 m) was defined around seven heavy, bright-colored cones with flags mounted on a 1.5-m pole, aligned in a straight line and set 3 m, 2 m, and 1 m apart from one another. Before starting the timed MWST, participants were positioned so that the front caster wheels of their wheelchair pointed backward and aligned with the start line marked on the floor with bright-colored tape. The participants were also invited to place their hands, palms down, on their thighs (starting position). Then, participants were instructed to propel their wheelchair at a self-selected maximum velocity to complete the trajectory as fast as pos-

sible until they crossed the finish line without disturbing the cones. To familiarize themselves with the MWST, participants completed the trajectory once at a slow pace before starting the test. The main outcome measures are the time needed to complete the MWST expressed in seconds. The timed MWST is a safe, reliable, and accurate performance-based outcome measure administered easily and quickly in individuals with SCI who rely on a manually propelled wheelchair for mobility [35]. Table 19 summarizes the papers' authors and languages and Table 20 shows the quality of the studies.

3.11 Obstacle Course Assessment of Wheelchair User Performance (OCAWUP)

Routhier et al. [36] proposed the OCAWUP to know what the wheelchair user is or cannot do to evaluate wheelchair user performance in poten-

Table 19 Characteristics of the studies of scale, test, or questionnaire with less than two validations

Scale, test, or questionnaire	Authors	Language	N	Age mean (SD, range) year	Gender % Female
MWST	Gagnon et al. [35]	French (Canadian)	15	40.7 (12.6)	n.a.
OCAWUP	Routhier et al. [36]	French (Canadian)	6	n.a.	n.a.
WPT	Askari et al. [4]	English	5	n.a.	n.a.
WPTTreadmill	Gauthier et al. [37]	French (Canadian)	22	35.3 (14.9)	3 (14)
MWPT	Gagnon et al. [38]	French (Canadian)	14	15.5 (6.63, 3–31)	n.a.
WCQc	Rispin et al. [39]	English	35 (cli)	15 (43)	n.a.
WUSPI	Curtis et al. [40]	English	80	41.9 (11.3, 21–68)	3 (4)
WMT-Q	Toro et al. [41]	English	38 (cli) 55 (w.s.)	n.a.	n.a.
QEWS	Gollan et al. [42]	English	100	37 (25–52)	15 (15)
Functional tasks for persons who self-propel a manual wheelchair	May et al. [43]	English	20	(19–70)	20 (100)
eMAST) 1.0	Friesen et al. [44]	English	32		11 (34)

n number of participants of the study, *n.a.* not available, *cli* (clinicians), *w.s.* (wheelchair users)

Table 20 Evaluation of quality and risk of bias

Authors	Item of COSMIN checklist									
	1	2	3	4	5	6	7	8	9	10
Gagnon et al. [35]	+	+	−	−	−	+	+	−	−	−
Routhier et al. [36]	?	?	−	−	−	+	−	+	+	−
Askari et al. [4]	+	+	−	−	−	+	−	+	+	−
Gauthier et al. [37]	?	+	−	−	−	+	+	−	−	−
Gagnon et al. [38]	?	+	−	−	−	−	−	+	+	−
Rispin et al. [39]	+	+	−	+	−	+	−	−	−	−
Curtis et al. [40]	?	?	−	−	+	+	−	+	+	−
Toro et al. [41]	+	+	−	−	+	+	−	−	−	+
Gollan et al. [42]	+	+	−	+	+	+	−	+	+	−
May et al. [43]	+	+	−	−	−	+	−	+	+	−
Friesen et al. [44]	?	?	−	+	−	+	−	+	+	−

Item 1 PROM development, *Item 2* content validity, *Item 3* structural validity, *Item 4* internal consistency, *Item 5* cross-cultural validity/measurement invariance, *Item 6* reliability, *Item 7* measurement error, *Item 8* criterion validity, *Item 9* hypothesis testing for construct validity, *Item 10* responsiveness, + sufficient, − insufficient, ? indeterminate

tially difficult environmental situations. This test was made in Quebec, Canada, and the participants were recruited at the Institut de Readaptation en Deficience Physique de Quebec (IRDPQ). It is designed for all propulsion methods and all client groups. In fact, the test can be applied to individuals that use one of the following three propulsion methods: hands (TH), one hand and one foot (OHOF), or a motorized wheelchair (MW). The OCAWUP consists of ten obstacles divided into four environmental categories. (driving and maneuvering while avoiding vertical obstacles; getting over a doorstep or onto a sidewalk; moving on different surfaces; going up and down an incline). Two variables are used to evaluate wheelchair user performance on each obstacle: execution time (Time) and degree of ease (DE). The time variable is measured in seconds (accurate to within 0.1 s) from when the rater tells the participant to start the task (overcoming obstacles) until it is completed, that is, when the individual crosses the finish line. The DE variable refers to the degree of success or failure in executing the task. It is measured on a four-level scale: total success (three points), success with difficulty (two points), partial failure (one point), and complete failure (zero points). Each obstacle has a specific scoring scale that tells the rater what events or behaviors may occur when they negotiate the particular obstacle. The DEs obtained on each obstacle are added to give

the global score of ease (GSE), varying from 0 to 30 [36]. Table 19 summarizes the authors and languages of the papers and Table 20 shows the quality of the studies.

3.12 Wheelchair Propulsion Test (WPT)

Askari et al. worked to develop a new WPT that evaluates the wheelchair mobility of manual wheelchair users. During 2011 and 2012, it was presented in part to the Rehabilitation Engineering and Assistive Technology Society of North America, Toronto, Canada, the Canadian Association of Physical Medicine and Rehabilitation, Victoria, Canada, and the Rehabilitation Engineering and Assistive Technology Society of North America, Baltimore [4]. It was published in 2013. The wheelchair user has to wheel 10 m on a smooth level surface from a stationary start. Then is evaluated the direction of travel (forward or backward), the limbs contributing to propulsion, steering, or braking, the limb used for counting cycles, time (to the nearest second), number of cycles (in whole cycles completed), and whether proper propulsion techniques were used. For participants who used one hand to propel forward, a correct contact phase was defined as when each hand generally began its contact with the hand–rim behind the top dead center of the rear wheel and remained on the hand–

rim until ahead top dead center. A correct recovery phase was defined as when each hand generally returned to the hand–rim using a path that was primarily beneath the hand–rim. If using one foot for propulsion and going forward, a correct foot propulsion cycle was defined as when the participant generally made initial foot contact with the knee flexed <90 from full extension and finished with the knee flexed >90 (or the opposite if going backward). Data were collected by observation and a stopwatch. Comments were recorded. Derived measures were speed (meters per second), push frequency (cycles per second), and effectiveness (meters per cycle). WPT is rapid to administer and inexpensive, requires little or no equipment, exhibits good measurement properties, requires minimal training for the tester, requires minimal time to analyze the data, generates a report, and applies to different rehabilitation populations. WPT appears to be a simple and inexpensive test with good measurement properties that can be used for people who use hand/or foot propulsion [4]. Table 19 summarizes the papers' authors and languages and Table 20 shows the quality of the studies.

3.13　Treadmill-Based Wheelchair Propulsion Test (WPTTreadmill)

The WPTTreadmill was developed to assess the cardiorespiratory fitness of manual wheelchair users (MWUs). It was validated in Canada. During its task-specific incremental test, individuals propel their own manual wheelchair (MW) over a motorized treadmill set at a different speed and slope combinations. The exercise intensity was gradually increased every minute until exhaustion, by changing the slope or speed according to a standardized protocol. This test allows for an assessment of cardiorespiratory fitness during MW propulsion and closely replicates everyday activity of MWUs [37]. Table 19 summarizes the paper's authors and languages and Table 20 shows the quality of the studies.

3.14　Manual Wheelchair Propulsion Tests (MWPT)

In Canada, Gagnon et al. quantified and compared the responsiveness and concurrent validity of three performance-based manual wheelchair propulsion tests among manual wheelchair users with subacute spinal cord injury [38].

1. 20-m Propulsion test: During this test, participants are instructed to propel their wheelchair at both a self-selected natural velocity and at a self-selected maximal velocity from a specified start line until they cross a finish line set 20 m further down the corridor. The average time required to complete the two trials expressed in seconds is calculated.

2. Slalom test: Participants are instructed to propel their wheelchair at a self-selected maximum velocity along a slalom trajectory defined by seven cones aligned in a straight line and set 3 m, 2 m, and 1 m apart from one another. The average time required to complete the two MWPTSLALOM, expressed in seconds, was the main outcome measure. The MWPTSLALOM was found to be reliable and precise.

3. Six-minute propulsion test: Participants are instructed to propel their wheelchair along a figure of eight trajectories. While doing so, they have to propel toward a cone, turn around it, and come back to the center of the trajectory, where they have to rapidly stop, before repeating this sequence in the other direction. The sequence is repeated as often as possible at a self-selected maximum velocity during a 6-min propulsion period. Participants are informed of the remaining time at 2, 4, and 6 min, respectively. The total distance traveled, recorded to the nearest meter, is the main outcome measure. The MWPT6min was found to be highly reliable and precise [38]. Table 19 summarizes the papers' authors and languages and Table 20 shows the quality of the studies.

3.15 Wheelchair Components Questionnaire for Condition (WCQc)

Rispin and colleagues worked to develop a professional report questionnaire to provide data specifically on the maintenance condition of a wheelchair. It was published in 2017 in the United States and Canada. The WCQc consists of 17 questions regarding the condition of wheelchair components. The questionnaire includes eight domain-specific questions intended for use as a stand-alone questionnaire. These questions cover components found in virtually every wheelchair and include a final question asking for an overall rating. The remaining nine extended questions concern components which may not be present on all wheelchairs and these questions are intended to be used only to accompany the domain-related questions. Each question utilizes a visual analog scale and includes an opportunity for qualitative explanatory comment. Questions are brief and include colored emotions to improve understanding and completion. Grade interpretation letters akin to school grades anchor the visual analog scale, providing a broadly understood calibration intended to improve inter-rater reliability and the intuitive understanding of results. The WCQc could be broadly applied to provide reliable data on maintenance condition. Informal observation indicated the WCQc takes from 15 to 20 min to complete depending on how much time was spent recording comments [39]. Table 19 summarizes the papers' authors and languages and Table 20 shows the quality of the studies.

3.16 Wheelchair User's Shoulder Pain Index (WUSPI)

In 1995, Curtis et al. contributed to examine the reliability and validity of the WUSPI, an instrument that measures shoulder pain associated with the functional activities of wheelchair users. The 15 items of WUSPI assess shoulder pain during transfers, self-care, wheelchair mobility, and general activities. The instrument is scored using a visual analog scale, with a minimum score of zero and a maximum score of 10 for each of the 15 items. Individual item scores are summed for the total index score. Thus, the total score index can range from 0 to 150. The WUSPI shows high levels of reliability and internal consistency and concurrent validity with loss of shoulder range of motion. As a valid and reliable instrument, this tool may be useful to both clinicians and researchers in documenting baseline shoulder dysfunction and for periodic measurement in longitudinal studies of musculoskeletal complications in wheelchair users. The instrument is also appropriate as an outcome measure to prevent pain and loss of function in the wheelchair using population [40]. Table 19 summarizes the paper's authors and languages and Table 20 shows the quality of the studies.

3.17 Wheelchair Maintenance Training Questionnaire (WMT-Q)

In 2016, Toro et al. collaborated to develop a Wheelchair Maintenance Training Programme (WMTP) as a tool for clinicians to teach wheelchair users (and caregivers when applicable) in a group setting to perform basic maintenance at home in the United States and to develop a Wheelchair Maintenance Training Questionnaire (WMT-Q) to evaluate wheelchair maintenance knowledge in clinicians, manual, and power wheelchair users. The WMT-Q is an acceptable instrument to measure pre- and post-training maintenance knowledge. Three versions (clinicians, manual wheelchair users, and power wheelchair users) of a knowledge-based WMT-Q were developed to evaluate whether the training impacted the knowledge and self-reported frequency of wheelchair maintenance performance among clinicians and wheelchair users [41]. Table 19 summarizes the papers' authors and languages and Table 20 shows the quality of the studies.

3.18 Queensland Evaluation of Wheelchair Skills (QEWS)

Gollan et al. published in 2015, in Australia, QEWS. The QEWS is an assessment tool of wheelchair skills for individuals with SCI. The QEWS consists of 5 items. Each item is scored on a 6-point scale ranging from 0 to 5 with a score of 0 indicating poor performance and a score of 5 indicating good performance. The scores for each item are tallied to a total possible score of 25. The QEWS is a valid and reliable tool for measuring wheelchair skills in individuals with SCI. The QEWS is efficient and practical to administer and does not require specialized equipment [42]. Table 19 summarizes the authors and languages of the papers and Table 20 shows the quality of the studies.

3.19 Functional Tasks for Persons Who Self-Propel a Manual Wheelchair

In Canada 2003, May et al. developed four functional tasks relevant to wheelchair seating for persons who Self-Propel a Manual Wheelchair. Tasks involve: (1) Timed forward wheeling; (2) Forward vertical reach; (3) Ramp ascent (forward wheeling); (4) One-stroke push [43]. Table 19 summarizes the papers' authors and languages and Table 20 shows the quality of the studies.

3.20 Electronic Mobile Shower Commode Assessment Tool (eMAST) 1.0

The eMAST 1.0 was developed in St Lucia, Australia, to test usability during mobile shower commode (MSC) design, assessment, and specification [44]. The eMAST1.0 measures the usability of MSCs from the perspective of adults with SCI. It contains 26 questions in three sections. The first section contains ten questions on MSC features, rated on a five-point Likert-type scale from 1 (very dissatisfied) to 5 (very satisfied). The second section contains 11 items covering MSC performance across key activities. Items

are measured on a five-point Likert-type scale from 1 (strongly disagree) to 5 (strongly agree). The third section comprises questions on the age of the MSC frame and seat (in years), and 2 items for users to list three positive and three negative aspects of their MSC [44]. Table 19 summarizes the papers' authors and languages and Table 20 shows the quality of the studies.

4 Conclusions

This chapter reports all assessment tools described in the literature to assess Assistive Devices Management aspects in people with SCI. Among the 22 tools included in this chapter resulted that most scales evaluate self-efficacy, mobility, and skill and that they are mainly performance tests. The most common assessment tools are the Wheelchair Circuit, which assesses manual wheelchair mobility, the Wheelchair Skills Test (WST), which consisted of 33 skills spanning the spectrum from skills as easy as applying the brakes to skills as difficult as performing a wheelie, and the Wheelchair use Confidence Scale (WheelCon), which is a measurement scale that assesses self-efficacy with manual wheelchair use in a physical environment, knowledge and problem-solving, and advocacy.

References

1. Kilkens OJ, Dallmeijer AJ, De Witte LP, Van Der Woude LH, Post MW. The wheelchair circuit: construct validity and responsiveness of a test to assess manual wheelchair mobility in persons with spinal cord injury. Arch Phys Med Rehabil. 2004. https://doi.org/10.1016/j.apmr.2003.05.006.
2. Passuni D, Dalzotto EF, Gath C, et al. Reliability of the Spanish version of the wheelchair skills test 4.2 for manual wheelchair users with spinal cord injury. Disabil Rehabil Assist Technol. 2019. https://doi.org/10.1080/17483107.2018.1463404.
3. Organization WH. Towards a common language for functioning, disability and health. ICF; 2002.
4. Askari S, Kirby RL, Parker K, Thompson K, O'Neill J. Wheelchair propulsion test: development and measurement properties of a new test for manual wheelchair users. Arch Phys Med Rehabil. 2013. https://doi.org/10.1016/j.apmr.2013.03.002.

5. Berardi A, De Santis R, Tofani M, et al. The Wheelchair Use Confidence Scale: Italian translation, adaptation, and validation of the short form. Disabil Rehabil Assist Technol. 2018;13(4):i. https://doi.org/10.1080/17483107.2017.1357053.

6. Fliess-Douer O, Van Der Woude LHV, Vanlandewijck YC. Reliability of the test of wheeled mobility (TOWM) and the short wheelie test. Arch Phys Med Rehabil. 2013. https://doi.org/10.1016/j.apmr.2012.09.023.

7. Moher D, Shamseer L, Clarke M, et al. Preferred reporting items for systematic review and meta-analysis protocols (PRISMA-P) 2015 statement. Rev Esp Nutr Human Diet. 2016. https://doi.org/10.1186/2046-4053-4-1.

8. Mokkink LB, Terwee CB, Patrick DL, et al. The COSMIN study reached international consensus on taxonomy, terminology, and definitions of measurement properties for health-related patient-reported outcomes. J Clin Epidemiol. 2010. https://doi.org/10.1016/j.jclinepi.2010.02.006.

9. Mokkink LB, de Vet HCW, Prinsen CAC, et al. COSMIN risk of bias checklist for systematic reviews of patient-reported outcome measures. Qual Life Res. 2018. https://doi.org/10.1007/s11136-017-1765-4.

10. Terwee CB, Prinsen CAC, Chiarotto A, et al. COSMIN methodology for evaluating the content validity of patient-reported outcome measures: a Delphi study. Qual Life Res. 2018. https://doi.org/10.1007/s11136-018-1829-0.

11. Miller WC, Garden J, Mortenson WB. Measurement properties of the wheelchair outcome measure in individuals with spinal cord injury. Spinal Cord. 2011. https://doi.org/10.1038/sc.2011.45.

12. Alimohammad S, Parvaneh S, Ghahari S, Saberi H, Yekaninejad MS, Miller WC. Translation and validation of the Farsi version of the wheelchair outcome measure (WhOM-Farsi) in individuals with spinal cord injury. Disabil Health J. 2016. https://doi.org/10.1016/j.dhjo.2015.09.004.

13. Kilkens OJ, Post MW, Van der Woude LH, Dallmeijer AJ, Van den Heuvel WJ. The wheelchair circuit: reliability of a test to assess mobility in persons with spinal cord injuries. Arch Phys Med Rehabil. 2002. https://doi.org/10.1053/apmr.2002.36066.

14. Cowan RE, Nash MS, De Groot S, Van Der Woude LH. Adapted manual wheelchair circuit: test-retest reliability and discriminative validity in persons with spinal cord injury. Arch Phys Med Rehabil. 2011. https://doi.org/10.1016/j.apmr.2011.03.010.

15. Ribeiro Neto F, Costa RRG, Lopes ACG, Carregaro RL. Cross-cultural validation of a Brazilian version of the adapted manual wheelchair circuit (AMWC-Brazil). Physiother Theory Pract. 2019. https://doi.org/10.1080/09593985.2018.1458356.

16. Fliess-Douer O, Vanlandewijck YC, Van Der Woude LHV. Reliability and validity of perceived self-efficacy in wheeled mobility scale among elite wheelchair-dependent athletes with a spinal cord injury. Disabil Rehabil. 2013. https://doi.org/10.3109/09638288.2012.712198.

17. Fliess-Douer O, Van Der Woude LHV, Vanlandewijck YC. Development of a new scale for perceived self-efficacy in manual wheeled mobility: a pilot study. J Rehabil Med. 2011. https://doi.org/10.2340/16501977-0810.

18. Dash S, Aikat R, Khanna N. Hindi translation, cross-cultural adaptation and validation of the "self-efficacy in wheeled mobility" (SEWM) scale in wheelchair users with spinal cord injury. Indian J Physiother Occup Ther An Int J. 2015. https://doi.org/10.5958/0973-5674.2015.00090.8.

19. Fliess-Douer O, Van Der Woude LH, Vanlandewijck YC. Test of wheeled mobility (TOWM) and a short wheelie test: a feasibility and validity study. Clin Rehabil. 2013. https://doi.org/10.1177/0269215512469118.

20. Kirby RL, Swuste J, Dupuis DJ, MacLeod DA, Monroe R. The wheelchair skills test: a pilot study of a new outcome measure. Arch Phys Med Rehabil. 2002. https://doi.org/10.1053/apmr.2002.26823.

21. Kirby RL, Worobey LA, Cowan R, et al. Wheelchair skills capacity and performance of manual wheelchair users with spinal cord injury. Arch Phys Med Rehabil. 2016. https://doi.org/10.1016/j.apmr.2016.05.015.

22. Demers L, Weiss-Lambrou R, Demers L, Ska B. Development of the Quebec user evaluation of satisfaction with assistive technology (QUEST). Assist Technol. 1996. https://doi.org/10.1080/10400435.1996.10132268.

23. Galeoto G, Colucci M, Guarino D, et al. Exploring validity, reliability, and factor analysis of the Quebec user evaluation of satisfaction with assistive Technology in an Italian Population: a cross-sectional study. Occup Ther Heal Care. 2018. https://doi.org/10.1080/07380577.2018.1522682.

24. Demers L, Weiss-Lambrou R, Ska. The Quebec user evaluation of satisfaction with assistive technology (QUEST 2.0): an overview and recent progress. Technol Disabil. 2002. https://doi.org/10.1080/10400435.1996.10132268.

25. Colucci M, Tofani M, Trioschi D, Guarino D, Berardi A, Galeoto G. Reliability and validity of the Italian version of Quebec user evaluation of satisfaction with assistive technology 2.0 (QUEST-IT 2.0) with users of mobility assistive device. Disabil Rehabil Assist Technol. 2019. https://doi.org/10.1080/17483107.2019.1668975.

26. Berardi A, Galeoto G, Lucibello L, Panuccio F, Valente D, Tofani M. Athletes with disability' satisfaction with sport wheelchairs: an Italian cross sectional study. Disabil Rehabil Assist Technol. 2020. https://doi.org/10.1080/17483107.2020.1800114.

27. Hwang WJ, Hwang S, Chung Y. Test-retest reliability of the Quebec user evaluation of satisfaction with assistive technology 2.0-Korean version for individuals with spinal cord injury. J Phys Ther Sci. 2015. https://doi.org/10.1589/jpts.27.1291.

28. Chan SCC, Chan APS. The validity and applicability of the Chinese version of the Quebec user evaluation of satisfaction with assistive technology for people with spinal cord injury. Assist Technol. 2006. https://doi.org/10.1080/10400435.2006.10131904.

29. Rushton PW, Miller WC, Kirby RL, Janice J. Measure for the assessment of confidence with manual wheelchair use (wheelcon-m) version 2.1: Reliability and validity. J Rehabil Med. 2013. https://doi.org/10.2340/16501977-1069.

30. Sakakibara BM, Miller WC, Rushton PW. Rasch analyses of the wheelchair use confidence scale. Arch Phys Med Rehabil. 2015. https://doi.org/10.1016/j.apmr.2014.11.005.

31. Rushton PW, Routhier F, Miller WC, Auger C, Lavoie MP. French-Canadian translation of the WheelCon-M (WheelCon-M-F) and evaluation of its validity evidence using telephone administration. Disabil Rehabil. 2015. https://doi.org/10.3109/09638288.2014.941019.

32. Scherer MJ, Cushman LA. Predicting satisfaction with assistive technology for a sample of adults with new spinal cord injuries. Psychol Rep. 2000. https://doi.org/10.2466/pr0.2000.87.3.981.

33. Scherer MJ, Cushman LA. Measuring subjective quality of life following spinal cord injury: a validation study of the assistive technology device predisposition assessment. Disabil Rehabil. 2001. https://doi.org/10.1080/09638280010006665.

34. Koumpouros Y, Papageorgiou E, Karavasili A, Alexopoulou D. Translation and validation of the assistive technology device predisposition assessment in Greek in order to assess satisfaction with use of the selected assistive device. Disabil Rehabil Assist Technol. 2017. https://doi.org/10.3109/17483107.2016.1161088.

35. Gagnon D, Décary S, Charbonneau MF. The timed manual wheelchair slalom test: a reliable and accurate performance-based outcome measure for individuals with spinal cord injury. Arch Phys Med Rehabil. 2011. https://doi.org/10.1016/j.apmr.2011.02.005.

36. Routhier F, Desrosiers J, Vincent C, Nadeau S. Reliability and construct validity studies of an obstacle course assessment of wheelchair user performance. Int J Rehabil Res. 2005. https://doi.org/10.1097/00004356-200503000-00007.

37. Gauthier C, Arel J, Brosseau R, Hicks AL, Gagnon DH. Reliability and minimal detectable change of a new treadmill-based progressive workload incremental test to measure cardiorespiratory fitness in manual wheelchair users. J Spinal Cord Med. 2017; https://doi.org/10.1080/10790268.2017.1369213.

38. Gagnon DH, Roy A, Verrier MC, Duclos C, Craven BC, Nadeau S. Do performance-based wheelchair propulsion tests detect changes among manual wheelchair users with spinal cord injury during inpatient rehabilitation in Quebec? Arch Phys Med Rehabil. 2016. https://doi.org/10.1016/j.apmr.2016.02.018.

39. Rispin K, Dittmer M, McLean J, Wee J. Preliminary reliability and internal consistency of the wheelchair components questionnaire for condition. Disabil Rehabil Assist Technol. 2017. https://doi.org/10.1080/17483107.2016.1277793.

40. Curtis KA, Roach KE, Applegate EB, et al. Reliability and validity of the wheelchair user's shoulder pain index (WUSPI). Paraplegia. 1995. https://doi.org/10.1038/sc.1995.126.

41. Toro ML, Bird E, Oyster M, et al. Development of a wheelchair maintenance training programme and questionnaire for clinicians and wheelchair users. Disabil Rehabil Assist Technol. 2017. https://doi.org/10.1080/17483107.2016.1277792.

42. Gollan EJ, Harvey LA, Simmons J, Adams R, McPhail SM. Development, reliability and validity of the Queensland evaluation of wheelchair skills (QEWS). Spinal Cord. 2015. https://doi.org/10.1038/sc.2015.82.

43. May LA, Butt C, Minor L, Kolbinson K, Tulloch K. Measurement reliability of functional tasks for persons who self-propel a manual wheelchair. Arch Phys Med Rehabil. 2003. https://doi.org/10.1053/apmr.2003.50021.

44. Friesen EL, Theodoros D, Russell TG. An instrument to measure mobile shower commode usability: the eMAST 1.0. J Assist Technol. 2016. https://doi.org/10.1108/JAT-12-2015-0037.

Measuring Walking and Balance in Spinal Cord Injury

Giulia Grieco, Francescaroberta Panuccio, Marina D'Angelo, Annamaria Servadio, and Giovanni Galeoto

1 Introduction

Many patients with spinal cord injury (SCI) suffer an incomplete lesion (e.g., sensory and/or motor preservation below the lesion level). Depending on the severity of the incomplete lesion, most patients will have the potential to recover walking function. Walking recovery is one of the patients' main goals after a spinal cord lesion; indeed, walking rates as the most important goal for patients with incomplete lesions. Therefore, the recovery of ambulation has become the target for several pharmacological and rehabilitative approaches, and a precise evaluation of ambulation in SCI patients has become mandatory [1].

Balance is an ability that persons with SCI must recover in order to walk. After SCI diagnosis, the balance automatism may be affected. SCI individuals begin to adopt new patterns of postural control. The decrease of sitting balance and postural control cannot be fully compensated by non-postural muscles, which only reduces functional disability partially. Thus, it is challenging to perform the trunk and upper limbs movements due to a lack of adequate postural stability after SCI [2].

Impaired balance is one of the many consequences of spinal cord injury (SCI). A fear of falling is associated with decreased quality of life, depression, anxiety, reduced participation in mobility and daily living activities, and physical and mental decline [3].

Also, the ability to sit unsupported is an important skill for wheelchair users with SCI to increase independence [4]. For example, transfers to/from a bed, car, toilet, tub, and daily living activities that commonly involve transfers, such as dressing, bathing often done out of the wheelchair require a certain amount of trunk stability and balance.

To make the subjects with SCI independent in their daily living to the maximum possible extent, therapists provide them balance training and walking training. To draft an appropriate and specific treatment, operators and therapists should know the exact assessment tools to evaluate the ability and skills of the person with SCI.

The objective of this study is to describe and evaluate the assessment tools on walking and balance in people with SCI through a systematic review of cross-sectional studies.

G. Grieco · F. Panuccio · M. D'Angelo
R.O.M.A. Rehabilitation Outcome Measures
Assessment, Non-Profit Organization, Rome, Italy

A. Servadio
Tor Vergata University of Rome, Rome, Italy

G. Galeoto (✉)
Department of Human Neurosciences, Sapienza
University of Rome, Rome, Italy
e-mail: giovanni.galeoto@uniroma1.it

2 Materials and Methods

This study was conducted by a research group composed of medical doctors and health professionals from the "Sapienza" University of Rome and the "Rehabilitation & Outcome Measure Assessment" (R.O.M.A.) association. In the last few years, the R.O.M.A. association has worked with several studies and validations of outcome measures in Italy for the Spinal Cord Injury population [5–18].

This chapter describes assessment tools regarding walking and balance resulted from a systematic review conducted on PubMed, Scopus, and Web of science. For specific methodology details, see Chapter 3 "Methodological Approach to Identifying Outcome Measures in Spinal Cord Injury." Eligibility criteria for considering studies for this chapter were validation studies and cross-cultural adaptation studies, studies about the quality of life, studies about tests, questionnaires, and self-reported and performance-based outcome measures, studies with a population of people with SCI and population ≥18 years old. Study selection: selection of studies was conducted in accordance with the 27-item PRISM Statement for Reporting Systematic Reviews [19]. For the data collection, the authors followed the recommendations from the COnsensus-based Standards for the selection of health Measurement Instruments (COSMIN) initiative [20]. Study quality and risk of bias were assessed using COSMIN checklist [21, 22].

3 Results

For this chapter, 47 papers were considered. The authors found 38 assessment tools that evaluate the walking and balance area in persons with SCI. In Fig. 1, a flow chart of included studies is reported [21, 22]. The assessment tools are described subsequently.

3.1 Walking Index for Spinal Cord Injury (WISCI) and WISCI II

The WISCI was introduced by Ditunno et al. in 2000 [23]. WISCI was validated in English [23, 24], Korean [23], Portuguese (Brazil) [23], Italian [23, 25, 26], Danish [26], German [26]. WISCI is a functional capacity scale developed as a research tool in clinical trials to measure ambulation improvements in persons with spinal cord injury. WISCI evaluates the amount of physical assistance, braces, or devices required to walk at 10 m. Participants are progressed systematically through a validated sequence of capacity levels, incorporating devices, and personal assistance, to their maximum walking capacity. The WISCI II ranks levels according to the severity of underlying impairment rather than the need for physical assistance, walking aids or braces, etc. It was validated in English [27, 28] Dutch [29], and Italian [27, 30]. For WISCI I, a score from 1 to 19 is assigned. Level 1: "patient ambulates in parallel bars, with braces and physical assistance of two persons, less than 10 meters" to level 19: "patient ambulates with no devices, no braces, and no physical assistance, 10 meters." For the WISCI II, a score from 0 to 20 is assigned. Level 0: "patient is unable to stand and/or participate in walking" to level 20: "ambulates with no devices, with a brace and no assistance." Table 1 summarizes the papers' authors and languages and Table 2 shows the quality of the studies.

3.2 10-M Walk Test (10MWT)

The validity and reliability of 10MWT were studied in many countries. It was validated in the Italian [1, 27], Thai [31–33], Hindi [34], and Dutch [29, 35]. The test is usually used to assess mobility and walking in incomplete SCI. In 2018, the 10MWT was also studied with motor-complete spinal cord injury in India. In fact, Rini et al. verified the test–retest reliability of 10MWT

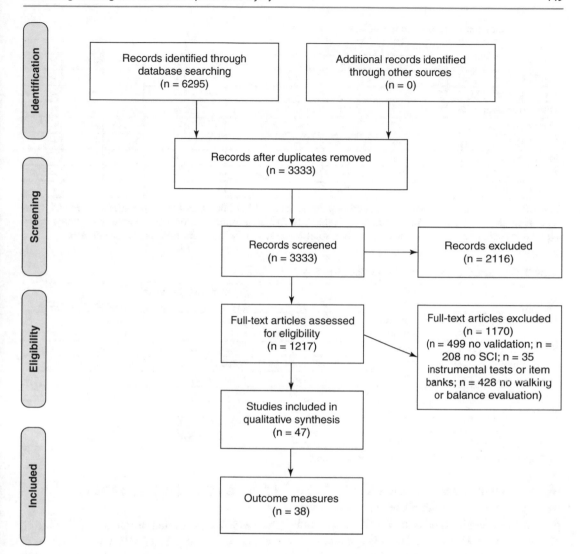

Fig. 1 Flow chart of included studies

Table 1 Characteristics of the studies validating WISCI and WISCI II

Scale, test, or questionnaire	Authors	Language	*n*	Age mean (SD, range) year	Gender % Female
WISCI	Ditunno Jr. et al. [23]	English Korean Portuguese (Brazil) Italian			
	Morganti et al. [25]	Italian	284	50.4 (19.3, 12–83)	100 (35)
	Ditunno Jr. et al. [24]	English	146	32 (16–69)	32 (22)
	Ditunno Jr. et al. [26]	Italian/Danish/ German	150		
WISCI II	Van Hedel et al. [29]	Dutch	22	45.59 (16.74)	4 (18.18)
	Marino et al. [27]	English Italian	26	46.4 (19.3)	10 (38.5)
	Burns et al. [28]	English	76	43.3 (13.8)	
	Scivoletto et al. [30]	Italian	33	44	5 (15.2)

n number of participants of the study, *n.a.* not available

Table 2 Evaluation of quality and risk of bias

| Authors | Item of COSMIN checklist | | | | | | | | | |
	1	2	3	4	5	6	7	8	9	10
Ditunno Jr. et al. [23]	+	+	−	−	−	−	−	−	−	−
Morganti et al. [25]	?	+	−	−	+	+	−	+	+	−
Ditunno Jr. et al. [24]	?	?	−	−	+	−	−	+	+	−
Ditunno Jr. et al. [26]	?	?	−	−	+	−	−	+	+	−
Van Hedel et al. [29]	?	?	−	−	−	−	−	+	+	+
Marino et al. [27]	?	+	−	−	−	+	−	+	+	−
Burns et al. [28]	?	−	−	−	−	+	−	+	+	−
Scivoletto et al. [30]	?	+	−	−	−	+	−	−	−	+

Item 1 PROM development, *Item 2* content validity, *Item 3* structural validity, *Item 4* internal consistency, *Item 5* cross-cultural validity/measurement invariance, *Item 6* reliability, *Item 7* measurement error, *Item 8* criterion validity, *Item 9* hypothesis testing for construct validity, *Item 10* responsiveness, + sufficient, − insufficient, ? indeterminate

Table 3 Characteristics of the studies validating 10MWT

Authors	Language	n	Age mean (SD, range) year	Gender % Female
Marino et al. [27]	English Italian	n.a.	n.a.	n.a.
Scivoletto et al. [1]	Italian	37	58.5 (19.67)	9 (24.3)
Poncumhak et al. [31]	Thai	66	30.9 (9.5)	20 (30.3)
Poncumhak et al. [32]	Thai	60	50.6 (9.68)	18 (30)
Amatachaya et al. [33]	Thai	94	n.a.	29 (30.8)
Rini et al. [34]	Hindi	25	n.a.	3 (12)
Van Hedel et al. [29]	Dutch	75	54 (29, 17–84)	4 (18.18)
Van Hedel et al. [35]	Dutch	22	45.59 (16.74)	4 (18.18)

n number of participants of the study, *n.a.* not available

with adults with a lower thoracic level of SCI who were trained to walk with bilateral solid polypropylene knee ankle–foot orthoses (KAFOs) and elbow crutches. During the 10MWT, people with SCI walk 10 m, and the time is measured using a stopwatch. Subjects walk with a preferred walking device at a comfortable pace along a 10-m walkway without any break to the end point. In order to minimize acceleration and deceleration effects, the test recorded the time required to cover the middle 4 m of the walkway. Then the time required over the 4 m was converted to walking speed. 10MWT is a quick and easily administered tool performed along a 10- to 14-m walkway. It is clinically interpretable and potentially modifiable, and hence the result is considered as a surrogate for the overall quality of gait and motor function. Table 3 summarizes the papers' authors and languages and Table 4 shows the quality of the studies.

3.3 6-Min Walk Test (6MWT)

The 6MWT was studied in Italian [1], Thai [33], and Dutch [29, 35]. The 6MWT is a measure of distance and represents the maximum distance walked in 6 min. Subjects are instructed to walk as far as possible in 6 min. The 6MWT indicates the global and integrated pulmonary, cardiovascular, and muscular systems; thus, they reflect the functional status for daily activities. However, the process of assessment is both area- and time-consuming (at least 6 min). Some studies measured the 6MWT by asking the subjects to walk up and down a walkway of a specific length, which allows the application of the test in a setting with limited area. Furthermore, the instruction and encouragement provided during the test have substantial impacts on the distance covered after 6 min; thus, the instruction should be rigorously standardized. Table 5 summarizes the

Table 4 Evaluation of quality and risk of bias

Authors	Item of COSMIN checklist									
	1	2	3	4	5	6	7	8	9	10
Marino et al. [27]	n.a.	n.a.	n.a.	n.a.	n.a.	n.a.	n.a.	n.a.	n.a.	n.a.
Scivoletto et al. [1]	?	+	−	−	−	+	−	−	−	−
Poncumhak et al. [31]	?	+	−	−	+	+	−	+	+	−
Poncumhak et al. [32]	?	?	−	−	−	+	−	+	+	−
Amatachaya et al. [33]	?	?	−	−	+	−	−	+	+	−
Rini et al. [34]	?	+	−	−	−	+	−	−	−	−
Van Hedel et al. [29]	?	+	−	−	−	+	−	+	+	−
Van Hedel et al. [35]	?	?	−	−	−	−	−	+	+	+

Item 1 PROM development, *Item 2* content validity, *Item 3* structural validity, *Item 4* internal consistency, *Item 5* cross-cultural validity/measurement invariance, *Item 6* reliability, *Item 7* measurement error, *Item 8* criterion validity, *Item 9* hypothesis testing for construct validity, *Item 10* responsiveness, + sufficient, − insufficient, ? indeterminate

Table 5 Characteristics of the studies validating 6MWT

Authors	Language	*n*	Age mean (SD, range) year	Gender % Female
Scivoletto et al. [1]	Italian	37	58.5 (19.67)	9 (24.3)
Amatachaya et al. [33]	Thai	94	n.a.	29 (30.8)
Van Hedel et al. [35]	Dutch	75	54 (29, 17–84)	30 (40)
Van Hedel et al. [29]	Dutch	22	45.59 (16.74)	4 (18.18)

n number of participants of the study, *n.a.* not available

Table 6 Evaluation of quality and risk of bias

Authors	Item of COSMIN checklist									
	1	2	3	4	5	6	7	8	9	10
Scivoletto et al. [1]	?	+	−	−	−	+	−	−	−	−
Amatachaya et al. [33]	?	?	−	−	+	−	−	+	+	−
Van Hedel et al. [35]	?	+	−	−	v	+	−	+	+	−
Van Hedel et al. [29]	?	?	−	−	−	−	−	+	+	+

Item 1 PROM development, *Item 2* content validity, *Item 3* structural validity, *Item 4* internal consistency, *Item 5* cross-cultural validity/measurement invariance, *Item 6* reliability, *Item 7* measurement error, *Item 8* criterion validity, *Item 9* hypothesis testing for construct validity, *Item 10* responsiveness, + sufficient, − insufficient, ? indeterminate

papers' authors and languages and Table 6 shows the quality of the studies.

3.4 Neuromuscular Recovery Scale (NRS)

The NRS is a measure specifically designed to assess recovery after SCI validated in English [36–39]. The NRS is an 11-item scale that compares sitting, standing, walking, and transfers relative to typical performance. The items focused on the trunk and lower extremity muscu-lature capacity to perform set tasks (Sit, Reverse Sit-up, Sit-up, Trunk extension, Sit-to-stand, Stand, Walking, Stand retraining, Stand adaptability, Step retraining, Step adaptability). The items represent a hierarchy of performance. The expectation that sitting and trunk-related items will be the "easiest" items and standing, and stepping items will be the "hardest" items. The time to complete the NRS ranged from approximately 30–50 min, depending on the degree of neuromuscular capacity. Table 7 summarizes the papers' authors and languages and Table 8 shows the quality of the studies.

Table 7 Characteristics of the studies validating NRS

Authors	Language	n	Age mean (SD, range) year	Gender % Female
Behrman et al. [37]	English	94	43 (17)	20 (21)
Basso et al. [38]	English	12	43 (18)	3 (25)
Velozo et al. [36]	English	188	39.3 (18.79)	41 (22)
Behrman et al. [39]	English	69	36 (15, 18–77)	12 (17)

n number of participants of the study, *n.a.* not available

Table 8 Evaluation of quality and risk of bias

Authors	Item of COSMIN checklist									
	1	2	3	4	5	6	7	8	9	10
Behrman et al. [37]	+	+	–	–	+	–	–	+	+	–
Basso et al. [38]	?	?	–	–	–	+	–	v	–	–
Velozo et al. [36]	?	?	+	+	+	+	–	–	–	–
Behrman et al. [39]	?	?	–	–	–	+	–	–	–	–

Item 1 PROM development, *Item 2* content validity, *Item 3* structural validity, *Item 4* internal consistency, *Item 5* cross-cultural validity/measurement invariance, *Item 6* reliability, *Item 7* measurement error, *Item 8* criterion validity, *Item 9* hypothesis testing for construct validity, *Item 10* responsiveness, + sufficient, – insufficient, *?* indeterminate

Table 9 Characteristics of the studies validating Trunk Control Test

Authors	Language	n	Age mean (SD, range) year	Gender % Female
Quinzaños-Fresnedo et al. [40]	Spanish	90	32.2 (12.8)	26 (28.9)
Quinzaños-Fresnedo et al. [41]	Spanish	531	38.1 (14.9, 16–81)	n.a.

n number of participants of the study, *n.a.* not available

Table 10 Evaluation of quality and risk of bias

Authors	Item of COSMIN checklist									
	1	2	3	4	5	6	7	8	9	10
Quinzaños-Fresnedo et al. [40]	?	+	–	–	+	–	–	–	–	–
Quinzaños-Fresnedo et al. [41]	?	+	+	–	+	+	–	+	+	–

Item 1 PROM development, *Item 2* content validity, *Item 3* structural validity, *Item 4* internal consistency, *Item 5* cross-cultural validity/measurement invariance, *Item 6* reliability, *Item 7* measurement error, *Item 8* criterion validity, *Item 9* hypothesis

3.5 Trunk Control Test

The Trunk Control Test was validated by J. Quinzanos et al. in 2014, in Mèxico in the Spanish language [40, 41]. In the scale, the static control was assessed by three elements that evaluate the maintenance of the sitting posture for 10 s with variations in the posture of the lower limbs. The dynamic control was divided into two parts: in the first dynamic control evaluates four elements for maintaining posture during activities (flexion of the trunk in a sitting position, in decubitus, and rolling), in the second dynamic control focused on performing activities with the upper extremities, which includes six elements that evaluate the maintenance of the sitting posture while carrying out activities in different positions using the upper extremities. The minimum score is 0 when the patient cannot perform any activity, and the maximum is 24. The average time for carrying out the test is 8 min. Table 9 summarizes the papers' authors and languages and Table 10 shows the quality of the studies.

3.6 Berg Balance Scale (BBS)

Originally developed to assess balance capacities for geriatric and stroke populations, clinicians applied the BBS to various conditions, including SCI. The BBS is validated for the SCI population in Swiss [42], French (Canada) [43], and Norwegian [44]. The ladder consists of a test that lasts 15–20 min and includes a series of 14 simple tasks related to balance ranging from getting up from a sitting position to standing on one foot. The degree of success in achieving each task is assigned a score from zero (incapable) to four (independent), and the final measure is the sum of all the scores. Depending on the performance, each task is rated from 0 (unable to perform the task) to 4 points (best performance), with a total score ranging from 0 to 56 points. Table 11 summarizes the papers' authors and languages and Table 12 shows the quality of the studies.

3.7 Mini-BEST

The Mini-BESTest is validated for the SCI population in Norwegian [44] and English in 2019 [45]. It is a 14-item test targeting dynamic balance by assessing four subsystems influencing balance control: anticipatory postural adjustments, postural responses, sensory orientation, and balance during gait. Each item is scored on an ordinal scale ranging from 0 to 2 (0 = unable; 2 = normal), with a total score of 28 points. Both sides are tested for 2 items (stand on one leg and compensatory stepping correction in a lateral direction), but only the lower score is included in the sum score. Assistive devices are permitted during testing, but using such devices lowers a participant's scores by 1 point on each item. Table 13 summarizes the papers' authors and languages and Table 14 shows the quality of the studies.

Table 11 Characteristics of the studies validating BBS

Authors	Language	n	Age mean (SD, range) year	Gender % Female
Lemay and Nadeau [43]	French (Canada)	32	47.9 (12.8, 20–75)	7 (21.9)
Wirz et al. [42]	Swiss	42	49.3 (11.5, 24–65)	9 (21.4)
Jørgensen et al. [44]	Norwegian	46	54.5 (17, 20–83)	14 (20)

n number of participants of the study, *n.a.* not available

Table 12 Evaluation of quality and risk of bias

Authors	Item of COSMIN checklist									
	1	2	3	4	5	6	7	8	9	10
Lemay and Nadeau [43]	?	+	–	–	+	–	–	+	+	–
Wirz et al. [42]	?	+	–	–	–	–	–	+	+	–
Jørgensen et al. [44]	?	+	+	+	+	–	–	+	+	–

Item 1 PROM development, *Item 2* content validity, *Item 3* structural validity, *Item 4* internal consistency, *Item 5* cross-cultural validity/measurement invariance, *Item 6* reliability, *Item 7* measurement error, *Item 8* criterion validity, *Item 9* hypothesis testing for construct validity, *Item 10* responsiveness, + sufficient, – insufficient, ? indeterminate

Table 13 Characteristics of the studies validating Mini-BEST

Authors	Language	n	Age mean (SD, range) year	Gender % Female
Jørgensen et al. [44]	Norwegian	46	54.5 (17, 20–83)	6 (20)
Chan et al. [54]	English	21	56.8 (14)	14 (66.6)

n number of participants of the study, *n.a.* not available

Table 14 Evaluation of quality and risk of bias

Authors	Item of COSMIN checklist									
	1	2	3	4	5	6	7	8	9	10
Jørgensen et al. [44]	?	+	+	+	+	–	–	+	+	–
Chan et al. [54]	?	?	–	–	–	+	–	+	+	–

Item 1 PROM development, *Item 2* content validity, *Item 3* structural validity, *Item 4* internal consistency, *Item 5* cross-cultural validity/measurement invariance, *Item 6* reliability, *Item 7* measurement error, *Item 8* criterion validity, *Item 9* hypothesis testing for construct validity, *Item 10* responsiveness, + sufficient, – insufficient, ? indeterminate

Table 15 Characteristics of the studies validating SCI-FAP and SCI FAI

Scale, test, or questionnaire	Authors	Language	*n*	Age mean (SD, range) year	Gender % Female
SCI-FAI	Field-Fote et al. [46]	English	22	32.6 (12.5)	5 (22.7)
SCI-FAP	Musselman et al. [47]	English	32	47.6 (14.2, 20–81)	8 (25)
	Musselman and Yang. [48]	English	22	32.6 (12.5)	5 (22.7)

n number of participants of the study, *n.a.* not available

Table 16 Evaluation of quality and risk of bias

Authors	Item of COSMIN checklist									
	1	2	3	4	5	6	7	8	9	10
Field-Fote et al. [46]	+	+	–	–	–	+	–	+	+	–
Musselman et al. [47]	+	+	+	+	–	+	–	+	+	–
Musselman and Yang [48]	–	+	–	–	–	–	+	+	+	+

Item 1 PROM development, *Item 2* content validity, *Item 3* structural validity, *Item 4* internal consistency, *Item 5* cross-cultural validity/measurement invariance, *Item 6* reliability, *Item 7* measurement error, *Item 8* criterion validity, *Item 9* hypothesis testing for construct validity, *Item 10* responsiveness, + sufficient, – insufficient, ? indeterminate

3.8 Spinal Cord Injury Functional Ambulation Inventory (SCI-FAI)

Field-Fote et al. developed SCI-FAI in 2001 in the United States [46]. It is a gait assessment test specific for people with spinal cord injury. The SCI-FAI can only be used with patients with SCI who can walk independently with or without braces and aids. The evaluation components into three parameters: gait, aid, mobility. Pace assessment occurs during weight transfer, step width, pace and step height, foot contact, and step length. The maximum score is 20 points, 10 points for each of the left and right sides. Walking or balancing aids include a stick, walker, parallel bars with a maximum score 14 points. The mobility on foot is evaluated on the distance traveled on foot, speed, frequency. The subjects are asked how often they walk on a scale from 0 to 5 (0 = I don't walk 5 = walks regularly in the commu-

nity). Table 15 summarizes the papers' authors and languages and Table 16 shows the quality of the studies.

3.9 Spinal Cord Injury Functional Ambulation Profile (SCI-FAP)

SCI-FAP measures functional walking in individuals with incomplete SCI through a variety of timed walking-related tasks. Kristin Musselman et al. based on the Modified Emory Functional Ambulation Profile (mEFAP), developed the SCI-FAP, in Canada [47, 48]. SCI-FAP evaluates ambulatory performance in people walking at low speed (i.e., <0.5 m/s) but without manual assistance. The SCI-FAP score is based on the time taken by a participant to complete each activity at a comfortable pace. Maximum times have been set for each activity. It contains seven timed walking tasks. The maximum score is

2100. Lower scores indicate higher functioning and reflect less time and less assistance to complete a task. Table 15 summarizes the papers' authors and languages and Table 16 shows the quality of the studies.

3.10 Timed up and Go Test (TUGT)

Poncumhak et al. investigated reliability, discriminative ability, and concurrent validity of the Timed Up and Go Test (TUGT) using the Functional Independence Measure Locomotor (FIM-L) scores as a standard criterion. TUGT was validated in the Thai [31, 32] and Dutch [35] languages. It measures balance control during upright and walking activities. Subjects get up from an armrest chair, walk around a traffic cone located 3 m away from the chair, and return to sit down on the chair at a maximum and safe speed. During the test, subjects can use a preferred walking device. The test recorded the time taken from the word "Go" until the subject's back was against the chair's backrest. Table 17 summarizes

the papers' authors and languages and Table 18 shows the quality of the studies.

3.11 Five Times Sit-to-Stand Test (FTSST)

Poncumhak et al. investigated the reliability, discriminative ability, and concurrent validity of the Five Times Sit-To-Stand Test (FTSST), using the Functional Independence Measure Locomotor (FIM-L) scores as a standard criterion. It was validated in the Thai language [31, 32, 49, 50]. Subjects sit on an armless chair with their arms at their sides, back upright, hip flexion 90°, and feet flat on the floor at 10 cm behind the knees. They are then instructed to stand up with the hips and knees in full extension and sit down five times as quickly and as safely as possible without using the arms. The test recorded the time from the command "Go" until the subject's back touched the chair's backrest on the fifth repetition. Table 19 summarizes the paper's authors and languages and Table 20 shows the quality of the studies.

Table 17 Characteristics of the studies validating TUGT

Authors	Language	n	Age mean (SD, range) year	Gender % Female
Poncumhak et al. [31]	Thai	66	30.9 (9.5)	20 (30.3)
Poncumhak et al. [32]	Thai	60	50.6 (9.68)	18 (30)
Van Hedel et al. [35]	Dutch	75	54 (29, 17–84)	30 (40)

n number of participants of the study, *n.a.* not available

Table 18 Evaluation of quality and risk of bias

Authors	Item of COSMIN Check List									
	1	2	3	4	5	6	7	8	9	10
Poncumhak et al. [31]	?	+	–	–	+	+	–	+	+	–
Poncumhak et al. [32]	?	?	–	–	–	+	–	+	+	–
Van Hedel et al. [35]	?	+	–	–	–	+	–	+	+	–

Item 1 PROM development, *Item 2* content validity, *Item 3* structural validity, *Item 4* internal consistency, *Item 5* cross-cultural validity/measurement invariance, *Item 6* reliability, *Item 7* measurement error, *Item 8* criterion validity, *Item 9* hypothesis testing for construct validity, *Item 10* responsiveness, + sufficient, – insufficient, ? indeterminate

Table 19 Characteristics of the studies validating FTSST

Authors	Language	n	Age mean (SD, range) year	Gender % Female
Poncumhak et al. [31]	Thai	66	30.9 (9.5)	20 (30.3)
Poncumhak et al. [32]	Thai	60	50.6 (9.68)	18 (30)
Khuna et al. [49]	Thai	82	52 (14.2)	13 (16)
Khuna et al. [50]	Thai	56	51 (15.2)	12 (21)

n number of participants of the study, *n.a.* not available

Table 20 Evaluation of quality and risk of bias

Authors	Item of COSMIN checklist									
	1	2	3	4	5	6	7	8	9	10
Poncumhak et al. [31]	?	+	–	–	+	+	–	+	+	–
Poncumhak et al. [32]	?	?	–	–	–	+	–	+	+	–
Khuna et al. [49]	?	?	–	–	+	+	–	+	+	–
Khuna et al. [50]	?	?	–	–	+	–	–	–	–	–

Item 1 PROM development, *Item 2* content validity, *Item 3* structural validity, *Item 4* internal consistency, *Item 5* cross-cultural validity/measurement invariance, *Item 6* reliability, *Item 7* measurement error, *Item 8* criterion validity, *Item 9* hypothesis testing for construct validity, *Item 10* responsiveness, + sufficient, – insufficient, ? indeterminate

3.12 Locomotor Stages in Spinal Cord Injury (LOSSCI)

Validated in 2016 for the German population [51], the LOSSCI is a five-point scale that tests the ability to control the body's position to carry out isolated, goal-directed movements of the arms. LOSSCI II tests the ability to upright the trunk against gravity in prone position and to perform isolated, goal-directed movement with one arm. LOSSCI III tests locomotion from a prone position using either the arms or the arms and legs (creeping—stomach remains in contact with the ground). LOSSCI IV tests the ability to move the body forward either by crawling (support on the hands and knees—stomach not on the ground) or by a verticalized bipedal gait with support through the arms of a walking aid, such as crutches or a wheeled walker. Substantial arm function is mandatory in LOSSCI IV, and its presence is the main discriminating factor between this stage and the highest stage. LOSSCI V represents the ability to walk bipedally without walking aids and the ability to perform a one-legged stand (this is considered a higher skill important for walking up and down the stairs independently). LOSSCI provides a reliable and valid clinical tool to assess locomotor function in SCI. Locomotor function is reflected by a wide range of motor skills, not only bipedal walking as in most other assessments in SCI. Table 21 summarizes the papers' authors and languages and Table 22 shows the quality of the studies.

3.13 The 6-Min Push Test (6MPT)

The 6MPT is validated in the United States [52]. 6MPT is a well-known field-based assessment of oxygen consumption (V˙O2) and functional change. It was initially developed to assess exercise capacity and functional status in persons with cardiorespiratory disorders. It has become one of the most widely applied assessments of function and functional capacity. 6MPT is done in a moderately busy hallway of an academic research center, and individuals were tested in their wheelchair. The course was a 30-m loop, marked by two cones spaced 15 m apart (30-m loop) with 2.8 m on either end to allow for turning. Two 180 turns were required to complete one 30-m loop. Beyond space, the only required equipment is a timer, a lap counter (or pen and paper), and pylons to mark the loop's ends. Finally, a method to quantify the distance traveled for any partially completed final lap is needed. The following testing order was used for each 6MPT: a 2-min self-selected slow velocity practice test, a 20-min rest, followed by the 6MPT. The 2-min practice test was completed on a shortened loop (15 m) to allow for more turning practice. For the practice test, participants were instructed to propel at comfortable velocity as if they were pushing around a grocery store, turning in the direction of their choice. Distance traveled in 6 min (m) was computed by multiplying the number of completed laps by 15 m and adding the distance traveled in the last lap. Table 21 summarizes the paper's authors and languages and Table 22 shows the quality of the studies.

Table 21 Characteristics of the studies of Scale, test, or questionnaire with less than two validations

Scale, test, or questionnaire	Authors	Language	n	Age mean (SD, range) year	Gender % Female
LOSSCI	Maurer-Burkhard et al. [51]	German	65	44.9 (16)	21 (33)
6MPT	Cowan et al. [52]	English	38	n.a.	4 (15)
ABLE scale	Ardolino et al. [53]	English	104	38.6 (14.9)	25 (24)
CB&M	Chan et al. [54]	English	30	38.5 (15.3)	7 (23.3)
ABC SCALE	Shah et al. [3]	English	26	59.7 (18.9)	6 (23.1)
THORACIC–LUMBAR CONTROL SCALE	Pastre et al. [2]	Portuguese (Brazil)	22	33.64 (11.02)	2 (9.1)
FIST	Abou et al. [4]	English	26	39 (15, 20–72)	16 (61.5)
FIST-SCI	Palermo et al. [55]	English	38	39.7 (11.79)	4 (10.5)
TTT	Pernot et al. [56]	Dutch	20	47.6 (12.5)	7 (35)
SBM	Wadhwa and Aikat [57]	Hindi	n.a.	n.a.	n.a.
FR	Sprigle et al. [58]	English	20	n.a.	n.a.
RA	Sprigle et al. [58]	English	20	n.a.	n.a.
BR	Sprigle et al. [58]	English	20	n.a.	n.a.
Upper-body sway	Boswell-Ruys et al. [59]	English	30	35 (11, 18–66)	6 (20)
Maximal balance range	Boswell-Ruys et al. [59]	English	30	35 (11, 18–66)	6 (20)
Coordinated stability	Boswell-Ruys et al. [59]	English	30	35 (11, 18–66)	6 (20)
Alternating reach test	Boswell-Ruys et al. [59]	English	30	35 (11, 18–66)	6 (20)
Seated reach distance	Boswell-Ruys et al. [59]	English	30	35 (11, 18–66)	6 (20)
T-shirt test	Boswell-Ruys et al. [59]	English	30	35 (11, 18 66)	6 (20)
LOS	Gao et al. [60]	Chinese (Hong Kong)	9	n.a.	n.a.
SWS	Gao et al. [60]	Chinese (Hong Kong)	9	n.a.	n.a.
MAS	Jørgensen et al. [61]	Norwegian	48	48 (18–69)	11 (22.9)
SBS	Jørgensen et al. [61]	Norwegian	48	48 (18–69)	12 (22.9)
TIC	Altmann et al. [62]	Dutch	20	n.a.	n.a.
SWAT	Musselman et al. [63]	English	34	n.a.	n.a.
SBASCI	Singh et al. [64]	Hindi	120	30.6 (10.7)	24 (20)

n number of participants of the study, *n.a.* not available

3.14 Activity-Based Balance-Level Evaluation (ABLE) Scale

The ABLE scale was validated in the United States, consisting of 30 items, which tests balance in sitting, standing, and walking [53]. The ABLE scale comprises 30 elements, which test the balance in people with SCI. It is divided into three sub-stairs: sitting position, standing position, and walking. The ladder can be administered entirely, or each subscale can be administered and separated. The person can be given the option to perform each task twice, taking the higher of the two marks as valid. The Sitting balance is composed of various tasks: the patient is asked to sit on a chair without back support, without armrests, and with their feet resting on the floor. They are asked to flex their trunk forward and then to lean sideways, first on one side and then on the other; to take a cup placed on the ground; to sit in the chair as far forward as possible without using a backrest to move; to move from the chair to the wheelchair; and, to hold a ball with both hands as high as possible. For the Standing position, the participant is asked to stand and sit without the help of their arms; to maintain balance in an upright position with eyes closed and then with feet together; to maintain balance while the evaluator pushes him/her; to lean forward; to grab an object on the ground; to rotate the trunk; to turn 180°. For

Table 22 Evaluation of quality and risk of bias

Authors	Item of COSMIN checklist									
	1	2	3	4	5	6	7	8	9	10
Maurer-Burkhard et al. [51]	?	+	−	−	+	+	−	+	+	−
Cowan et al. [52]	?	+	−	−	−	+	−	+	+	−
Ardolino et al. [53]	+	+	+	−	+	−	−	+	+	−
Chan et al. [54]	?	−	−	+	+	−	−	+	+	−
Shah et al. [3]	?	+	−	−	+	+	−	+	+	−
Pastre et al. [2]	?	+	−	−	−	+	−	−	−	−
Abou et al. [4]	?	?	−	+	−	+	−	+	+	−
Palermo et al. [55]	+	+	+	+	−	−	+	−	−	−
Pernot et al. [56]	?	?	−	−	+	−	−	+	+	−
Wadhwa and Aikat [57]	+	+	−	−	+	−	−	−	−	−
Sprigle et al. [58]	+	+	−	−	+	+	−	+	+	−
Sprigle et al. [58]	+	+	−	−	+	+	−	+	+	−
Sprigle et al. [58]	+	+	−	−	+	+	−	+	+	−
Boswell-Ruys et al. [59]	?	?	−	−	−	+	−	+	+	−
Boswell-Ruys et al. [59]	?	?	−	−	−	+	−	+	+	−
Boswell-Ruys et al. [59]	?	?	−	−	−	+	−	+	+	−
Boswell-Ruys et al. [59]	?	?	−	−	−	+	−	+	+	−
Boswell-Ruys et al. [59]	?	?	−	−	−	+	−	+	+	−
Boswell-Ruys et al. [59]	?	?	−	−	−	+	−	+	+	−
Gao et al. [60]	+	+	−	−	−	+	−	+	+	−
Gao et al. [60]	+	+	−	−	−	+	−	+	+	−
Jørgensen et al. [61]	+	+	−	−	−	+	−	+	+	−
Jørgensen et al. [61]	+	+	−	−	−	+	−	+	+	−
Altmann et al. [62]	?	?	−	−	−	+	−	−	−	−
Musselman et al. [63]	+	+	−	−	−	−	−	−	−	−
Singh et al. [64]	+	+	−	+	−	+	−	+	+	−

Item 1 PROM development, *Item 2* content validity, *Item 3* structural validity, *Item 4* internal consistency, *Item 5* cross-cultural validity/measurement invariance, *Item 6* reliability, *Item 7* measurement error, *Item 8* criterion validity, *Item 9* hypothesis testing for construct validity, *Item 10* responsiveness, + sufficient, − insufficient, ? indeterminate

walking, the participant is asked to walk on a flat surface; to turn their head 90° while walking; to change direction; to walk avoiding objects on the ground; to carry an object with two hands; to go down and upstairs; go up and down a ramp. Table 21 summarizes the papers' authors and languages and Table 22 shows the quality of the studies.

3.15 Community Balance and Mobility Scale (CB&M)

In 2017, K Chan et al. validated CB&M, individuals with incomplete spinal cord injury (iSCI), in Canada [54]. CB&M initially has been validated in traumatic brain injury and used in the following conditions: pediatric acquired brain injury, older adults, children, strokes, individuals with knee osteoarthritis, and hemophilia. It is completed using a set 8-m measured track, and a full flight of stairs is required. This test requires approximately 20–30 min to administer. The CB&M is comprised of 13 items, and 6 of the tasks are to be performed bilaterally. Scoring is based on a scale of 0–5, with a score of 0 reflecting complete inability to perform the task and a score of 5 reflecting the most successful completion of the task possible. CB&M scores range from 0 to 96, and items are scored upon completion of the first trial of an item. The only exceptions are if it is clear that the individual did not understand the task, in which case re-instruction and a second trial are allowed. Items are to be completed without using a gait aid, except for item 12, although orthoses are allowed to be worn. If the patient cannot complete the task or the therapist deems the task would not be safe for the patient to complete, a score of zero should be recorded. The items are: Unilateral Stance, Tandem Walking,180 Tandem Pivot, Lateral Foot Scooting, Hopping Forward, Crouch and Walk, Lateral Dodging, Walking and Looking, Running with Controlled Stop, Forward to Backward Walking, Walk, Look and Carry, Descending Stairs, Step-Ups × 1 Step. Table 21 summarizes the papers' authors and languages and Table 22 shows the quality of the studies.

3.16 Activities-Specific Balance Confidence (ABC) Scale

In 2017, Shah et al. evaluated the test–retest reliability, convergent validity, and discriminative validity of the ABC scale in individuals with incomplete spinal cord injury (iSCI). The scale was originally used in older adults, and has been used also with the SCI population in English [3]. Individuals rate how confident they are to maintain their balance while performing 16 standing and walking tasks, such as walking around the house and sweeping the floor. The majority of these tasks involved functional variations of walking, such as climbing up and down the stairs or walking on a ramp. The respondent rates his/her confidence in performing each activity without losing balance by selecting a value between 0% (no confidence) and 100% (completely confident). The ABC scale is a valid and reliable measure of balance confidence in community-dwelling, ambulatory individuals with chronic iSCI. It is an appropriate measure for clinicians and researchers to use with this sub-group of SCI. Table 21 summarizes the papers' authors and languages and Table 22 shows the quality of the studies.

3.17 Thoracic–Lumbar Control Scale

The Thoracic–Lumbar Control Scale was developed in the United States. In 2011, the Brazilian

Portuguese version of Thoracic–Lumbar Control Scale was published for people with SCI [2]. The scale measures trunk dysfunction level of patients' post-SCI. This instrument assesses ten tasks in the supine, prone, sitting, and standing positions and the patients' ability to perform activities in these positions. The 10 items to assess: trunk extension in prone, the elevation of the pelvis, trunk flexion in supine, trunk rotation, sit to supine, supine to sit, sitting posture, trunk extension in sitting, sitting balance, and standing balance. The tasks are scored according to the patients' ability to perform them with minimal effort, ranging 0–5 points. Scores decrease as the use of compensatory strategies increase. If the patient must change their position to perform the task, grades vary 3–0. In some cases, contractile activity is detected or assistance is given from the therapist in the greatest part of the movement, the task is graded 1. In the absence of movement and muscle contraction, or assistance given to perform the task fully, the patient score is 0. Table 21 summarizes the papers' authors and languages and Table 22 shows the quality of the studies.

3.18 Function in Sitting Test (FIST)

The FIST was originally developed to assess functional sitting balance among adults with stroke and validated for nonambulatory individuals with multiple sclerosis. In 2019, Abou et al. assessed the reliability and validity of the 14-item FIST among nonambulatory individuals with SCI in the United States [4]. The FIST quantifies static, proactive, reactive, and sensory integration of sitting balance systems during 14 everyday functional activities. It describes sitting balance at the activity level of the International Classification of Functioning, Disability, and Health (ICF). Activities included in the FIST comprise, but are not limited to, quiet sitting with eyes open and closed for 30 s, self-initiated activities, and reactive nudges. The FIST administration takes less than 10 min, is simple, at a low cost, and it requires minimal training. Each of the 14 items on the FIST is scored on a scale from 0 to 4. Participants score 0 when they cannot complete the sitting task even with assistance, 1 indicates that they need physical assistance, and 2 indicates that they use UE assistance to complete the task. Participants score 3 when they need verbal cues or more time and 4 when they complete the task independently. A total score ranging from 0 to 56 is obtained, where 0 equates to the inability to perform any of the sitting tasks, and 56 equates to the full ability to perform all of the tasks. In 2020, Palermo et al. developed a modified version specific for SCI (FIST-SCI) [55] Table 21 summarizes the papers' authors and languages, and Table 22 shows the quality of the studies.

3.19 Test–Table–Test (TTT)

TTT was introduced in 1985 for the first time and later adapted by The International Paralympic Committee (IPC) classifiers. In 2011, HFM Pernot et al. worked to assess the interrater reliability and validity of the TTT with which paralympic sports participants involved in Nordic sit-ski sports may be classified, in Dutch [56]. The TTT is a functional test testing sitting ability and trunk stability. During the TTT, the participant is strapped on a stable board with supporting cushions under the knees and feet. The participant is asked to accomplish four tasks: movements of 45° flexion, 45° backward inclination, lifting a ball above the head, and maximum trunk rotation are required. The score goes from 0 to 3 with "0" = no function; score "1" = weak function; score "2" = fair function; score "3" = normal function. Table 21 summarizes the papers' authors and languages and Table 22 shows the quality of the studies.

3.20 Sitting Balance Measure (SBM)

In 2015, G Wadhwa et al. developed SBM to assess the sitting balance of subjects with SCI, in India [57]. SBM is a performance-based scale that includes 16 items being scored by the examiner on an ordinal scale of 0–3. A score of "0" indicates minimum balance ability, and "3" indicates maximum balance ability. The equipment

required for the SBM administration is one hospital bed/plinth, one chair without armrests, a measuring tape, a stopwatch, and a footstool. SBM measures a number of components that are considered to be essential when measuring sitting balance. These include the ability to control sitting balance statically during quiet sitting (steady-state control), move oneself in sitting while maintaining seated postural control (proactive control), and maintain seated postural control during external perturbations (reactive control). Thus, SBM items have been designed to assess maximum components related to various aspects of sitting balance. The SBM provides a measure for rehabilitation professionals and other clinicians for documenting the sitting balance of the subjects with SCI objectively and comprehensively. Table 21 summarizes the papers' authors and languages and Table 22 shows the quality of the studies.

3.21 Functional Reach (FR)

In 2006, Stephen Sprigle et al. worked in Georgia and in Pennsylvania to develop simple postural stability tests that relate to the performance of activities of daily living (ADL) [58]. The FR measure is a unilateral forward reach. A sliding peg was mounted on a horizontal bar mounted to a tripod. The starting position of the peg was placed at the end of the flexed hand as an investigator passively extended the dominant UE with the subjects back against the backrest of the wheelchair. Subjects were instructed to reach as far forward as possible without losing balance. This distance was recorded as FR. The contralateral hand was placed on the umbilicus, negating any UE compensatory stabilization. Table 21 summarizes the papers' authors and languages and Table 22 shows the quality of the studies.

3.22 Reach Area (RA)

In 2006, Stephen Sprigle et al. worked in Georgia and in Pennsylvania to develop simple postural stability tests that relate to the performance of activities of daily living (ADL) [58]. RA is a unilateral task that measures the total area encompassed while reaching lateral, forward, and contralateral directions. A digital tape measure secured to a tripod was placed in front of the subject, far enough away to not interfere with a forward reach. A tape measure was secured to the subjects' wrists on their dominant UE, and the tape measure was zeroed out with the subjects sitting upright in the wheelchair, their back against the backrest of the wheelchair, and their reaching arm flexed forward 90°. Subjects were instructed to reach in a random order as far as possible without losing their balance in four directions: laterally (0°), diagonally to the ipsilateral side (45°), forward (90°), and across their bodies (1 35°), and the maximum distance reached was recorded. The area encompassed by these reaches was calculated using a trigonometric algorithm, and this area was normalized to the area defined by sweeping the arm through a range of 135° without any trunk rotation or flexion. During reach, subjects placed the contralateral hand on the umbilicus to negate UE compensatory stabilization. Three trials were recorded with the median entered into the analysis. RA reliability from a test chair has been previously reported as 0.902. Table 21 summarizes the papers' authors and languages and Table 22 shows the quality of the studies.

3.23   Bilateral Reach (BR)

In 2006, Stephen Sprigle et al. worked in Georgia and in Pennsylvania to develop simple postural stability tests that relate to the performance of activities of daily living (ADL) [58]. Bilateral reach (BR) measures the maximum forward distance that the subject can perform during a bilateral task without loss of balance. Subjects were asked to depress switches positioned in front of each arm with their distances normalized to arm length (measured from acromioclavicular joint to styloid process). Targets were placed at a minimum forward distance of 70% of arm's length and progressively moved outward by 10%. The task was to sequentially depress each of the switches for 5 s, moving from one switch to the next within 1 s. This 1-s time limit between switches ensured that the action was not a sequence of unilateral tasks allowing the subject to use excessive arm swing to prevent loss of balance. Results were the final normalized distance at which successful completion was achieved without loss of balance. BR has been found to have test–retest reliability of 0.905 when performed from a test chair. Table 21 summarizes the papers' authors and languages and Table 22 shows the quality of the studies.

3.24   Upper Body Sway

It was validated in the English language [59]. The test measured participants' abilities to sit unsupported and remain as still as possible for 30 s. The Lord sway meter, which was originally designed to measure total body sway while attempting to stand still, was used to measure upper body sway. It consisted of a 40-cm hinged rod that was fastened by a firm belt to the participants' chest at the level of the axilla and extended in a horizontal plane from the body. For this test, the rod was positioned to extend in the posterior direction. A ballpoint pen mounted vertically at the end of the rod recorded the movements of the upper body on a sheet of graph paper that was fixed to the top of a height-adjustable table. The tip of the pen was placed on the graph paper when the participants had commenced unsupported sitting. The resultant trace was measured in three components: maximal lateral displacement, maximal AP displacement, and the total length of the sway path (number of square mm traversed by the pen). Small displacement and length indicated better performance. The test was performed three times, and the mean was derived. Table 21 summarizes the papers' authors and languages and Table 22 shows the quality of the studies.

3.25 Maximal Balance Range

It was validated in the English language [59]. The test was adapted from a standing test. Participants were asked to lean as far forward as they could without falling and then return to their starting position. They were then asked to lean back as far as possible without falling and then return to their starting position. The maximal AP distance traversed was measured by using the sway meter described earlier. However, the rod was positioned to extend in the anterior plane for visual feedback. The pen attached to the end of the rod recorded the anterior and posterior movements of the participants on a sheet of graph paper fastened to the top of a height-adjustable table. The participants had two attempts at the test, with the longer distance taken as the test result. The score recorded was the maximal AP distance moved. A long distance was considered a better performance but corrected for body height (score % mean height/participants' height) measuring from the center of the sway meter strap to the top of the seat. Table 21 summarizes the papers' authors and languages and Table 22 shows the quality of the studies.

3.26 Coordinated Stability

It was validated in the English language [59]. The coordinated stability test was also adapted from a standing test. It measured participants' abilities to adjust their sitting posture in a steady and coordinated way when near or at the limits of their postural equilibrium. The sway meter was again attached to the participants, with the rod extending in the anterior plane for visual feedback. The participants were asked to adjust their posture by bending or rotating the upper body so that the sway meter pen tip followed and remained within a convoluted track. Two tracks were tested: the original version from the standing test (test A) and a simpler version (test B). Each track was marked on a piece of paper attached to the top of a height-adjustable table. In order to complete test A without errors, the sway meter pen had to remain within the track, which was 1.5-cm

wide, and the participant had to be capable of adjusting the position of the pen 25 cm laterally and 18 cm in the AP plane. Test B comprised a less convoluted track and required smaller displacements of the pen (14 cm lateral and 12 cm anteroposterior). In both test versions, a total error score was calculated by summing (1) the number of occasions the pen failed to stay within the path (1 error point), (2) the number of track corners cut (3 error points), and (3) the number of times the participants used their hands for support (5 points). Participants attempted each test twice, with the lesser score (better performance) taken as the test result. Table 21 summarizes the papers' authors and languages and Table 22 shows the quality of the studies.

3.27 Alternating Reach Test

Validated in the English language [59], the alternating reach test measured participant abilities to tap a table eight times as fast as possible by using alternate arms upon each repetition. The test was similar to item 12 of the Berg Balance Scale. A table was positioned at the height of the participants' axilla with the closest edge an arm's length away. The participants were tested under two conditions: supported, with their nonmoving hand grasping their thigh, and unsupported, with their nonmoving hand beside their body (shoulder at $0°$ and elbow at $90°$ flexion). The time taken to perform the tests was recorded using a stopwatch. A short time indicated better performance. Table 21 summarizes the papers' authors and languages and Table 22 shows the quality of the studies.

3.28 Seated Reach Distance

It was validated in the English language [59]. The test measured the participants' abilities to reach in different directions as far as possible without falling. This test was similar to the one used in the stroke population. A large table was positioned with its closest edge in line with the greater trochanters of the participants and at the height of their iliac crests. A semicircle was cut out of the table to accommodate the participants' abdomens. The table was covered with a large paper sheet with 5 pre-drawn lines. The directions of the lines were (1) lateral right (3 o'clock), (2) lateral left (9 o'clock), (3) 45° right (1.30 o'clock), (4) 45° left (10.30 o'clock), and (5) forwards (12 o'clock). A marker pen was taped into the thumb web spaces of the participants' two hands. Without holding on for support, the participants were asked to reach sideways, as far as possible, with the right hand, to make a light mark across the lateral right line before returning to the starting position. The exercise was then performed with the left hand on the lateral left line. This was repeated for each direction; those on the right side of the body with the right hand and those on the left side of the body with the left hand. The greatest reach distance for each direction was measured from the point of confluence of the lines. Arm length was measured from the acromion process to the position of the pen in the thumb web space. The seated reach distance was calculated as a proportion of the length of the participants' arms (greatest reach distance/arm length); a high proportion indicated better performance. A perpendicular measure from the top of the seat to the acromion process was used to correct the score for body height (score % mean height/participants' height). Table 21 summarizes the papers' authors and languages and Table 22 shows the quality of the studies.

3.29 T-Shirt Test

The t-shirt test measures the time taken for participants to put on and take off a t-shirt [59]. The test was designed to be similar to that reported by Chen et al., except it was performed in a short sitting as previously described. A table was positioned with its closest edge aligned with the participants' knees and at the height of their iliac crests. A pullover t-shirt was spread out flat on the table face down. Standardized t-shirts were supplied and were one size larger than the participants would normally wear. No harness was worn during this test, but a research assistant was ready

to support the participants if they were at risk of falling. The participants were required to put on and take off the t-shirt, resting between each maneuver. The test was repeated twice, with the average times calculated for each component (on, off, and total time). Short times indicated better performance. Table 21 summarizes the papers' authors and languages and Table 22 shows the quality of the studies.

3.30 Balance Tests (LOS/SWS)

K.L. Gao et al. collaborated to develop a reliable and valid tool for measuring the dynamic sitting balance of wheelchair users with SC. They worked in Hong Kong in 2014 to develop limits of stability (LOS) and sequential weight shifting (SWS) [60]. The balance tests measure participants' volitional weight shifting in multiple directions within their base of support. Their mobility scores on the Spinal Cord Independence Measure III (SCIM III) correlated with the balance test results. The LOS results showed moderate to excellent test-retest reliability for both the wheelchair and the unsupported sitting. The SWS results showed moderate to excellent reliability. The tests encompass temporal and spatial domains and involve both diagonal and orthogonal displacements. Fast reaction, maximal weight shifting, and accurate movement control are required for the functional aspects of daily living. Table 21 summarizes the papers' authors and languages and Table 22 shows the quality of the studies.

3.31 Sequential Weight Shifting

The sitting positions were the same as those used in the LOS test developed by Gao et al. in Hong Kong [60]. As soon as a target appeared, participants were asked to shift their COP to move the screen trace to the target quickly as possible without losing their balance. Twelve targets appeared sequentially. When each target was hit, it disappeared, and another appeared. The 12 targets appeared above, left, below, and right of the center. The distance from the center to each target was 75% of that patient's maximal excursion, as determined in the LOS test. The participants had continuous visual feedback about their COP position from the screen as they performed the weight shifts. The total time and directional control for participants to hit the 12 targets sequentially were computed. Table 21 summarizes the papers' authors and languages and Table 22 shows the quality of the studies.

3.32　Limits of Stability (LOS)

For the LOS test in sitting condition, the traditional standing protocol, which has widely been used in both research and clinical studies, was adopted [60]. The test measured the intentional weight shifting ability in multiple directions within their base of support. The initial COP was displayed at the center of the screen, together with eight target positions: in front, right front, right, right back, back, left back, left, and left front. The participants were required to move the COP trace on the screen toward one of eight selected target positions by shifting their weight within their LOS as quickly and as smoothly as possible when one of the visual targets appeared. There was a 20-s rest period between trials to minimize fatigue that might affect performance. The participants wore a safety harness connected to an overhead suspension frame during the unsupported sitting tests. The investigator was beside the participant for safety. There was a 2-s baseline measurement of COP sway before the appearance of the visual target. Each direction was repeated three times, and the results were averaged. A computer program was developed to record the following parameters: (1) reaction timed the time from the appearance of a target to the onset of the voluntary shifting of the COP; (2) maximum excursion the maximum displacement of the COP in the target direction; (3) directional controlled comparison of the amount of movement of the COP in the on-target direction with the amount of off-target displacement. In the supported trials, the data from both the eight directions and the "combined forward" direction,

which consisted of data of forward, right forward, and left forward targets only, were captured for data analysis. The "combined forward" direction was analyzed because the other five directions could, to some extent, be affected by the wheelchair's armrests and back support. Table 21 summarizes the papers' authors and languages and Table 22 shows the quality of the studies.

3.33　Motor Assessment Scale (MAS)

The MAS consists of six different items. It is a six-point ordinal scale where the scores of each item are ranked in order of difficulty. The patient is scored on the best of three attempts. It assesses static and proactive sitting balance control and takes B10 min to perform, less if the patient cannot perform all tasks. For SCI patients, item 3 was modified [61]. Table 21 summarizes the papers' authors and languages and Table 22 shows the quality of the studies.

3.34　Sitting Balance Score (SBS)

The SBS is a four-point ordinal scale to test static and reactive balance control and was originally constructed for stroke rehabilitation prognosis. The test takes two min to perform. For SCI patients, item 3 was modified [61]. Table 21 summarizes the papers' authors and languages and Table 22 shows the quality of the studies.

3.35　Trunk Impairment Classification System (TIC)

The TIC includes all five neuromusculoskeletal impairment types that can affect the trunk and which are also considered eligible impairments for Paralympic sport: muscle strength, ROM, coordination (defined as the ability to control voluntary movements), limitations in leg or trunk length, and limb deficiency [62]. Table 21 summarizes the papers' authors and languages and Table 22 shows the quality of the studies.

3.36 The Standing and Walking Assessment Tool (SWAT)

The use of the SWAT involves two steps. First, an individual's walking ability is staged on an ordinal scale. Stages 1, 2, and 3 are further subdivided based on either the level of assistance required and/or the maximum walking distance achievable. Second, the measures of walking and balance associated with the assigned SWAT stage are completed. The core set of measures include: (1) BBS = Berg Balance Scale, 5 (2) mTUG = the modified Timed Up and Go (mTUG) (3) ABC Scale = Activities-specific Balance Confidence Scale (4) 10MWT = 10-m Walk Test (5) 6MWT = 6-min Walk Test. It was validated in the English language [63]. Table 21 summarizes the papers' authors and languages and Table 22 shows the quality of the studies.

3.37 Standing Balance Assessment for Spinal Cord Injury (SBASCI)

The developed SBASCI scale is a performance-based ordinal scale that includes 22 items. Each item has a score ranging from 0 to 4, with 0 indicating the lowest function level and 4 indicating the highest functional level. Each item has a maximum score of 4, indicating the subject's ability to perform the activity independently (based on time constraints, physical assistance required, or distance/range required) and a minimum score of zero, indicating the inability to do the activity. The minimum and maximum score of SBASCI is 0 and 88.2, respectively. It was validated in the Hindi language in 2020 [64]. Table 21 summarizes the papers' authors and languages and Table 22 shows the quality of the studies.

4 Conclusions

This chapter reports all assessment tools described in the literature to assess walking and balance aspects in people with SCI. Results

among the 38 tools included in this chapter show that most scales evaluate assistance and distance and are mainly performance tests. The most common assessment tools are the functional capacity Walking Index for Spinal Cord Injury (WISCI) to measure improvements in ambulation evaluating the amount of physical assistance, braces or devices required to walk at 10 m; the 6-min Walking Test (6MWT) to measure of distance and represents the maximum distance walked in 6 min; the 11-item Neuromuscolar Recovery Scale (NRS) that compares sitting, standing, walking, and transfers relative to typical performance; and, the Berg Balance Scale (BBS) which consists of a test that lasts 15–20 min and includes a series of 14 simple tasks related to balance, ranging from getting up from a sitting position to standing on one foot.

References

1. .Scivoletto G, Tamburella F, Laurenza L, Foti C, Ditunno JF, Molinari M. Validity and reliability of the 10-m walk test and the 6-min walk test in spinal cord injury patients. Spinal Cord 2011. https://doi.org/10.1038/sc.2010.180.
2. Pastre CB, Lobo AM, Oberg TD, Pithon KR, Yoneyama SM, Lima NMFV. Validation of the Brazilian version in Portuguese of the thoracic-lumbar control scale for spinal cord injury. Spinal Cord 2011. https://doi.org/10.1038/sc.2011.86.
3. Shah G, Oates AR, Arora T, Lanovaz JL, Musselman KE. Measuring balance confidence after spinal cord injury: the reliability and validity of the activities-specific balance confidence scale. J Spinal Cord Med 2017. https://doi.org/10.1080/10790268.2017.1369212.
4. Abou L, Sung JH, Sosnoff JJ, Rice LA. Reliability and validity of the function in sitting test among non-ambulatory individuals with spinal cord injury. J Spinal Cord Med 2019. https://doi.org/10.1080/10790268.2019.1605749.
5. Castelnuovo G, Giusti EM, Manzoni GM, et al. What is the role of the placebo effect for pain relief in neurorehabilitation? Clinical implications from the Italian consensus conference on pain in neurorehabilitation. Front Neurol 2018. https://doi.org/10.3389/fneur.2018.00310.
6. Marquez MA, De Santis R, Ammendola V, et al. Cross-cultural adaptation and validation of the "spinal cord injury-falls concern scale" in the Italian population. Spinal Cord. 2018;56(7):712–8. https://doi.org/10.1038/s41393-018-0070-6.

7. Berardi A, De Santis R, Tofani M, et al. The Wheelchair Use Confidence Scale: Italian translation, adaptation, and validation of the short form. Disabil Rehabil Assist Technol. 2018;13(4):i. https://doi.org/10.1080/17483107.2017.1357053.

8. Anna B, Giovanni G, Marco T, et al. The validity of rasterstereography as a technological tool for the objectification of postural assessment in the clinical and educational fields: pilot study. In: Advances in intelligent systems and computing. 2020. https://doi.org/10.1007/978-3-030-23884-1_8.

9. Panuccio F, Berardi A, Marquez MA, et al. Development of the pregnancy and motherhood evaluation questionnaire (PMEQ) for evaluating and measuring the impact of physical disability on pregnancy and the management of motherhood: a pilot study. Disabil Rehabil. 2020;2020:1–7. https://doi.org/10.1080/09638288.2020.1802520.

10. Amedoro A, Berardi A, Conte A, et al. The effect of aquatic physical therapy on patients with multiple sclerosis: a systematic review and meta-analysis. Mult Scler Relat Disord. 2020. https://doi.org/10.1016/j.msard.2020.102022.

11. Dattoli S, Colucci M, Soave MG, et al. Evaluation of pelvis postural systems in spinal cord injury patients: outcome research. J Spinal Cord Med. 2018;43:185–92.

12. Berardi A, Galeoto G, Guarino D, et al. Construct validity, test-retest reliability, and the ability to detect change of the Canadian occupational performance measure in a spinal cord injury population. Spinal Cord Ser Cases 2019. https://doi.org/10.1038/s41394-019-0196-6.

13. Ponti A, Berardi A, Galeoto G, Marchegiani L, Spandonaro C, Marquez MA. Quality of life, concern of falling and satisfaction of the sit-ski aid in sit-skiers with spinal cord injury: observational study. Spinal Cord Ser Cases 2020. https://doi.org/10.1038/s41394-020-0257-x.

14. Panuccio F, Galeoto G, Marquez MA, et al. General sleep disturbance scale (GSDS-IT) in people with spinal cord injury: a psychometric study. Spinal Cord 2020. https://doi.org/10.1038/s41393-020-0500-0.

15. Monti M, Marquez MA, Berardi A, Tofani M, Valente D, Galeoto G. The multiple sclerosis intimacy and sexuality questionnaire (MSISQ-15): validation of the Italian version for individuals with spinal cord injury. Spinal Cord 2020. https://doi.org/10.1038/s41393-020-0469-8.

16. Galeoto G, Colucci M, Guarino D, et al. Exploring validity, reliability, and factor analysis of the Quebec user evaluation of satisfaction with assistive Technology in an Italian Population: a cross-sectional study. Occup Ther Heal Care 2018. https://doi.org/10.1080/07380577.2018.1522682.

17. Colucci M, Tofani M, Trioschi D, Guarino D, Berardi A, Galeoto G. Reliability and validity of the Italian version of Quebec user evaluation of satisfaction with assistive technology 2.0 (QUEST-IT 2.0) with users of mobility assistive device. Disabil Rehabil Assist Technol 2019. https://doi.org/10.1080/17483107.2019.1668975.

18. Berardi A, Galeoto G, Lucibello L, Panuccio F, Valente D, Tofani M. Athletes with disability' satisfaction with sport wheelchairs: an Italian cross sectional study. Disabil Rehabil Assist Technol 2020. https://doi.org/10.1080/17483107.2020.1800114.

19. Moher D, Shamseer L, Clarke M, et al. Preferred reporting items for systematic review and meta-analysis protocols (PRISMA-P) 2015 statement. Rev Esp Nutr Human Diet. 2016. https://doi.org/10.1186/2046-4053-4-1.

20. Mokkink LB, Terwee CB, Patrick DL, et al. The COSMIN study reached international consensus on taxonomy, terminology, and definitions of measurement properties for health-related patient-reported outcomes. J Clin Epidemiol 2010. https://doi.org/10.1016/j.jclinepi.2010.02.006.

21. Terwee CB, Prinsen CAC, Chiarotto A, et al. COSMIN methodology for evaluating the content validity of patient-reported outcome measures: a Delphi study. Qual Life Res 2018. https://doi.org/10.1007/s11136-018-1829-0.

22. Mokkink LB, de Vet HCW, Prinsen CAC, et al. COSMIN risk of bias checklist for systematic reviews of patient-reported outcome measures. Qual Life Res 2018. https://doi.org/10.1007/s11136-017-1765-4.

23. Ditunno JF, Ditunno PL, Graziani V, et al. Walking index for spinal cord injury (WISCI): an international multicenter validity and reliability study. Spinal Cord 2000. https://doi.org/10.1038/sj.sc.3100993.

24. Ditunno JF, Barbeau H, Dobkin BH, et al. Validity of the walking scale for spinal cord injury and other domains of function in a multicenter clinical trial. Neurorehabil Neural Repair 2007. https://doi.org/10.1177/1545968307301880.

25. Morganti B, Scivoletto G, Ditunno P, Ditunno JF, Molinari M. Walking index for spinal cord injury (WISCI): criterion validation. Spinal Cord 2005. https://doi.org/10.1038/sj.sc.3101658.

26. Ditunno JF, Scivoletto G, Patrick M, Biering-Sorensen F, Abel R, Marino R. Validation of the walking index for spinal cord injury in a US and European clinical population. Spinal Cord 2008. https://doi.org/10.1038/sj.sc.3102071.

27. Marino RJ, Scivoletto G, Patrick M, et al. Walking index for spinal cord injury version 2 (WISCI-II) with repeatability of the 10-m walk time: inter- and intrarater reliabilities. Am J Phys Med Rehabil 2010. https://doi.org/10.1097/PHM.0b013e3181c560eb.

28. Burns AS, Delparte JJ, Patrick M, Marino RJ, Ditunno JF. The reproducibility and convergent validity of the walking index for spinal cord injury (WISCI) in chronic spinal cord injury. Neurorehabil Neural Repair 2011. https://doi.org/10.1177/1545968310376756.

29. Van Hedel HJA, Wirz M, Curt A. Improving walking assessment in subjects with an incomplete spinal cord injury: responsiveness. Spinal Cord 2006. https://doi.org/10.1038/sj.sc.3101853.

30. Scivoletto G, Tamburella F, Laurenza L, Torre M, Molinari M, Ditunno JF. Walking index for spinal cord injury version II in acute spinal cord injury: reliability and reproducibility. Spinal Cord 2014. https://doi.org/10.1038/sc.2013.127.

31. Poncumhak P, Saengsuwan J, Kamruecha W, Amatachaya S. Reliability and validity of three functional tests in ambulatory patients with spinal cord injury. Spinal Cord 2013. https://doi.org/10.1038/sc.2012.126.

32. Poncumhak P, Saengsuwan J, Amatachaya S. Ability of walking without a walking device in patients with spinal cord injury as determined using data from functional tests. J Spinal Cord Med 2014. https://doi.org/10.1179/2045772313Y.0000000160.

33. Amatachaya S, Naewla S, Srisim K, Arrayawichanon P, Siritaratiwat W. Concurrent validity of the 10-meter walk test as compared with the 6-minute walk test in patients with spinal cord injury at various levels of ability. Spinal Cord 2014. https://doi.org/10.1038/sc.2013.171.

34. Rini D, Senthilvelkumar T, Noble K, Magimairaj H. Test–retest reliability of the 10-meter walk test in ambulatory adults with motor-complete spinal cord injury. Int J Ther Rehabil 2018. https://doi.org/10.12968/ijtr.2018.25.7.335.

35. Van Hedel HJ, Wirz M, Dietz V. Assessing walking ability in subjects with spinal cord injury: validity and reliability of 3 walking tests. Arch Phys Med Rehabil 2005. https://doi.org/10.1016/j.apmr.2004.02.010.

36. Velozo C, Moorhouse M, Ardolino E, et al. Validity of the neuromuscular recovery scale: a measurement model approach. Arch Phys Med Rehabil 2015. https://doi.org/10.1016/j.apmr.2015.04.004.

37. Behrman AL, Ardolino E, Vanhiel LR, et al. Assessment of functional improvement without compensation reduces variability of outcome measures after human spinal cord injury. Arch Phys Med Rehabil 2012. https://doi.org/10.1016/j.apmr.2011.04.027.

38. Basso DM, Velozo C, Lorenz D, Suter S, Behrman AL. Interrater reliability of the neuromuscular recovery scale for spinal cord injury. Arch Phys Med Rehabil 2015. https://doi.org/10.1016/j.apmr.2014.11.026.

39. Behrman AL, Velozo C, Suter S, Lorenz D, Basso DM. Test-retest reliability of the neuromuscular recovery scale. Arch Phys Med Rehabil 2015. https://doi.org/10.1016/j.apmr.2015.03.022.

40. Quinzaños-Fresnedo J, Villa AR, Flores AA, Pérez R. Proposal and validation of a clinical trunk control test in individuals with spinal cord injury. Spinal Cord 2014. https://doi.org/10.1038/sc.2014.34.

41. Quinzaños-Fresnedo J, Fratini-Escobar PC, Almaguer-Benavides KM, et al. Prognostic validity of a clinical trunk control test for independence and walking in individuals with spinal cord injury. J Spinal Cord Med 2020. https://doi.org/10.1080/10790268.2018.1518124.

42. Wirz M, Müller R, Bastiaenen C. Falls in persons with spinal cord injury: validity and reliability of the berg balance scale. Neurorehabil Neural Repair 2010. https://doi.org/10.1177/1545968309341059.

43. Lemay JF, Nadeau S. Standing balance assessment in ASIA D paraplegic and tetraplegic participants: concurrent validity of the Berg balance scale. Spinal Cord 2010. https://doi.org/10.1038/sc.2009.119.

44. Jørgensen V, Opheim A, Halvarsson A, Franzén E, Roaldsen KS. Comparison of the berg balance scale and the mini-BESTest for assessing balance in ambulatory people with spinal cord injury: validation study. Phys Ther 2017. https://doi.org/10.1093/ptj/pzx030.

45. Chan K, Unger J, Lee JW, et al. Quantifying balance control after spinal cord injury: reliability and validity of the mini-BESTest. J Spinal Cord Med 2019. https://doi.org/10.1080/10790268.2019.1647930.

46. Field-Fote EC, Fluet GG, Schafer SD, et al. The spinal cord injury functional ambulation inventory (SCI-FAI). J Rehabil Med 2001. https://doi.org/10.1080/165019701750300645.

47. Musselman K, Brunton K, Lam T, Yang J. Spinal cord injury functional ambulation profile: a new measure of walking ability. Neurorehabil Neural Repair 2011. https://doi.org/10.1177/1545968310381250.

48. Musselman KE, Yang JF. Spinal cord injury functional ambulation profile: a preliminary look at responsiveness. Phys Ther 2014. https://doi.org/10.2522/ptj.20130071.

49. Khuna L, Thaweewannakij T, Wattanapan P, Amatachaya P, Amatachaya S. Five times sit-to-stand test for ambulatory individuals with spinal cord injury: a psychometric study on the effects of arm placements. Spinal Cord 2020. https://doi.org/10.1038/s41393-019-0372-3.

50. Khuna L, Phadungkit S, Thaweewannakij T, Amatachaya P, Amatachaya S. Outcomes of the five times sit-to-stand test could determine lower limb functions of ambulatory people with spinal cord injury only when assessed without hands. J Spinal Cord Med August. 2020;2020:1–8. https://doi.org/10.1080/10790268.2020.1803658.

51. Maurer-Burkhard B, Smoor I, Von Reumont A, et al. Validity and reliability of a locomotor stage-based functional rating scale in spinal cord injury. Spinal Cord 2016. https://doi.org/10.1038/sc.2015.223.

52. Cowan RE, Callahan MK, Nash MS. The 6-min push test is reliable and predicts low fitness in spinal cord injury. Med Sci Sports Exerc 2012. https://doi.org/10.1249/MSS.0b013e31825cb3b6.

53. Ardolino EM, Hutchinson KJ, Zipp GP, Clark MA, Harkema SJ. The ABLE scale: the development and psychometric properties of an outcome measure for the spinal cord injury population. Phys Ther 2012. https://doi.org/10.2522/ptj.20110257.

54. Chan K, Guy K, Shah G, et al. Retrospective assessment of the validity and use of the community balance and mobility scale among individuals with subacute spinal cord injury. Spinal Cord 2017. https://doi.org/10.1038/sc.2016.140.

55. Palermo AE, Cahalin LP, Garcia KL, Nash MS. Psychometric testing and clinical utility of a

modified version of the function in sitting test for individuals with chronic spinal cord injury. In: Arch Phys Med Rehabil 2020. https://doi.org/10.1016/j. apmr.2020.06.014.

56. Pernot HFM, Lannem AM, Geers RPJ, Ruijters EFG, Bloemendal M, Seelen HAM. Validity of the test-table-test for Nordic skiing for classification of paralympic sit-ski sports participants. Spinal Cord 2011. https://doi.org/10.1038/sc.2011.30.

57. Wadhwa G, Aikat R. Development, validity and reliability of the "sitting balance measure" (SBM) in spinal cord injury. Spinal Cord 2016. https://doi. org/10.1038/sc.2015.148

58. Sprigle S, Maurer C, Holowka M. Development of valid and reliable measures of postural stability. J Spinal Cord Med 2007. https://doi.org/10.1080/1079 0268.2007.11753913.

59. Boswell-Ruys CL, Sturnieks DL, Harvey LA, Sherrington C, Middleton JW, Lord SR. Validity and reliability of assessment tools for measuring unsupported sitting in people with a spinal cord injury. Arch Phys Med Rehabil 2009. https://doi.org/10.1016/j. apmr.2009.02.016.

60. Gao KL, Chan KM, Purves S, Tsang WWN. Reliability of dynamic sitting balance tests and their correlations with functional mobility for wheelchair users with chronic spinal cord injury. J Orthop Transl 2015. https://doi.org/10.1016/j.jot.2014.07.003.

61. Jørgensen V, Elfving B, Opheim A. Assessment of unsupported sitting in patients with spinal cord injury. Spinal Cord 2011. https://doi.org/10.1038/ sc.2011.9.

62. Altmann VC, Groen BE, Groenen KH, Vanlandewijck YC, Van Limbeek J, Keijsers NL. Construct validity of the trunk impairment classification system in relation to objective measures of trunk impairment. Arch Phys Med Rehabil 2016. https://doi.org/10.1016/j. apmr.2015.10.096.

63. Musselman KE, Lemay JF, Walden K, Harris A, Gagnon DH, Verrier MC. The standing and walking assessment tool for individuals with spinal cord injury: a qualitative study of validity and clinical use. J Spinal Cord Med 2019. https://doi.org/10.1080/107 90268.2019.1616148.

64. Singh M, Sarkar A, Kataria C. Development and validation of the standing balance assessment for individuals with spinal cord injury (SBASCI) – a new outcome measure. NeuroRehabilitation. 2020;47(2):161–9. https://doi.org/10.3233/NRE-203148.

Measuring Pediatric Spinal Cord Injury

Donatella Valente, Maurizio Sabbadini,
Enrico Castelli, and Marco Tofani

1 Introduction

Spinal cord injury (SCI) is a devastating event with lasting implications for children and families. Physical and psychosocial well-being is challenged, creating a range of needs for intervention from rehabilitation services. Because these needs are dynamic, resulting from SCI interaction with growth and development, the rehabilitation and habilitation of children and adolescents with an SCI must be developmentally based and respond to an individual's changing needs as they grow. Rehabilitation programs should take into account findings on adult outcomes in pediatric-onset SCI. So rehabilitation programs must focus on reducing medical complications, achieving functional independence, facilitating access to education, preparing for work, enabling and encouraging community participation (in such productive activities as hobbies, social activities, and travel within the community), and facilitating preparation for significant personal relationships with, for example, future spouses or children [1].

Children as young as 6 years of age learn to manage their bladder and begin participating in their bowel program. Children with an SCI are taught skills for independent dressing, body transfers, and upright and wheeled mobility [2].

This line is important as much as the adult evaluation, the evaluation for children and adolescents. Many scales exist to evaluate the different variables of the adult with SCI; in the same way, assessment tools for SCI adolescents should exist.

This study's objective was to describe and evaluate scales of the assessment tools on pediatric SCI through a systematic review of cross-sectional studies.

2 Materials and Methods

This study was conducted by a research group composed of medical doctors and health professionals from the "Sapienza" University of Rome and the "Rehabilitation & Outcome Measure Assessment" (R.O.M.A.) association. In the last few years, the R.O.M.A. association has engaged several studies and the validation of many outcome measures in Italy for the Spinal Cord Injury population [3–16].

This chapter describes all assessment tools regarding Pediatric SCI resulting from a system-

D. Valente
Department of Human Neurosciences, Sapienza
University of Rome, Rome, Italy

M. Sabbadini · E. Castelli ·
Department of Neurorehabilitation and Robotics,
Bambino Gesù Paediatric Hospital University,
Vatican City, Italy

M. Tofani (✉)
Department of Neurorehabilitation and Robotics,
Bambino Gesù Paediatric Hospital,
Rome, Italy
e-mail: marco.tofani@uniroma1.it

atic review conducted on PubMed, Scopus, CINALH, and Web of Science. For specific details on methodology, see chapter "Methodological Approach to Identifying Outcome Measures in Spinal Cord Injury."

Eligibility criteria for considering studies for this chapter were validation studies and cross-cultural adaptation studies, studies about pediatrics, studies about tests, questionnaires, self-reported and performance-based outcome measures, studies with a population of people with SCI, and populations <18 years old. Study selection: the selection of studies was conducted in accordance with the 27-item PRISM Statement for Reporting Systematic Reviews [17]. For the data collection, the authors followed the recommendations from the COnsensus-based Standards for the selection of health Measurement Instruments (COSMIN) initiative [18]. Study quality and risk of bias were assessed using COSMIN Checklist [19, 20].

3   Results

For this chapter, 20 papers were considered. The authors found 15 assessment tools that evaluate children and adolescents with SCI. In Fig. 1, a flow chart of included studies is reported.

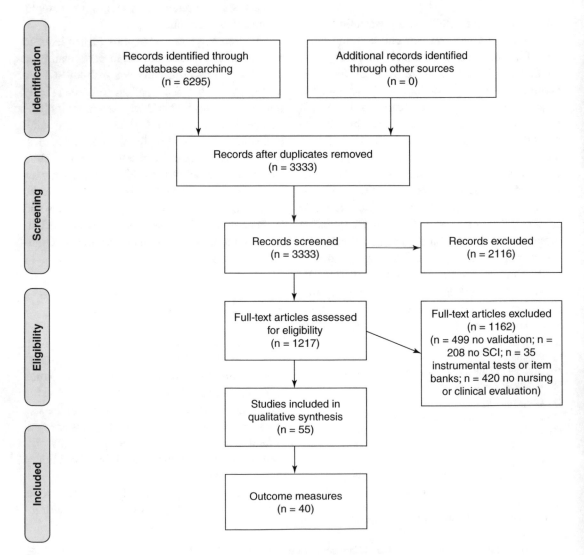

Fig. 1 Flow chart of included studies

3.1 Walking Index for Spinal Cord Injury II (WISCI II)

The Walking Index for Spinal Cord Injury II (WISCI II) is an ordinal scale (0–20) consisting of 21 items reflecting various walking ability levels, taking into account the use of assistive devices, orthotic devices, and physical assistance. The individual assessed walks 10 m, which is a distance often correlated with household ambulation. The WISCI II scale is a measure of walking capacity and was developed for use in clinical trials to document a change in functional capacity resulting from an intervention [21]. In 2012, C.L. Calhoun and Mulcahey evaluated the reliability of WISCI II in children and adolescents with spinal cord injury, in Philadelphia, PA, USA. They worked with ten children with SCI and six trained physical therapist raters. In 2016, also C. Calhoun Thielen et al. examined the construct validity, and established reliability of the WISCI-II related to its use in children with spinal cord injury (SCI), in the United States, and they demonstrated and supported the use of the WISCI-II in children

with SCI [22]. Table 1 summarizes the papers' authors and languages and Table 2 shows the quality of the studies.

3.2 Spinal Cord Independence Measure (SCIM)

The Spinal Cord Independence Measure (SCIM) is a functional outcomes tool developed specifically for the assessment of individuals with SCI. The SCIM evaluates self-care, respiratory and sphincter management, and mobility. The SCIM has been shown to be reliable and a more sensitive measure to a functional change in adults with SCI. In 2012, Calhoun and Mulcahey evaluated SCIM indoor mobility item 12 in children and adolescents with spinal cord injury in Philadelphia, PA, USA. In 2016, they evaluated the validity of the SCIM-III Self-Report for pediatric utilization in the United States [2, 21, 23]. In 2018, the same authors validated the SCIM III [2, 21, 23]. Table 3 summarizes the papers' authors and languages and Table 4 shows the quality of the studies.

Table 1 Characteristics of the studies validating WISCI II

Authors	Language	n	Age mean (SD, range) year	Gender % Female
Calhoun and Mulcahey [21]	English (American)	10	9, 2 (2, 8, 5–13)	2 (20)
Calhoun et al. [22]	English (American)	52	n.a.	30 (57,7)

n number of participants of the study, *n.a.* not available

Table 2 Evaluation of quality and risk of bias

Authors	Item of COSMIN checklist									
	1	2	3	4	5	6	7	8	9	10
Calhoun and Mulcahey [21]	?	?	–	–	+	+	–	+	+	–
Calhoun et al. [22]	?	?	–	–	+	+	–	–	–	–

Item 1 PROM development, *Item 2* content validity, *Item 3* structural validity, *Item 4* internal consistency, *Item 5* cross-cultural validity/measurement invariance, *Item 6* reliability, *Item 7* measurement error, *Item 8* criterion validity, *Item 9* hypothesis testing for construct validity, *Item 10* responsiveness, + sufficient, – insufficient, ? indeterminate

Table 3 Characteristics of the studies validating SCIM indoor mobility item (12) and SCIM-III-Self-report

Scale, test, or questionnaire	Authors	Language	N	Age mean (SD, range) year	Gender % Female
SCIM indoor mobility item (12)	Calhoun and Mulcahey [21]	English	10	9, 2 (2, 8, 5–13)	2 (20)
SCIM III self-report	Mulcahey et al. [2]	English	16	11, 3 (2, 7, 7–15)	7 (43,75)
	Mulcahey et al. [23]	English	124	10.8 (2–18)	57 (46)

n number of participants of the study, *n.a.* not available

Table 4 Evaluation of quality and risk of bias

| Authors | Item of COSMIN checklist | | | | | | | | | |
	1	2	3	4	5	6	7	8	9	10
Calhoun and Mulcahey [21]	?	?	–	–	+	–	–	–	–	–
Mulcahey et al. [2]	?	+	–	–	+	+	–	+	+	–
Mulcahey et al. [23]	?	–	+	–	+	+	–	–	–	–

Item 1 PROM development, *Item 2* content validity, *Item 3* structural validity, *Item 4* internal consistency, *Item 5* cross-cultural validity/measurement invariance, *Item 6* reliability, *Item 7* measurement error, *Item 8*: criterion validity, *Item 9* hypothesis testing for construct validity, *Item 10* responsiveness, + sufficient, – insufficient, ? indeterminate

Table 5 Characteristics of the studies validating NRS

Authors	Language	N	Age mean (SD, range) year	Gender % Female
Behrman et al. [25]	English	32	6 (3, 2–12)	15 (46.9)
Ardolino et al. [24]	English	5	n.a.	n.a.

n number of participants of the study, *n.a.* not available

Table 6 Evaluation of quality and risk of bias

| Authors | Item of COSMIN checklist | | | | | | | | | |
	1	2	3	4	5	6	7	8	9	10
Behrman et al. [25]	?	?	n.a.	n.a.	n.a.	n.a.	n.a.	n.a.	n.a.	n.a.
Ardolino et al. [24]	+	+	–	–	+	–	–	–	–	–

Item 1: PROM development, *Item 2* content validity, *Item 3* structural validity, *Item 4* internal consistency, *Item 5* cross-cultural validity/measurement invariance, *Item 6* reliability, *Item 7* measurement error, *Item 8* criterion validity, *Item 9* hypothesis testing for construct validity, *Item 10* responsiveness, + sufficient, – insufficient, ? indeterminate

3.3 Neuromuscular Recovery Scale (NRS)

The Neuromuscular Recovery Scale (NRS) was developed to assess neuromuscular capacity to perform specific functional tasks without compensation in adults with SCI.2 The NRS assesses the ability to perform a series of functional tasks, movements, and transitions (e.g., sit, sit to stand, and walk) using preinjury movement patterns and disallows compensation for weakened or paralyzed muscles by stronger muscles, substitutions, or devices. Based on the performance across 14 items, an overall "phase" score is calculated ranging from a low level to a high neuromuscular recovery level. In 2016, NRS was validated in pediatric SCI in the English language [24, 25]. Table 5 summarizes the papers' authors and languages and Table 6 shows the quality of the studies.

3.4 Shriners Pediatric Instrument for Neuromuscular Scoliosis (SPINS)

The Shriners Pediatric Instrument for Neuromuscular Scoliosis (SPINS) (originally titled the Paralytic Spine Deformity Outcomes Questionnaire [PSDOQ]) was developed with the ultimate goal of measuring the impact of bracing and/or surgery on the HRQOL of children with SCI and neuromuscular scoliosis. The development of the SPINS began with the identification of the following related domains by a physiatrist with several years of clinical experience working with children with neuromuscular conditions: sitting balance, activities of daily living (ADLs)/self-care, bowel and bladder management, mobility, sports/recreation/leisure, pain, pulmonary, self-esteem/self-concept, cosmesis, skin integrity, and surgical intervention. It was validated in the English language [26]. Table 7 summarizes the papers' authors and languages and Table 8 shows the quality of the studies.

3.5 Capabilities of Upper Extremity Test (CUE-T)

The CUE-T version 1.0 is composed of 17 items: six arm items (each arm), nine hand function items (each hand), and two bilateral items. The raw scores for each item are based on one of three types of actions: (1) repetitive actions—number of repetitions completed within a specific time frame; (2) progressive actions—weight moved;

(3) timed actions—amount of time required for task completion. The raw scores were then converted to a 5-point scale ranging from 0 to 4, where 0 = unable/complete difficulty and 4 = no difficulty. It was validated in children with SCI in 2018 [27]. Table 7 summarizes the papers' authors and languages and Table 8 shows the quality of the studies.

3.6 Moorong Self-Efficacy Scale (MSES)

The Moorong Self-Efficacy Scale (MSES) was developed to measure the unique impact of SCI's

Table 7 Characteristics of the studies of scale, test, or questionnaire with less than two validations

Scale, test or Questionnaire	Authors	Language	n	Age mean (SD, range) year	Gender % Female
ChNAC	Webster and Kennedy [1]	English	33	8.45 (4.27, 2–16)	13 (39)
STAMP	Wong et al. [33]	English	62	(1–18)	24 (39.4)
GRASSP	Mulcahey et al. [23]	Swedish	35	13 (37)	
SPINS	Hunter et al. [26]	English	14	(6–17)	4 (28.6)
CUE	Dent et al. [27]	English	39	21.3 (3–17)	15 (39)
MSES	De Paula et al. [28]	Dutch	n.a.	n.a.	n.a.
ISNCSCI	Mulcahey et al. [29]	English	181	14.5 (4.2)	72 (39.78)
Peds QL	Hwang et al. [30]	English	22	n.a.	13 (59.1)
PEDI-SCI AM	Slavin et al. [31]	English	381	15.5 (3.5)	171 (45)
SATCo	Argetsinger et al. [32]	English	21	n.a.	n.a.
GRT	Mulcahey et al. [2]	English	19	(7–20)	n.a.

n number of participants of the study, *n.a.* not available

Table 8 Evaluation of quality and risk of bias

Authors	Item of COSMIN checklist									
	1	2	3	4	5	6	7	8	9	10
Webster and Kennedy [1]	?	+	−	−	+	−	−	−	−	−
Wong et al. [33]	?	+	−	−	+	+	−	+	+	−
Mulcahey et al. [23]	?	−	+	−	+	+	−	−	−	−
Hunter et al. [26]	+	+	−	−	−	+	−	−	−	−
Dent et al. [27]	?	+	−	−	+	−	−	+	+	−
De Paula et al. [28]	+	+	−	−	−	−	−	−	−	−
Mulcahey et al. [29]	?	+	−	−	−	+	−	−	−	−
Hwang et al. [30]	+	+	−	−	+	−	−	−	−	−
Slavin et al. [31]	?	+	−	+	+	+	−	−	−	−
Argetsinger et al. [32]	?	+	−	−	+	−	−	−	−	+
Mulcahey et al. [2]	?	+	−	−	+	+	−	+	+	+

Item 1: PROM development, *Item 2* content validity, *Item 3* structural validity, *Item 4* internal consistency, *Item 5*: cross-cultural validity/measurement invariance, *Item 6* reliability, *Item 7* measurement error, *Item 8* criterion validity, *Item 9*: hypothesis testing for construct validity, *Item 10* responsiveness, + sufficient; −: insufficient, ? indeterminate

medical and functional complications. The MSES contains 16 items across domains of Daily Activities and Social Functioning. Items are measured on a 7-point Likert-type scale, ranging from 1 (very uncertain) to 7 (very certain). Higher ratings indicate higher levels of perceived self-efficacy (5, 6). It was validated for the pediatric population in 2015 in the Dutch language [28]. Table 7 summarizes the papers' authors and languages and Table 8 shows the quality of the studies.

3.7 International Standards for Neurological and Functional Classification of Spinal Cord Injury (ISCSCI)

The International Standards for Neurological Classification of Spinal Cord Injury (ISNCSCI) was developed in 1982 by the American Spinal Injuries Association (ASIA). The ISNCSCI examination and classification provide a common language to describe the extent of motor and sensory dysfunction due to SCI. It was validated in 2011 in the pediatric population [29]. Table 7 summarizes the papers' authors and languages and Table 8 shows the quality of the studies.

3.8 Pediatric Quality of Life Inventory (PedsQL)

The Pediatric Quality of Life Inventory version 4.0 (PedsQLTM 4.0) Generic Core Scales is a reliable and valid measure of HRQoL that spans childhood and adolescence, with versions for self-reporting by the Young Child (ages 5–7), Child (ages 8–12), Teen (ages 13–18), and also Parent Proxy versions for the same age groups and Toddler (ages 2–4). It was validated in the English language in 2020 [30]. Table 7 summarizes the papers' authors and languages and Table 8 shows the quality of the studies.

3.9 Pediatric Spinal Cord Injury Activity Measure (PEDI-SCI AM)

The Pediatric Spinal Cord Injury Activity Measure (PEDI-SCI AM) was developed to assess activity outcomes in youth with SCI, providing an alternative to generic pediatric outcome measures. The PEDI-SCI AM includes activities important to youth with SCI, and items assess a wide range of abilities in the following domains: general mobility, daily routines, wheeled mobility, and ambulation. It was validated in English [31]. Table 7 summarizes the papers' authors and languages and Table 8 shows the quality of the studies.

3.10 Segmental Assessment of Trunk Control (SATCo)

For SATCo testing, the patient was positioned in short sit with hips, knees, and ankles flexed to 90°. Manual support was provided to maintain neutral, vertical pelvis as an alternative to pelvis/leg strapping to prevent skin breakdown. It was validated for the SCI population in 2018 [32]. Table 7 summarizes the papers' authors and languages and Table 8 shows the quality of the studies.

3.11 Child Needs Assessment Checklist (ChNAC)

The ChNAC was developed in 2007 for use with children and adolescents younger than 17 years of age. The ChNAC is a practical tool for planning young people's rehabilitation after SCI and assessing rehabilitation outcomes [1]. It provides a developmentally sensitive way to assess and address young people's needs within the context of their family and community. It is a behavioral checklist consisting of key indicators in the following areas of need: Activities of Daily Living (17 specific indicators), Skin Management

(10 indicators), Bladder Management (7 indicators), Bowel Management (11 indicators), Knowledge of Spine and Promoting Healthy Growth (15 indicators), Mobility (11 indicators), Wheelchair and Equipment (36 indicators), Community and Education (20 indicators), Discharge Coordination (28 indicators), and Psychological Issues (26 indicators for ages 0–6 years and 28 indicators for ages 7–16 years). Table 7 summarizes the authors and languages of the papers and Table 8 shows the quality of the studies.

3.12 Screening Tool for the Assessment of Malnutrition in Pediatrics (STAMP)

In 2013, S Wong et al. validated the STAMP in pediatric spinal cord injury (SCI) patients admitted to a tertiary SCI center in the United Kingdom. STAMP was developed in the United Kingdom, specifically for use by members of a multidisciplinary team. The STAMP incorporates three components, all of which are recognized indices or symptoms of undernutrition: the presence of a clinical diagnosis with nutritional implications, estimated current nutritional intake, and differences in weight/height centile chart. Each component carries a score of up to 3, and the total score reflects the risk of undernutrition. A score of 2 or 3 indicates medium risk, and >4 indicates high risk [33]. Table 7 summarizes the papers' authors and languages and Table 8 shows the quality of the studies.

3.13 Grasp and Release Test

The GRT (30) was designed to assess FES outcomes on the hand function of persons with C5- and weak C6-level tetraplegia (ICSHT motor groups 0-2). The GRT consists of six objects that vary in size and weight. The peg and block are the lightest of objects (0.1 Newton Meters [N] and 0.02 N, respectively) and represent finger food. The paperweight (2 .59 N), can (2 .1 N), and videotape (3.49 N) represent medium-sized objects such as a book or a soda can. The fork object simulates stabbing food or writing and requires 4.4 N to depress the handle to an indicator line, which is the force required to stab fruit, cooked vegetables, or meat. It was validated in the English language in 2004 [34]. Table 7 summarizes the papers' authors and languages and Table 8 shows the quality of the studies.

4 Conclusions

This chapter reports all assessment tools described in the literature to assess children and adolescents with SCI. Among the 15 tools included in this chapter resulted that most scales evaluate activities of daily living. The most common assessment tools are the Walking Index for Spinal Cord Injury (WISCI II), which is an ordinal scale consisting of 21 items reflecting various levels of walking ability, the Spinal Cord Independence Measure (SCIM) III Self-Report, which evaluates self-care, respiratory, sphincter management, and mobility, and the Pediatric Neuromuscular Recovery Scale (NRS), which assesses a child's neuromuscular capacity to perform 13 everyday tasks without behavioral compensation, physical assistance, or assistive device/orthotics.

References

1. Webster G, Kennedy P. Addressing children's needs and evaluating rehabilitation outcome after spinal cord injury: the child needs assessment checklist and goal-planning program. J Spinal Cord Med. 2007. https://doi.org/10.1080/10790268.2007.11754592.
2. Mulcahey MJ, Calhoun CL, Sinko R, Kelly EH, Vogel LC. The spinal cord independence measure (SCIM)-III self report for youth. Spinal Cord. 2016;54(3):204–12. https://doi.org/10.1038/sc.2015.103.
3. Castelnuovo G, Giusti EM, Manzoni GM, et al. What is the role of the placebo effect for pain relief in neurorehabilitation? Clinical implications from the Italian consensus conference on pain in neurorehabilitation. Front Neurol. 2018. https://doi.org/10.3389/fneur.2018.00310.

4. Marquez MA, De Santis R, Ammendola V, et al. Cross-cultural adaptation and validation of the "spinal cord injury-falls concern scale" in the Italian population. Spinal Cord. 2018;56(7):712–8. https://doi.org/10.1038/s41393-018-0070-6.

5. Berardi A, De Santis R, Tofani M, et al. The Wheelchair Use Confidence Scale: Italian translation, adaptation, and validation of the short form. Disabil Rehabil Assist Technol. 2018;13(4):i. https://doi.org/10.1080/17483107.2017.1357053.

6. Anna B, Giovanni G, Marco T, et al. The validity of rasterstereography as a technological tool for the objectification of postural assessment in the clinical and educational fields: pilot study. In: Advances in intelligent systems and computing. 2020. https://doi.org/10.1007/978-3-030-23884-1_8.

7. Panuccio F, Berardi A, Marquez MA, et al. Development of the pregnancy and motherhood evaluation questionnaire (PMEQ) for evaluating and measuring the impact of physical disability on pregnancy and the management of motherhood: a pilot study. Disabil Rehabil. 2020:1–7. https://doi.org/10.1080/09638288.2020.1802520.

8. Amedoro A, Berardi A, Conte A, et al. The effect of aquatic physical therapy on patients with multiple sclerosis: a systematic review and meta-analysis. Mult Scler Relat Disord. 2020. https://doi.org/10.1016/j.msard.2020.102022.

9. Dattoli S, Colucci M, Soave MG, et al. Evaluation of pelvis postural systems in spinal cord injury patients: outcome research. J Spinal Cord Med. 2018;43:185–92.

10. Berardi A, Galeoto G, Guarino D, et al. Construct validity, test-retest reliability, and the ability to detect change of the Canadian occupational performance measure in a spinal cord injury population. Spinal Cord Ser Cases. 2019. https://doi.org/10.1038/s41394-019-0196-6.

11. Ponti A, Berardi A, Galeoto G, Marchegiani L, Spandonaro C, Marquez MA. Quality of life, concern of falling and satisfaction of the sit-ski aid in sit-skiers with spinal cord injury: observational study. Spinal Cord Ser Cases. 2020. https://doi.org/10.1038/s41394-020-0257-x.

12. Panuccio F, Galeoto G, Marquez MA, et al. General sleep disturbance scale (GSDS-IT) in people with spinal cord injury: a psychometric study. Spinal Cord. 2020. https://doi.org/10.1038/s41393-020-0500-0.

13. Monti M, Marquez MA, Berardi A, Tofani M, Valente D, Galeoto G. The multiple sclerosis intimacy and sexuality questionnaire (MSISQ-15): validation of the Italian version for individuals with spinal cord injury. Spinal Cord. 2020. https://doi.org/10.1038/s41393-020-0469-8.

14. Galeoto G, Colucci M, Guarino D, et al. Exploring validity, reliability, and factor analysis of the Quebec user evaluation of satisfaction with assistive Technology in an Italian Population: a cross-sectional study. Occup Ther Heal Care. 2018. https://doi.org/10.1080/07380577.2018.1522682.

15. Colucci M, Tofani M, Trioschi D, Guarino D, Berardi A, Galeoto G. Reliability and validity of the Italian version of Quebec user evaluation of satisfaction with assistive technology 2.0 (QUEST-IT 2.0) with users of mobility assistive device. Disabil Rehabil Assist Technol. 2019. https://doi.org/10.1080/17483107.2019.1668975.

16. Berardi A, Galeoto G, Lucibello L, Panuccio F, Valente D, Tofani M. Athletes with disability' satisfaction with sport wheelchairs: an Italian cross sectional study. Disabil Rehabil Assist Technol. 2020. https://doi.org/10.1080/17483107.2020.1800114.

17. Moher D, Shamseer L, Clarke M, et al. Preferred reporting items for systematic review and meta-analysis protocols (PRISMA-P) 2015 statement. Rev Esp Nutr Human Diet. 2016. https://doi.org/10.1186/2046-4053-4-1.

18. Mokkink LB, Terwee CB, Patrick DL, et al. The COSMIN study reached international consensus on taxonomy, terminology, and definitions of measurement properties for health-related patient-reported outcomes. J Clin Epidemiol. 2010. https://doi.org/10.1016/j.jclinepi.2010.02.006.

19. Terwee CB, Prinsen CAC, Chiarotto A, et al. COSMIN methodology for evaluating the content validity of patient-reported outcome measures: a Delphi study. Qual Life Res. 2018. https://doi.org/10.1007/s11136-018-1829-0.

20. Mokkink LB, de Vet HCW, Prinsen CAC, et al. COSMIN risk of bias checklist for systematic reviews of patient-reported outcome measures. Qual Life Res. 2018. https://doi.org/10.1007/s11136-017-1765-4.

21. Calhoun CL, Mulcahey MJ. Pilot study of reliability and validity of the walking index for spinal cord injury II (WISCI-II) in children and adolescents with spinal cord injury. J Pediatr Rehabil Med. 2012. https://doi.org/10.3233/PRM-2012-00224.

22. Calhoun Thielen C, Sadowsky C, Vogel LC, et al. Evaluation of the walking index for spinal cord injury II (WISCI-II) in children with spinal cord injury (SCI). Spinal Cord. 2017;55(5):478–82. https://doi.org/10.1038/sc.2016.142.

23. Mulcahey MJ, Thielen CC, Sadowsky C, et al. Despite limitations in content range, the SCIM-III is reproducible and a valid indicator of physical function in youths with spinal cord injury and dysfunction. Spinal Cord. 2018. https://doi.org/10.1038/s41393-017-0036-0.

24. Ardolino EM, Mulcahey MJ, Trimble S, et al. Development and initial validation of the pediatric neuromuscular recovery scale. Pediatr Phys Ther. 2016. https://doi.org/10.1097/PEP.0000000000000285.

25. Behrman AL, Trimble SA, Argetsinger LC, et al. Interrater reliability of the pediatric neuromuscular recovery scale for spinal cord injury. Top Spinal Cord Inj Rehabil. 2019. https://doi.org/10.1310/sci2502121.

26. Hunter L, Molitor F, Chafetz RS, et al. Development and pilot test of the Shriners pediatric instrument for neuromuscular scoliosis (SPNS): a quality of life

questionnaire for children with spinal cord injuries. J Spinal Cord Med. 2007. https://doi.org/10.1080/1079 0268.2007.11754594.

27. Dent K, Grampurohit N, Thielen CC, et al. Evaluation of the capabilities of upper extremity test (CUE-T) in children with tetraplegia. Top Spinal Cord Inj Rehabil. 2018. https://doi.org/10.1310/sci2403-239.

28. de Paula B, Friesen B, Chapman B, et al. Initial development and face validation of the Moorong Self-Efficacy Scale for adolescents (MSES-A). Int J Child Adolesc Health. 2017;10(1):43–7.

29. Mulcahey MJ, Gaughan JP, Chafetz RS, Vogel LC, Samdani AF, Betz RR. Interrater reliability of the international standards for neurological classification of spinal cord injury in youths with chronic spinal cord injury. Arch Phys Med Rehabil. 2011. https:// doi.org/10.1016/j.apmr.2011.03.003.

30. Hwang M, Zebracki K, Vogel LC, Mulcahey MJ, Varni JW. Development of the Pediatric quality of life Inventory™ spinal cord injury (PedsQL™ SCI) module: qualitative methods. Spinal Cord. 2020. https:// doi.org/10.1038/s41393-020-0450-6.

31. Slavin MD, Mulcahey MJ, Calhoun Thielen C, et al. Measuring activity limitation outcomes in youth with spinal cord injury. Spinal Cord. 2016. https://doi.org/10.1038/sc.2015.194.

32. Argetsinger LC, Trimble SA, Roberts MT, Thompson JE, Ugiliweneza B, Behrman AL. Sensitivity to change and responsiveness of the segmental assessment of trunk control (SATCo) in children with spinal cord injury. Dev Neurorehabil. 2019. https://doi.org/1 0.1080/17518423.2018.1475429.

33. Wong S, Graham A, Hirani SP, Grimble G, Forbes A. Validation of the screening tool for the assessment of malnutrition in paediatrics (STAMP) in patients with spinal cord injuries (SCIs). Spinal Cord. 2013. https://doi.org/10.1038/sc.2012.166.

34. Mulcahey MJ, Smith BT, Betz RR. Psychometric rigor of the grasp and release test for measuring functional limitation of persons with tetraplegia: a preliminary analysis. J Spinal Cord Med. 2004. https://doi.org/10.1080/10790268.2004.11753729.

Measuring Caregiver in Spinal Cord Injury

Marina D'Angelo, Giulia Grieco, Francescaroberta Panuccio, and Anna Berardi

1   Introduction

A caregiver is a person who provides support and assistance, formal or informal, through various means and activities for people with disabilities and long-term conditions, or elders. Caregivers provide different types of support including emotional, physical, financial, and hands-on help with different daily activities [1]. Despite a lack of any formal or informal training, the caregiver becomes responsible for providing professional support such as giving medications, guiding rehabilitation, or attending to medical emergencies. Typically, people responsible for caring and supporting individuals with spinal cord injury (SCI) are close family members or other relative [2].

Thus, caregiving is intricately tied to the well-being of the individual with SCI, which can lead to depression, high levels of stress, and diminished quality of life due to high levels of physical, emotional, and social burdens on many caregivers. Reversely, the behavior of a person who is receiving care is a factor that can increase the amount of stress and strain in the caregiver [3].

However, there is limited evidence about the quality of life and its effective factors on caregivers for patients with SCI, which seems to result from lack of an appropriate assessment tool. It is crucial to identify risks for burnout and other factors such as burden and depression via a valid assessment tool to prevent them.

Caregiver burden is the emotional, physical, and financial demands, in addition to other responsibilities, that are placed on family members, friends, or others outside the health care system [1].

This chapter aims to describe and evaluate assessment tools on quality of life for people with SCI through a systematic review.

2   Materials and Methods

This study was conducted by a research group composed of medical doctors and health professionals from the "Sapienza" University of Rome and the "Rehabilitation & Outcome Measure Assessment" (R.O.M.A.) association. The R.O.M.A. association in the last few years has dealt with several studies and validated several outcome measures in Italy for the spinal cord injury population [4–17]. This chapter describes all assessment tools regarding caregiving resulting from a systematic review conducted on PubMed, Scopus, and web of science. For specific details on methodology, see chapter

M. D'Angelo · G. Grieco · F. Panuccio
R.O.M.A. Rehabilitation Outcome Measures Assessment, Non-Profit Organization, Rome, Italy

A. Berardi (✉)
Department of Human Neurosciences, Sapienza University of Rome, Rome, Italy
e-mail: anna.berardi@uniroma1.it

"Methodological Approach to Identifying Outcome Measures in Spinal Cord Injury." Eligibility criteria for considering studies for this chapter were validation studies and cross-cultural adaptation studies, studies about the caregiver, studies about tests, questionnaires, and self-reported and performance-based outcome measures, studies with a population of people of SCI and population ≥18 years old. Study selection: the selection of studies was conducted in accordance with the 27-item PRISM Statement for Reporting Systematic Reviews [18]. For the data collection, the authors followed the recommendations from the COnsensus-based Standards for the selection of health Measurement Instruments (COSMIN) initiative [19]. Study quality and risk of bias were assessed using COSMIN checklist [20, 21].

3   Results

For this chapter, four papers were considered. The authors found four assessment tools that evaluate the caregiving area for persons with SCI. In Fig. 1, a flow chart of included studies is reported. The assessment tools are described subsequently.

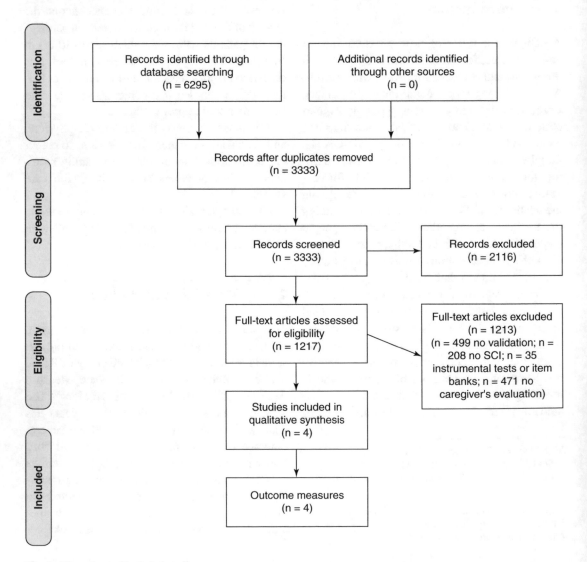

Fig. 1 Flow chart of included studies

3.1 Caregiver Burden Scale (CBS)

CBS is a modified scale of the original scale developed by Oremark, used to assess the caregivers of chronic patients. It was translated into Persian [1]. The original version included 20 items; however, two more items were added using exploratory factor analysis of 150 caregivers. The scale is a multidimensional scale assessing the subjective impact of the burden of taking care of people with chronic diseases. It includes 22 items and is divided into five domains: general strain (8 items), isolation (3 items), disappointment (5 items), emotional involvement (3 items), and environment (3 items). Each item is rated on a scale of 1–4 (1¼ not at all, 2¼ seldom, 3¼ sometimes, and 4¼ often), with a higher value representing greater perceived burden. The individual score is either calculated separately to determine the domain value or jointly (the total value of the 22 items), which can be reported as a raw total or mean score of items. The overall score is obtained by calculating the arithmetic mean of 22 items. The score for each domain is obtained through the arithmetic average of the value of each item comprising that domain. Table 1 summarizes the papers' authors and languages and Table 2 shows the quality of the studies.

3.2 Zarit Caregiver Burden Interview Short Form (ZBI)

Zarit et al. validated the 22-item version of the ZBI in 1985. It is the instrument most consistently used in dementia caregiving research. This version evolved from the original 29-item version published in 1980. Hébert and colleagues proposed a shorter version based on 12 items. It was validated in Persian in 2015 [3]. The short version of the ZBI has consisted of 12 items in two domains, personal strain, and role strain. Each question is scored on a five-point Likert-type scale from 0 to 4 (never to almost always). A high score represents a higher feeling of burden. Range of summed score is 0–48. Table 1 summarizes the papers' authors and languages and Table 2 shows the quality of the studies.

Table 1 Characteristics of the studies validating caregiver scale, test, or questionnaire

Scale, test, or questionnaire	Authors	Language	n	Age mean (SD, range) year	Gender % Female
CBS	Farajzadeh et al. [1]	Persian	110	37.61 (12.10)	50 (45.5)
CBI	Conti et al. [23]	Italian	176	56.2 (14.6)	146 (83)
ZBI	Rajabi-Mashhadi et al. [3]	Persian	72	44.7 (6.5, 31–69)	72 (100)
FNQ	Meade et al. [22]	English		36 (19–81)	

n number of participants of the study, n.a. not available

Table 2 Evaluation of quality and risk of bias

Authors	Item of COSMIN checklist									
	1	2	3	4	5	6	7	8	9	10
Farajzadeh et al. [1]	?	+	+	+	−	+	−	+	+	−
Conti et al. [23]	?	+	+	+	+	−	−	+	+	−
Rajabi-Mashhadi et al. [3]	-	+	+	+	−	+	−	+	+	−
Meade et al. [22]	?	+	−	−	−	−	−	−	−	−

Item 1 PROM development, *Item 2* content validity, *Item 3* structural validity, *Item 4* internal consistency, *Item 5* cross-cultural validity/measurement invariance, *Item 6* reliability, *Item 7* measurement error, *Item 8* criterion validity, *Item 9* hypothesis testing for construct validity, *Item 10* responsiveness, + sufficient, − insufficient, ? indeterminate

3.3 Family Needs Questionnaire (FNQ)

The FNQ is a 40-item self-report questionnaire developed initially for use with families of patients with brain injury to assess their perceived needs. The statements were designed to address diverse psychosocial and educational needs apparent in the acute and post-acute phases after injury. Family members rate the extent to which needs are perceived as important on a 1–4 scale of values ranging from not important, slightly important, important, and very important. Respondents also rate the degree to which each need has been met (not met, partly met, or met) [22]. Table 1 summarizes the papers' authors and languages and Table 2 shows the quality of the studies.

3.4 Caregiver Burden Inventory in Spinal Cord Injuries (CBI-SCI)

This self-reported questionnaire was developed in 1989 and is composed of five subscales assessing the impact of the burden on different domains: time-dependent burden (T/dep-B), evaluating strain caused by restriction of individual personal time; developmental burden (Dev-B), indicating the sense of failing about one's intentions and hopes; physical burden (Phys-B), assessing the bodily strain and physical disorders; social burden (Soc-B), produced by striving to achieve the roles connected to the caregiver's job or family; and, emotional burden (Emot-B), referring to any shaming or humiliation caused by the assisted people. All subscales except Phys-B include 5 items with scores ranging from 0 (strongly disagree) to 4 (strongly agree), and an overall score ranging from 0 to 20 for each dimension. Since Phys-B incorporates 4 items, a correction factor of 1.25 was applied to allow comparisons with the other subscales. Thus, the total CBI score was assessed starting from a minimum of 0, showing no burden, to a maximum of 100, indicating the highest achievable burden level. It was validated in the Italian

language for the SCI population [23]. Table 1 summarizes the papers' authors and languages and Table 2 shows the quality of the studies.

4 Conclusions

This chapter reports all assessment tools described in the literature to evaluate caregiving for people with SCI. The four resulted scales evaluate caregiver burden and family needs. These are the Caregiver Burden Scale (CBS), the Caregiver Burden Index (CBI), the Zarit Caregiver Burden Interview Short Form (ZBI), and the Family Needs Questionnaire (FNQ). Specifically, CBS assesses the subjective impact of the burden of taking care of people with chronic diseases. The ZBI assesses the tension perceived by the caregiver.

References

1. Farajzadeh A, Akbarfahimi M, Maroufizadeh S, Rostami HR, Kohan AH. Psychometric properties of Persian version of the caregiver burden scale in Iranian caregivers of patients with spinal cord injury. Disabil Rehabil. 2018. https://doi.org/10.1080/09638288.2016.1258738.
2. Gajraj-Singh P. Psychological impact and the burden of caregiving for persons with spinal cord injury (SCI) living in the community in Fiji. Spinal Cord. 2011. https://doi.org/10.1038/sc.2011.15.
3. Rajabi-Mashhadi MT, Mashhadinejad H, Ebrahimzadeh MH, Golhasani-Keshtan F, Ebrahimi H, Zarei Z. The Zarit caregiver burden Interview short form (ZBI-12) in spouses of veterans with chronic spinal cord injury, validity and reliability of the Persian version. Arch Bone Joint Surg. 2015. https://doi.org/10.22038/abjs.2015.3795.
4. Castelnuovo G, Giusti EM, Manzoni GM, et al. What is the role of the placebo effect for pain relief in neurorehabilitation? Clinical implications from the Italian consensus conference on pain in neurorehabilitation. Front Neurol. 2018. https://doi.org/10.3389/fneur.2018.00310
5. Marquez MA, De Santis R, Ammendola V, et al. Cross-cultural adaptation and validation of the "spinal cord injury-falls concern scale" in the Italian population. Spinal Cord. 2018;56(7):712–8. https://doi.org/10.1038/s41393-018-0070-6.
6. Berardi A, De Santis R, Tofani M, et al. The Wheelchair Use Confidence Scale: Italian translation, adaptation, and validation of the short form. Disabil

Rehabil Assist Technol. 2018;13(4):i. https://doi.org/10.1080/17483107.2017.1357053.

7. Anna B, Giovanni G, Marco T, et al. The validity of rasterstereography as a technological tool for the objectification of postural assessment in the clinical and educational fields: pilot study. In: Advances in intelligent systems and computing. 2020. https://doi.org/10.1007/978-3-030-23884-1_8.

8. Panuccio F, Berardi A, Marquez MA, et al. Development of the pregnancy and motherhood evaluation questionnaire (PMEQ) for evaluating and measuring the impact of physical disability on pregnancy and the management of motherhood: a pilot study. Disabil Rehabil. 2020;2020:1–7. https://doi.org/10.1080/09638288.2020.1802520.

9. Amedoro A, Berardi A, Conte A, et al. The effect of aquatic physical therapy on patients with multiple sclerosis: a systematic review and meta-analysis. Mult Scler Relat Disord. 2020. https://doi.org/10.1016/j.msard.2020.102022.

10. Dattoli S, Colucci M, Soave MG, et al. Evaluation of pelvis postural systems in spinal cord injury patients: outcome research. J Spinal Cord Med. 2018;43:185–92.

11. Berardi A, Galeoto G, Guarino D, et al. Construct validity, test-retest reliability, and the ability to detect change of the Canadian occupational performance measure in a spinal cord injury population. Spinal Cord Ser Cases. 2019. https://doi.org/10.1038/s41394-019-0196-6.

12. Ponti A, Berardi A, Galeoto G, Marchegiani L, Spandonaro C, Marquez MA. Quality of life, concern of falling and satisfaction of the sit-ski aid in sit-skiers with spinal cord injury: observational study. Spinal Cord Ser Cases. 2020. https://doi.org/10.1038/s41394-020-0257-x.

13. Panuccio F, Galeoto G, Marquez MA, et al. General sleep disturbance scale (GSDS-IT) in people with spinal cord injury: a psychometric study. Spinal Cord. 2020. https://doi.org/10.1038/s41393-020-0500-0.

14. Monti M, Marquez MA, Berardi A, Tofani M, Valente D, Galeoto G. The multiple sclerosis intimacy and sexuality questionnaire (MSISQ-15): validation of the Italian version for individuals with spinal cord injury. Spinal Cord. 2020. https://doi.org/10.1038/s41393-020-0469-8.

15. Galeoto G, Colucci M, Guarino D, et al. Exploring validity, reliability, and factor analysis of the Quebec user evaluation of satisfaction with assistive Technology in an Italian Population: a cross-sectional study. Occup Ther Heal Care. 2018. https://doi.org/10.1080/07380577.2018.1522682.

16. Colucci M, Tofani M, Trioschi D, Guarino D, Berardi A, Galeoto G. Reliability and validity of the Italian version of Quebec user evaluation of satisfaction with assistive technology 2.0 (QUEST-IT 2.0) with users of mobility assistive device. Disabil Rehabil Assist Technol. 2019. https://doi.org/10.1080/17483107.2019.1668975.

17. Berardi A, Galeoto G, Lucibello L, Panuccio F, Valente D, Tofani M. Athletes with disability' satisfaction with sport wheelchairs: an Italian cross sectional study. Disabil Rehabil Assist Technol. 2020. https://doi.org/10.1080/17483107.2020.1800114.

18. Moher D, Shamseer L, Clarke M, et al. Preferred reporting items for systematic review and meta-analysis protocols (PRISMA-P) 2015 statement. Rev Esp Nutr Human Diet. 2016. https://doi.org/10.1186/2046-4053-4-1.

19. Mokkink LB, Terwee CB, Patrick DL, et al. The COSMIN study reached international consensus on taxonomy, terminology, and definitions of measurement properties for health-related patient-reported outcomes. J Clin Epidemiol. 2010. https://doi.org/10.1016/j.jclinepi.2010.02.006.

20. Terwee CB, Prinsen CAC, Chiarotto A, et al. COSMIN methodology for evaluating the content validity of patient-reported outcome measures: a Delphi study. Qual Life Res. 2018. https://doi.org/10.1007/s11136-018-1829-0.

21. Mokkink LB, de Vet HCW, Prinsen CAC, et al. COSMIN risk of bias checklist for systematic reviews of patient-reported outcome measures. Qual Life Res. 2018. https://doi.org/10.1007/s11136-017-1765-4.

22. Meade MA, Taylor LA, Kreutzer JS, Marwitz JH, Thomas V. A preliminary study of acute family needs after spinal cord injury: analysis and implications. Rehabil Psychol. 2004. https://doi.org/10.1037/0090-5550.49.2.150.

23. Conti A, Clari M, Garrino L, et al. Adaptation and validation of the caregiver burden inventory in spinal cord injuries (CBI-SCI). Spinal Cord. 2019. https://doi.org/10.1038/s41393-018-0179-7.

Nursing and Clinical Evaluation in Spinal Cord Injury

Donatella Valente, Azzurra Massimi, Giulia Grieco,
Francescaroberta Panuccio, Marina D'Angelo,
Julita Sansoni, and Giovanni Galeoto

1 Introduction

Spinal cord injury (SCI) is a complicated condition that can change many aspects of daily life. For this reason, nursing and clinical evaluation are essential in these persons. This evaluation should be a global evaluation that should assess the body structure and function and the impact on routine, social life, sleep, and quality of life. The nurses and clinicians have to know the skin sensitivity, organ function, and general health to take care of the person with SCI correctly and professionally. In relation to this, many aspects have to be considered during a correct nursing and clinical evaluation. For example, individuals with SCI are taught preventive skin care behaviors but often perform them inconsistently, particularly after discharge to the community. Adherence to a skin care regimen requires integrating new habits into one's lifestyle, presenting a challenge to clinicians to promote behavior change [1].

Also, neurogenic bowel dysfunction (NBD) and malnutrition are a common problem in most patients with SCI. Colorectal transit times are usually prolonged, and anorectal sensibility and voluntary control of the external anal sphincter are reduced or lost. Constipation, fecal incontinence, and abdominal pain or discomfort are the symptoms of NBD. Recent research reported that 50% of patients with SCI had moderate to severe NBD symptoms and that NBD is associated with health-related quality of life [2]. Malnutrition is both a cause and a consequence of illness, particularly in vulnerable patient groups such as those with SCI. It leads to poorer clinical outcomes such as infection, extended hospital stay, reduced quality of life, and increased healthcare costs [3].

Also, fatigue, sleep, and pain should be considered during the clinical evaluation because these factors can grow the symptoms. Fatigue is a universal human experience that can negatively affect participation in daily tasks, recreation, and work, and the fatigue may create an additional barrier to community reintegration [4]. Finally, nurses and clinicians have to know the most common tests, questionnaires, or scales that assess the many aspects of SCI people to help and take care of these individuals.

The objective of this study is to describe and evaluate the assessment tools on nursing and clinical evaluation in people with SCI through a systematic review of cross-sectional studies.

D. Valente · G. Galeoto (✉)
Department of Human Neurosciences, Sapienza
University of Rome, Rome, Italy
e-mail: giovanni.galeoto@uniroma1.it

A. Massimi · J. Sansoni
Department of Public Health and Infectious Disease,
Sapienza University of Rome, Rome, Italy

G. Grieco · F. Panuccio · M. D'Angelo
R.O.M.A. Rehabilitation Outcome Measures
Assessment, Non-Profit Organization, Rome, Italy

2   Materials and Methods

This study was conducted by a research group composed of medical doctors and health professionals from the "Sapienza" University of Rome and "Rehabilitation & Outcome Measure Assessment" (R.O.M.A.) association. In the last few years, the R.O.M.A. association has worked with several studies and validations of outcome measures in Italy for the Spinal Cord Injury population [5–18].

This chapter describes all assessment tools regarding nursing and clinical evaluation resulting from a systematic review conducted on PubMed, Scopus, and Web of science. For specific details on methodology, see chapter "Methodological Approach to Identifying Outcome Measures in Spinal Cord Injury." Eligibility criteria for considering studies for this chapter were validation studies and cross-cultural adaptation studies, studies about the nursing and clinic, studies about tests, questionnaires, and self-reported and performance-based outcome measures, studies with a population of people of SCI and population ≥18 years old. Study selection: the selection of studies was conducted in accordance with the 27-item PRISM Statement for Reporting Systematic Reviews [19]. For the data collection, the authors followed the recommendations from the COnsensus-based Standards for the selection of health Measurement Instruments (COSMIN) initiative [20]. Study quality and risk of bias were assessed using COSMIN checklist [21, 22].

3   Results

For this chapter, 59 papers were considered. The authors found 40 assessment tools that evaluate nursing and clinical aspects for persons with SCI. In Fig. 1, a flow chart of included studies is reported.

3.1   Skin Management Needs Assessment Checklist (SMnac)

The Skin Management needs assessment checklist (SMnac) is a self-administered questionnaire listing the physical medicine and rehabilitation (PM&R) objectives of persons with SCI. The questionnaire was validated for people with SCI in English in 2003 [23], and in French in 2011 [24]. SMnac corresponds to the skin management area and aims to evaluate the self-reported prevention measures of persons with SCI and their knowledge regarding SCI-related skin disorders. SMnac is highly relevant because it was designed and focused on assessing a patient's knowledge and self-reported prevention measures in terms of skin lesions. It includes 12 questions divided into three different categories: skin checks, preventing pressure ulcers (PUs), and preventing wounds. The 12th question relates to buying a mirror for skin checks, but it is not computed into the final score. Each item is scored from 0 to 3 (0 = completely dependent, never does to; 3 = completely independent, always does or instructs someone to). The total score is expressed as a percentage. The revised SMnac version was elaborated during translation and transcultural adaptation in the French language. For the revised version, six new items were added focused on detecting the early onset [25]. Table 1 summarizes the papers' authors and languages and Table 2 shows the quality of the studies.

3.2   Spinal Cord Impairment Pressure Ulcer Monitoring Tool (SCI-PUMT)

In 2014, Thomason et al. worked to provide support for the validity and reliability of SCI-PUMT to assess pressure ulcer (PrU) healing in veterans with SCI, in Tampa, FL, USA [26]. SCI-PUMT contains 7 items. The first group of items is named "Geometric Factor" because these items

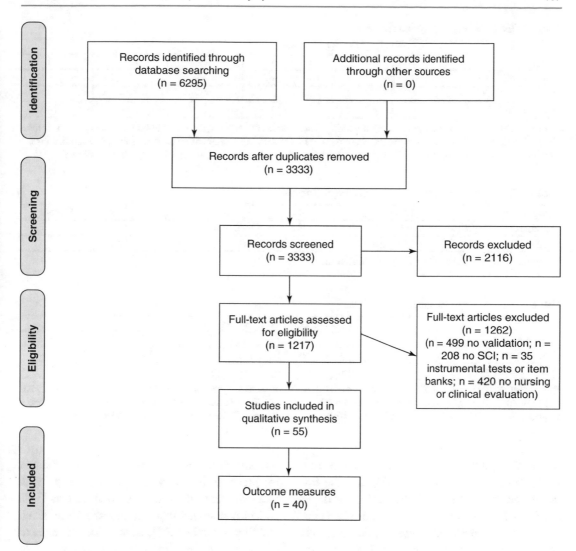

Fig. 1 Flow chart included studies

Table 1 Characteristics of the studies validating SMnac and revised SMnac

Scale, test, or questionnaire	Authors	Language	n	Age mean (SD, range) year	Gender % Female
SMnac	Berry et al. [23]	English	317	41 (17.4)	73 (23)
	Gélis et al. [24]	French	138	45.9 (14.9, 19–82)	35 (25)
Revised SMnac	Gélis et al. [25]	French	132	45.9 (14.9)	35 (25)

n number of participants of the study, *n.a.* not available

characterize the ulcer's shape. These items include surface area (length × width), depth, edges, tunneling, and undermining. The second group is named "Substance Factor" because they reflect ulcer contents (i.e., exudate type and necrotic tissue amount). The SCI-PUMT total score is the sum of the 7-item scores with a maximum score of 26. Higher scores indicate more

Table 2 Evaluation of quality and risk of bias

| Authors | Item of COSMIN checklist | | | | | | | | | |
	1	2	3	4	5	6	7	8	9	10
Berry et al. [23]	?	?	–	+	+	–	–	–	–	+
Gélis et al. [24]	?	+	–	–	+	+	–	–	–	–
Gélis et al. [25]	+	+	–	+	–	–	–	+	+	–

Item 1 PROM development, *Item 2* content validity, *Item 3* structural validity, *Item 4* internal consistency, *Item 5* cross-cultural validity/measurement invariance, *Item 6* reliability, *Item 7* measurement error, *Item 8* criterion validity, *Item 9* hypothesis testing for construct validity, *Item 10* responsiveness, + sufficient, – insufficient, ? indeterminate

Table 3 Characteristics of the studies validating SCI-PMUT

Authors	Language	n	Age mean (SD, range) year	Gender % Female
Thomason et al. [26]	English	66	59.8 (9.8)	1 (2)
Thomason et al. [26]	English	43	n.a.	n.a.

n number of participants of the study, *n.a.* not available

Table 4 Evaluation of quality and risk of bias

| Authors | Item of COSMIN checklist | | | | | | | | | |
	1	2	3	4	5	6	7	8	9	10
Thomason et al. [26]	+	+	+	–	–	+	–	+	+	–
Thomason et al. [26]	+	+	–	–	–	–	–	–	–	–

Item 1 PROM development, *Item 2* content validity, *Item 3* structural validity, *Item 4* internal consistency, *Item 5* cross-cultural validity/measurement invariance, *Item 6* reliability, *Item 7* measurement error, *Item 8* criterion validity, *Item 9* hypothesis testing for construct validity, *Item 10* responsiveness, + sufficient, – insufficient, ? indeterminate

severe PrUs. The SCI-PUMT was designed to be completed weekly for each PrU, and the total score can be used to track the healing or degeneration of the ulcer over time. The SCI-PUMT provides a common language and definitions for team members to describe the PrU (location, bodyside, orientation) and standard patient positioning during the assessment (flexion of the upper leg when turned, dependent side) [27]. Table 3 summarizes the papers' authors and languages and Table 4 shows the quality of the studies.

3.3 Spinal Cord Injury Pressure Ulcer Scale (SCIPUS)

The Salzberg Scale or SCIPUS is a 15-item risk assessment created to specifically evaluate the risk for pressure ulcer development in the SCI population. It was validated in the United States and Canada. The total scores range from 0 (no

risk) to 25. It was developed to measure the risk for pressure ulcer development for people with SCI who are in a rehabilitation center. Each patient is assessed in 15 domains: activity level; mobility; complete SCI; urinary incontinence or constant humidity; autonomous dysreflexia or severe spasticity; age; use of tobacco/smoking; lung disease; heart disease blood glucose levels: >110 mg/dL; kidney disease; impaired cognitive function; if the patient is in a nursing home or hospital; albumin <3.4 or T, protein <6.4; hematocrit <36.0% [28–30]. Table 5 summarizes the papers' authors and languages and Table 6 shows the quality of the studies.

3.4 Neurogenic Bowel Dysfunction (NBD) Score

The NBD score is a symptom-based score that has been developed by Krogh et al. [31] to evaluate the severity of colorectal dysfunction clinically in

Table 5 Characteristics of the studies validating SCI-PMUT

Authors	Language	n	Age mean (SD, range) year	Gender % Female
Delparte et al. [28]	English	759	53.9 (18.5)	247 (33)
Krishnan et al. [29]	English	17	35.5 (14.9)	3 (17.6)
Higgins et al. [30]	French (Canadian)	886	56 (28)	363 (41)

n number of participants of the study, *n.a.* not available

Table 6 Evaluation of quality and risk of bias

Authors	Item of COSMIN checklist									
	1	2	3	4	5	6	7	8	9	10
Delparte et al. [28]	?	?	–	–	+	–	–	+	+	–
Krishnan et al. [29]	?	?	–	–	–	–	–	+	+	–
Higgins et al. [30]	?	+	+	–	+	–	–	–	–	–

Item 1 PROM development, *Item 2* content validity, *Item 3* structural validity, *Item 4* internal consistency, *Item 5* cross-cultural validity/measurement invariance, *Item 6* reliability, *Item 7* measurement error, *Item 8* criterion validity, *Item 9* hypothesis testing for construct validity, *Item 10* responsiveness, + sufficient, – insufficient, ? indeterminate

Table 7 Characteristics of the studies validating NBD

Authors	Language	n	Age mean (SD, range) year	Gender % Female
Krogh et al. [31]	Danish	424	41 (8–88)	124 (29)
Mallek et al. [32]	Arabic	23	40.79 (9.16)	n.a.
Erdem et al. [2]	Turkish	42	39 (16)	8 (19)

n number of participants of the study, *n.a.* not available

patients with SCI. The NBD score is a questionnaire consisting of 10 items associated with impaired QoL caused by bowel symptoms, including frequency of defecation (0–6 points), time used for each defecation (0–7 points), uneasiness or headache or perspiration during defecation (0–2 points), regular use of tablets against constipation (0–2 points), regular use of drops against constipation (0–2 points), digital stimulation or evacuation of the anorectum (0–6 points), frequency of fecal incontinence (0–13 points), medication against fecal incontinence (0–4 points), flatus incontinence (0–2 points), and perianal skin problems (0–3 points). The overall NBD score ranges between 0 and 47 points. A higher score indicates more severe bowel symptoms. The severity level of NBD is divided into four subgroups based on the scores: very minor NBD (0–6); minor NBD; 7–9 moderate NBD; 10–13 and severe NBD (14 and more). The NBD score has been added to the International SCI Bowel Function Basic Data Set (Version 2.0) a simple, standardized tool developed for collecting and

reporting a minimal amount of information on bowel function in daily practice and research. The NBD score was translated in 2017 in Turkish [2], and in 2016 in Arabic [32]. Table 7 summarizes the papers' authors and languages and Table 8 shows the quality of the studies.

3.5 Spinal Cord Injury Secondary Conditions Scale (SCI-SCS)

It was first published in 2007 and adapted the generic Seekins Secondary Condition Questionnaire for people with injury-related disabilities. SCI-SCS is validated in the United States and Australia. It is a 16-item questionnaire that covers common health conditions related to SCI. Some of the items focus on the skin, musculoskeletal system, pain, bowel function, bladder function, and the cardiovascular system. Patients rate each item on a 0–3 scale, where a score of 0 indicates that the condition has not been experienced or has not been a significant problem in the

Table 8 Evaluation of quality and risk of bias

Authors	Item of COSMIN checklist									
	1	2	3	4	5	6	7	8	9	10
Krogh et al. [31]	+	+	−	−	+	−	−	+	+	−
Mallek et al. [32]	?	+	−	+	−	−	−	−	−	−
Erdem et al. [2]	?	+	−	+	+	+	+	+	+	−

Item 1 PROM development, *Item 2* content validity, *Item 3* structural validity, *Item 4* internal consistency, *Item 5* cross-cultural validity/measurement invariance, *Item 6* reliability, *Item 7* measurement error, *Item 8* criterion validity, *Item 9* hypothesis testing for construct validity, *Item 10* responsiveness, + sufficient, − insufficient, ? indeterminate

Table 9 Characteristics of the studies validating SCI-SCS

Authors	Language	n	Age mean (SD, range) year	Gender % Female
Kalpakjian et al. [33]	English	65	43.8 (13.4)	19 (29.2)
Arora et al. [34]	English	40	n.a.	8 (20)
Conti et al. [35]	Italian	156	50.17 (14.44)	30 (19.2)

n number of participants of the study, *n.a.* not available

Table 10 Evaluation of quality and risk of bias

Authors	Item of COSMIN checklist									
	1	2	3	4	5	6	7	8	9	10
Kalpakjian et al. [33]	+	+	−	+	+	+	−	+	+	−
Arora et al. [34]	?	+	−	−	−	−	+	−	−	−
Conti et al. [35]	?	+	+	+	−	+	−	+	+	−

Item 1 PROM development, *Item 2* content validity, *Item 3* structural validity, *Item 4* internal consistency, *Item 5* cross-cultural validity/measurement invariance, *Item 6* reliability, *Item 7* measurement error, *Item 8* criterion validity, *Item 9* hypothesis testing for construct validity, *Item 10* responsiveness, + sufficient, − insufficient, ? indeterminate

last 3 months. A score of 3 indicates that the condition is chronic and/ or a serious problem. A total score is derived by adding the scores for each item to a total possible score of 48. A higher score indicates more severe secondary conditions compared with a lower score [33, 34]. It was validated in the Italian language in 2020 [35]. Table 9 summarizes the papers' authors and languages and Table 10 shows the quality of the studies.

3.6 Brief Pain Inventory (BPI)

The Brief Pain Inventory (BPI) is a well-validated instrument for pain assessment. It measures both pain intensity and pain interference with different domains of life. Its simplicity enables patients to complete it in a short time. Cleeland et al. initially developed it in English to assess cancer pain. It was subsequently used to evaluate different types of chronic pain for post-SCI neuro-

pathic pain in English [36, 37] and Persian [38]. The BPI is a multidimensional measurement tool. It contains a figure of the body on which patients can mark their painful sites. The BPI asks the patients to rate their pain intensity at its worst, least, and average during the last 24 hours and also at the time of the interview on an 11-point NRS. The "0" corresponds to no pain, and the "10" shows the worst imaginable pain. It also assesses the interference of pain with different personal life domains, including general activity, mood, walking ability, work, relations with other people, sleep, and enjoyment of life. Again, patients answer these questions on an 11-point NRS ("0" corresponds to no interference, and "10" shows complete interference). Additionally, it asks the patients to specify their pain sites on a body diagram, their pain treatments, and subsequent pain relief. Table 11 summarizes the papers' authors and languages and Table 12 shows the quality of the studies.

Table 11 Characteristics of the studies validating BPI

Authors	Language	n	Age mean (SD, range) year	Gender % Female
Raichle et al. [37]	English	127	48.56 (12.99, 21–88)	35 (27.6)
Majedi et al. [38]	Persian	201	n.a.	122 (60.6)
Hand et al. [36]	English	876	50.1 (16.39)	244 (27.9)

n number of participants of the study, *n.a.* not available

Table 12 Evaluation of quality and risk of bias

Authors	Item of COSMIN checklist									
	1	2	3	4	5	6	7	8	9	10
Raichle et al. [37]	?	+	–	+	–	–	–	+	+	–
Majedi et al. [38]	?	+	–	–	+	+	–	+	+	–
Hand et al. [36]	?	+	+	–	–	–	–	–	–	–

Item 1 PROM development, *Item 2* content validity, *Item 3* structural validity, *Item 4* internal consistency, *Item 5* cross-cultural validity/measurement invariance, *Item 6* reliability, *Item 7* measurement error, *Item 8* criterion validity, *Item 9* hypothesis testing for construct validity, *Item 10* responsiveness, + sufficient, – insufficient, ? indeterminate

Table 13 Characteristics of the studies validating MPRCQ and MPRCQ2

Scale, test, or questionnaire	Authors	Language	n	Age mean (SD, range) year	Gender % Female
MPRCQ	Nielson et al. [39]	English	127	n.a.	n.a.
MPRCQ2	Nielson et al. [40]	English	93	45.4 (20–72)	91 (98)

n number of participants of the study, *n.a.* not available

3.7 Multidimensional Pain Readiness to Change Questionnaire (MPRCQ) and Multidimensional Pain Readiness to Change Questionnaire (MPRCQ2)

In 2008, Nielson et al. developed a revised version of the MPRCQ, the MPRCQ2. They worked with fibromyalgia syndrome, arthritis, acquired amputation, and spinal cord injury in Canada and the United States. The Multidimensional Pain Readiness to Change Questionnaire (MPRCQ) [39] was specifically designed to measure the degree of readiness to change a wide range of coping behaviors typically addressed in multidisciplinary chronic pain management programs (e.g., exercise, relaxation techniques, activity pacing). This measure is based on the idea that patients can and do vary in their readiness to adopt each of these different pain management strategies. Several modifications to the original version of the MPRCQ were made to enhance the measure's sensitivity in detecting the degree of readiness to adopt specific pain-coping behaviors, the clarity of the item content, and the reliability and discriminant validity of the individual subscales.

A revised Multidimensional Pain Readiness to Change Questionnaire (MPRCQ2) [40] was developed from an initial item pool of 81 questions, each of which was designed to measure one of the ten readiness to change domains. These included items that assessed readiness beliefs related to Exercise, Task Persistence, Relaxation, Cognitive Control (with Diverting Attention, Coping Self-Statements, Reinterpreting Sensations, Avoid Catastrophizing, and Ignoring Pain subscales), Pacing, Avoid Pain Contingent Rest, Avoid Asking for Assistance, Assertive Communication, Proper Body Mechanics, and Avoid Guarding. Respondents are asked to indicate how ready they are to engage in each activity on a scale from 1 to 7. The MPRCQ2 is divided into two sections, one containing an item describing adaptive coping behaviors and the other maladaptive coping behaviors. Table 13 summarizes the papers' authors and languages and Table 14 shows the quality of the studies.

Table 14 Evaluation of quality and risk of bias

Authors	Item of COSMIN checklist									
	1	2	3	4	5	6	7	8	9	10
Nielson et al. [39]	+	+	+	+	+	−	−	+	+	−
Nielson et al. [40]	+	+	+	−	−	−	−	+	+	−

Item 1 PROM development, *Item 2* content validity, *Item 3* structural validity, *Item 4* internal consistency, *Item 5* cross-cultural validity/measurement Invariance, *Item 6* reliability, *Item 7* measurement error, *Item 8* criterion validity, *Item 9* hypothesis testing for construct validity, *Item 10* responsiveness, + sufficient, − insufficient, *?* indeterminate

Table 15 Characteristics of the studies validating SCIPI

Authors	Language	n	Age mean (SD, range) year	Gender % Female
Bryce et al. [41]	English	36	41.9 (12.6)	10 (27.8)
Franz et al. [42]	German	88	53.9 (16.5, 18–97)	33 (37.5)

n number of participants of the study, *n.a.* not available

Table 16 Evaluation of quality and risk of bias

Authors	Item of COSMIN checklist									
	1	2	3	4	5	6	7	8	9	10
Bryce et al. [41]	+	+	−	−	+	−	−	+	+	−
Franz et al. [42]	−	+	−	−	−	−	−	+	+	−

Item 1 PROM development, *Item 2* content validity, *Item 3* structural validity, *Item 4* internal consistency, *Item 5* cross-cultural validity/measurement invariance, *Item 6* reliability, *Item 7* measurement error, *Item 8* criterion validity, *Item 9* hypothesis testing for construct validity, *Item 10* responsiveness, + sufficient, − insufficient, *?* indeterminate

3.8 SCI Pain Instrument (SCIPI)

SCIPI was developed by Bryce et al. in 2014, and it was validated in 2017 in the United States, Switzerland, Germany, and Malaysia. The SCIPI was designed as a 7-item questionnaire mainly including items commonly associated with Neuropathic pain (NeuP) characteristics in SCI. The SCIPI contains unique items with regard to interview-based or self-reported NeuP questionnaires, such as the presence of pain related to movement (item #5), the incessant character of NeuP (item #6), and pain distribution in body regions with impaired sensory function (item #7) [41]. In 2017, S. Franz et al. validated SCIPI in German, and in the preliminary validation, the SCIPI was reduced from 7 items to 4 items (items #1–3 and #7). These items were found to be the most relevant indicating the presence of NeuP [42]. Table 15 summarizes the papers' authors and languages and Table 16 shows the quality of the studies.

3.9 PainDETECT Questionnaire (PD-Q)

The PD-Q was specifically developed to detect neuropathic pain components in adult patients with low back pain. It was validated for the SCI population by Franz et al. [42] in German and in 2017 in English language [43]. The questionnaire consists of seven questions that address the quality of neuropathic pain symptoms; the patient completes it, and no physical examination is required. Table 17 summarizes the papers' authors and languages and Table 18 shows the quality of the studies.

3.10 International Spinal Cord Injury Pain Basic Data Set (Version 1.1), (Version 2.0) and (ISCIPEDS/ISCIPDS:B)

The ISCIPEDSB/ISCIPDBS (version 1.1) was developed in 2008 by a working group consisting of individuals with published evidence of

Table 17 Characteristics of the studies validating PD-Q

Authors	Language	n	Age mean (SD, range) year	Gender % Female
Franz et al. [42]	German	88	53.9 (16.5, 18–97)	33 (37.5)
Packham et al. [43]	English	97	n.a.	n.a.

n number of participants of the study, *n.a.* not available

Table 18 Evaluation of quality and risk of bias

Authors	Item of COSMIN checklist									
	1	2	3	4	5	6	7	8	9	10
Franz et al. [42]	–	+	–	–	–	–	–	+	+	–
Packham et al. [43]	?	+	+	–	–	–	–	+	+	–

Item 1 PROM development, *Item 2* content validity, *Item 3* structural validity, *Item 4* internal consistency, *Item 5* cross-cultural validity/measurement invariance, *Item 6* reliability, *Item 7* measurement error, *Item 8* criterion validity, *Item 9* hypothesis testing for construct validity, *Item 10* responsiveness, + sufficient, – insufficient, *?* indeterminate

Table 19 Characteristics of the studies validating ISCIBPDS:B, ISCIBPDS:B SR, and ISCIBPDS:B 2.0

Scale, test, or questionnaire	Authors	Language	n	Age mean (SD, range) year	Gender % Female
ISCIBPDS:B	Widerström-Noga et al. [44]	English	n.a.	n.a.	n.a.
	Stampacchia et al. [45]	Italian	66	53.4 (16.0)	13 (19.7)
ISCIBPDS:B SR	Jensen et al. [46]	English	184	54.4 (21–87)	46.9 (25.5)
	Kim et al. [47]	Korean	115	48.4 (14.1)	28 (24.3)
ISCIBPDS:B 2.0	Widerström-Noga et al. [48]	English	n.a.	n.a.	n.a.

n number of participants of the study, *n.a.* not available

expertise in SCI-related pain regarding taxonomy, psychophysics, psychology, epidemiology, and assessment, and one representative of the Executive Committee of the International SCI Standards and Data Sets. The ISCIPDS:B is validated in the United States, Denmark, Australia, and Italy. The items in the ISCIPBDS investigate pain type, average pain intensity and interference, location, frequency, duration, and their impact on physical, social, and emotional functions, and sleep. It provides information on pain intensity, and the pain impact on day-to-day activities, mood, and sleep interference [44, 45]. The ISCIPDS:B evaluates any present, chronic and intermittent pain, and it defines the number of different pain problems an individual perceives that he/she has experienced during the last 7 days. The ISCIPDS:B asks the description of the three worst pain problems, the location(s) of pain, the types of pain, and the average pain intensity in the last week. The self-report version was validated by Jensen et al. in English [46] and Kim HR et al. in Korean [47].

The ISCIPBDS (version 2.0) [48] is validated in the United States and Australia, in 2014. In 2016, E Widerström-Noga et al. developed the ISCIPEDS (version 1.0) [49] in the United States and Australia. Table 19 summarizes the papers' authors and languages and Table 20 shows the quality of the studies.

3.11 Needs Assessment Checklist (NAC)

The NAC consists of nine specific SCI rehabilitation domains, each with key indicators of independence and attainment: ADL (29 indicators); Skin Management (14 indicators); Bladder Management (10 indicators); Bowel Management (7 indicators); Mobility (17 indicators); Wheelchair and Equipment (33 indicators); Community Preparation (24 indicators);

Table 20 Evaluation of quality and risk of bias

Authors	Item of COSMIN checklist									
	1	2	3	4	5	6	7	8	9	10
Widerström-Noga et al. [44]	+	+	−	−	−	−	−	−	−	−
Stampacchia et al. [45]	?	+	−	−	−	+	−	−	−	−
Jensen et al. [46]	?	+	+	+	+	+	−	+	+	−
Kim et al. [47]	?	+	−	−	−	+	−	−	−	−
Widerström-Noga et al. [48]	+	+	−	−	−	−	−	−	−	−

Item 1 PROM development, *Item 2* content validity, *Item 3* structural validity, *Item 4* internal consistency, *Item 5* cross-cultural validity/measurement invariance, *Item 6* reliability, *Item 7* measurement error, *Item 8* criterion validity, *Item 9* hypothesis testing for construct validity, *Item 10* responsiveness, + sufficient, − insufficient, *?* indeterminate

Table 21 Characteristics of the studies validating NAC and PMnac

	Authors	Language	n	Age mean (SD, range) year	Gender % Female
NAC	Berry et al. [50]	English	43	42.19 (14.6)	5 (11.6)
	Kennedy et al. [51]	English	193	n.a.	n.a.
PMnac	Kennedy et al. [52]	English	261	40.79 (17.49, 16–85)	57 (21)

n number of participants of the study, *n.a.* not available

Table 22 Evaluation of quality and risk of bias

Authors	Item of COSMIN checklist									
	1	2	3	4	5	6	7	8	9	10
Berry et al. [50]	?	?	−	+	+	+	−	+	+	−
Kennedy et al. [51]	?	?	−	+	−	−	−	+	+	−
Kennedy et al. [52]	+	+	−	+	+	−	−	−	−	+

Item 1 PROM development, *Item 2* content validity, *Item 3* structural validity, *Item 4* internal consistency, *Item 5* cross-cultural validity/measurement invariance, *Item 6* reliability, *Item 7* measurement error, *Item 8* criterion validity, *Item 9* hypothesis testing for construct validity, *Item 10* Responsiveness, + sufficient, − insufficient, *?* indeterminate

Discharge Coordination (32 indicators); and Psychological Issues (19 indicators). The NAC was developed to incorporate patient perceptions, and each patient rates his/her level of independence for each task/item using an interview, lasting approximately 1 hour. Each item receives a score from 0 to 3 (0 1/4 completely dependent; 1 1/4 mostly dependent, 2 1/4 moderately dependent, or 3 1/4 completely independent or not applicable). Item scores for each subscale are totaled and a "percentage achieved" score is derived, reflecting the patient's level of independence in each rehabilitation area. Thus, for each NAC subscale, total scores range between 0% and 100%, with higher NAC scores indicating greater independence levels. It was validated in the English language [50]. The Perceived Manageability Scale (PMnac) lies within the NAC's psychology domain, alongside a scale assessing mood and questions relating to sexual issues. The PMnac contains 6 items and aims to measure how manageable the individual believes their injury and new situation to be [52]. Table 21 summarizes the papers' authors and languages and Table 22 shows the quality of the studies.

3.12 Barthel Index (BI) and Modified Barthel Index (MBI)

The BI was validated for the SCI population in 2004 in English [53] and 1995 in Dutch [54]. The BI has 10 items. The values assigned to each item are based on the amount of physical assistance required to perform the task, being summed to give a total score ranging from 0 to 100 (0: fully dependent; 100: fully independent). In the original version, each item is scored in three steps. A modified Barthel Index (MBI) with a five-step scoring system, developed by Shah et al., was found to achieve greater sensitivity and improved reliability than the original version. It was validated in the Turkish language for people with SCI [55]. Table 23 summarizes the papers' authors and languages and Table 24 shows the quality of the studies.

3.13 Northwick Park Dependency Score (NPDS)

The NPDS was designed for application in neurological rehabilitation, and its validity was tested in patient groups with severe and complex disabilities arising from brain injury or stroke and SCI. It was validated in Dutch for the SCI

population in 2006 [56]. The NPDS consists of two domains of needs, namely the "Basic care needs" (BCN) and the "Special nursing needs" (SNN). The BCN section reflects information needed to predict care needs and is therefore mainly determined by the number of helpers needed (at the level of supervision or physical help) and the time taken to complete each task. The BCN consists of 16 items. Each item's scale varies between 3 and 5 depending on the number of possibilities (e.g., washing and grooming may require two helpers while drinking requires only one), which summates to a maximum of 65. The SNN section comprises 7 items reflecting the needs for nursing care specific to the therapeutic environment, and each item is associated with a substantial workload. Items are assessed as dichotomous variables with a score of either 0 or 5 with a maximum score of 35.6. The total composite NPDS score ranges between 0 and 100. It was validated in English in 2013 [57]. Table 25

Table 23 Characteristics of the studies validating BI and MBI

Scale, test, or questionnaire	Authors	Language	n	Age mean (SD, range) year	Gender % Female
BI	Post et al. [54]	Dutch	318	(18–65)	
	O'Connor et al. [53]	English	254		
MBI	Küçükdeveci et al. [55]	Turkish	50	31.5	28 (56)

n number of participants of the study, *n.a.* not available

Table 24 Evaluation of quality and risk of bias

Authors	Item of COSMIN checklist									
	1	2	3	4	5	6	7	8	9	10
Post et al. [54]	?	+	-	+	+	n.a.	n.a.	n.a.	n.a.	n.a.
O'Connor et al. [53]	?	+	–	–	+	–	–	–	–	+
Küçükdeveci et al. [55]	?	+	+	–	+	+	–	+	+	–

Item 1 PROM development, *Item 2* content validity, *Item 3* structural validity, *Item 4* internal consistency, *Item 5* cross-cultural validity/measurement invariance, *Item 6* reliability, *Item 7* measurement error, *Item 8* criterion validity, *Item 9* hypothesis testing for construct validity, *Item 10* responsiveness, + sufficient, – insufficient, ? indeterminate

Table 25 Characteristics of the studies validating NPDS

Authors	Language	n	Age mean (SD, range) year	Gender % Female
Plantinga et al. [56]	Dutch	17	n.a.	n.a.
Alexandrescu et al. [57]	English	191	n.a.	n.a.

n number of participants of the study, *n.a.* not available

Table 26 Evaluation of quality and risk of bias

Authors	Item of COSMIN checklist									
	1	2	3	4	5	6	7	8	9	10
Plantinga et al. [56]	?	?	–	–	–	–	–	+	+	–
Alexandrescu et al. [57]	?	+	+	–	+	–	–	+	+	+

Item 1 PROM development, *Item 2* content validity, *Item 3* structural validity, *Item 4* internal consistency, *Item 5* cross-cultural validity/measurement invariance, *Item 6* reliability, *Item 7* measurement error, *Item 8* criterion validity, *Item 9* hypothesis testing for construct validity, *Item 10* responsiveness, + sufficient, – insufficient, ? indeterminate

Table 27 Characteristics of the studies validating MPI

Authors	Language	n	Age mean (SD, range) year	Gender % Female
Soler et al. [58]	Spanish	126	49 (13.8)	48 (38.1)
Widerström-Noga et al. [59]	English	161	43.5 (13.4)	23 (14)

n number of participants of the study, *n.a.* not available

Table 28 Evaluation of quality and risk of bias

Authors	Item of COSMIN checklist									
	1	2	3	4	5	6	7	8	9	10
Soler et al. [58]	?	?	+	+	–	–	–	+	+	–
Widerström-Noga et al. [59]	?	?	+	+	+	+	–	+	+	–

Item 1 PROM development, *Item 2* content validity, Item 3 structural validity, *Item 4* internal consistency, *Item 5* cross-cultural validity/measurement invariance, *Item 6* reliability, *Item 7* measurement error, *Item 8* criterion validity, *Item 9* hypothesis testing for construct validity, *Item 10* responsiveness, + sufficient, – insufficient, ? indeterminate

summarizes the papers' authors and languages and Table 26 shows the quality of the studies.

3.14 Multidimensional Pain Inventory (MPI)

The MPI was validated in Spain [58] and the United States [59]. It is a 60-item questionnaire based on the cognitive-behavioral perspective on chronic pain answered on a 7-point Likert-type scale. It comprises Section 1 (pain impact), Section 2 (responses by significant others), and Section 3 (common activities) with subscales assessing pain severity, pain interference, affective distress, control over life, support from significant others, responses by significant others (negative, distracting, and solicitous responses) and the performance of common, general activities (Table 1). The MPI-SCI2 is a modified version of the MPI developed to be used in persons with SCI, where Section 3 asks about pain-specific inter-

ference. Table 27 summarizes the papers' authors and languages and Table 28 shows the quality of the studies.

3.15 Modified Fatigue Impact Scale Spinal Cord Injury (MFIS-SCI)

In 2012, B. Imam et al. validated a telephone-administered version of the MFIS among individuals with a traumatic SCI at 6 months post-discharge from rehabilitation [60]. MFIS is a multidimensional scale that captures information regarding the fatigue's impact on an individual's life. The MFIS-SCI aims to capture the physical, cognitive, and psychosocial impact of fatigue on daily function. The MFIS-SCI is a 21-item questionnaire consisting of Cognitive subscale (11 items); Physical subscale (7 items), and Psychosocial subscale (3 items). The three scores create a total MFIS-SCI score. Table 29 summarizes the papers' authors and languages and Table 30 shows the quality of the studies.

Table 29 Characteristics of the studies of scale, test, or questionnaire with less than two validations

Scale, test, or questionnaire	Authors	Language	n	Age mean (SD, range) year	Gender % Female
MFIS-SCI	Imam et al. [60]	English	42	48 (19)	10 (23.8)
FSS	Hubert et al. [4]	English	48	40.4 (12.6)	17 (35)
FI	Palimaru et al. [61]	English	464	45 (12)	242 (52)
Spinal cord injury (SCI) sacral sparing self-report questionnaire	Liu et al. [62]	Chinese	102	46	19 (19)
SCBS	King et al. [1]	English	406	n.a.	106 (26)
International spinal cord injury bowel function basic and extended data sets	Juul et al. [63]	English Italian Danish	73	20–81	17 (23)
SNST	Wong et al. [3]	English	150	n.a.	46 (30.7)
NRS	Jensen et al. [64]	English	10	46.1 (12.6, 22–66)	3 (30)
GCP disability scale	Raichle et al. [37]	English	127	48.56 (12.99, 21–88)	35 (27.6)
PMQ	Hand et al. [65]	English	971	50.5 (16.37)	209 (28.1)
ISCIPEDS (version 1.0)	Widerström-Noga et al. [48]	English	n.a.	n.a.	n.a.
ISCIP	Bryce et al. [41]	English	n.a.	n.a.	n.a.
PMEQ	Panuccio et al. [9]	Italian	5	n.a.	n.a.
PPRQ	Lindberg et al. [66]	German	268	(18–80)	40 (28.4)
SCAT	Boss et al. [67]	French (Canadian)	n.a.	n.a.	n.a.
NPCS	Siegert et al. [68]	English	38	n.a.	n.a.
PCAT	Turner-Stokes et al. [69]	English	486	n.a.	n.a.
NPSI	Wong et al. [70]	English	72	n.a.	13 (18)
PrU	Liu et al. [71]	English	48	n.a.	23 (48)
SCIPROBE	Burns et al. [72]	English	138	n.a.	38 (53)

n number of participants of the study, *n.a.* not available

3.16 Fatigue Severity Scale (FSS)

In 2007, Anton et al. evaluated the psychometric properties of the FSS in persons with SCI in Canada [4]. The Fatigue Severity Scale (FSS) is a measure originally developed for use in multiple sclerosis (MS). It has been extensively validated in other settings and might be the most widely used measure of fatigue in neurologic disorders. The FSS is easy to use both in clinical practice and research settings. It was designed to measure fatigue and fatigue effects on function, which makes its use in rehabilitation settings particularly appealing. The FSS is a 9-item measure of the severity of fatigue. It requires the participant to choose the degree of agreement on a 7-point ordinal scale ranging from 1 (strongly disagree) to 7 (strongly agree). Scores are calculated by

deriving an arithmetic mean. Table 29 summarizes the papers' authors and languages and Table 30 shows the quality of the studies.

3.17 Fatigability Index (FI)

The FI was validated for people with SCI in the United States [61]. The Index highlights the causes of fatigue and areas requiring immediate intervention. The Index has 82 items separating physical and mental fatigue, with four areas of fatigability: (1) health problems, (2) problems in the home environment, (3) activities in the home, and (4) activities away from home (which may be more demanding, with varying degrees of logistical challenges and physical exertion). The index asks, separately, about the level of physical and

Table 30 Evaluation of quality and risk of bias

Authors	Item of COSMIN Check List									
	1	2	3	4	5	6	7	8	9	10
Imam et al. [60]	?	+	−	+	+	−	−	+	+	−
Hubert et al. [4]	?	+	−	+	−	+	−	+	+	−
Palimaru et al. [61]	+	+	+	−	+	−	−	+	+	−
Liu et al. [62]	?	+	−	−	+	−	−	+	+	−
King et al. [1]	+	+	+	+	+	−	−	+	+	−
Juul et al. [63]	?	+	−	−	+	+	−	−	−	−
Wong et al. [3]	?	+	−	−	+	+	−	+	+	−
Jensen et al. [64]	?	+	−	+	+	+	−	−	−	+
Raichle et al. [37]	?	+	−	+	−	−	−	+	+	−
Hand et al. [65]	?	+	+	−	−	+	−	−	−	−
Widerström-Noga et al. [48]	+	+	−	−	−	−	−	−	−	−
Bryce et al. [41]	+	+	−	−	−	−	−	−	−	−
Panuccio et al. [9]	+	+	−	+	−	−	−	−	−	−
Lindberg et al. [66]	+	+	−	+	+	−	−	+	+	−
Boss et al. [67]	+	+	−	−	−	−	−	−	−	−
Siegert et al. [68]	?	+	+	−	+	+	−	−	−	−
Turner-Stokes et al. [69]	?	+	+	−	+	−	−	+	+	−
Wong et al. [70]	?	?	−	−	+	+	−	+	+	−
Liu et al. [71]	+	+	+	+	−	+	−	+	+	−
Burns et al. [72]	+	+	−	−	+	−	−	−	−	−

Item 1 PROM development, *Item 2* content validity, *Item 3* structural validity, *Item 4* internal consistency, *Item 5* cross-cultural validity/measurement invariance, *Item 6* reliability, *Item 7* measurement error, *Item 8* criterion validity, *Item 9* hypothesis testing for construct validity, *Item 10* responsiveness, + sufficient, − insufficient, ? indeterminate

mental fatigue associated with 41 activities, using the following response scale: 0 (no fatigue), 1 (mild fatigue), 2 (moderate fatigue), and 3 (extreme fatigue). Table 29 summarizes the papers' authors and languages of the papers and Table 30 shows the quality of the studies.

3.18 Spinal Cord Injury (SCI) Sacral Sparing Self-Report Questionnaire

In 2017, N. Liu et al. developed a self-administered tool for assessing sacral sparing after spinal cord injury (SCI) and testing its validity in individuals with SCI in Beijing, China [62]. A SCI sacral sparing self-report questionnaire was developed based on events that most patients experience during their regular bowel routine. The questionnaire evaluates S4-5 sensory and motor function. The questions regard the sensation of light touch (LT), pinprick (PP), deep anal pressure (DAP), and voluntary anal contraction (VAC). Five questions comprise the questionnaire: Q1 (perceiving the tissue) and Q2 (identifying the water temperature as warm or cold) designed for the evaluation of sensation at S4-5 dermatome, Q3 (perceiving the inserted finger) and Q4 (perceiving the inserted enema tube) for testing of the DAP, and Q5 (holding the enema for more than 1 minute) for evaluation of the VAC. Three options are offered for each question: Yes, No, and Not Applicable (NA), and only one of them could be chosen. Table 29 summarizes the papers' authors and languages and Table 30 shows the quality of the studies.

3.19 Skin Care Belief Scales (SCBS)

In 2012, R.B. King et al. worked to develop and validate a measure of skincare beliefs and describe the skincare behaviors of persons with SCI, in Chicago, IL, USA [1]. SCBS has 146 items. The items include generic belief concepts (severity, susceptibility, and self-efficacy) and behavior-specific items for the barriers and benefits. Self-efficacy items include the concept that caregivers may be responsible for some care behaviors. All items use a Likert-type, 5-point response scale (strongly disagree, disagree, neutral, agree, and strongly agree). Higher values indicate greater agreement with the belief. The health belief concepts are defined below: (1) Susceptibility reflects the risk of developing a pressure ulcer when care is not performed. (2) Severity includes beliefs about the physical, social, and psychological consequences of not preventing a pressure ulcer. (3) Benefit is the belief that skincare will prevent pressure ulcers. (4) Barriers include perceptions of the cost or negative aspects of completing skincare. (5) Self-efficacy is the belief that the individual or a caregiver has the ability to perform preventive activities. Table 29 summarizes the papers' authors and languages and Table 30 shows the quality of the studies.

3.20 International Spinal Cord Injury Bowel Function Basic and Extended Data Sets

The International SCI Bowel Function Data Sets, developed by a working group of experts appointed by the American Spinal Injury Association and International Spinal Cord Society (ISCoS), was published in 2009. The International SCI Bowel Function Basic Data Set consists of 12 items and the International SCI Bowel Function Extended Data Set of 26 items. The combined data sets contain information for computation of the Cleveland Constipation Score, Wexner Fecal Incontinence Score, and NBD Score (uneasiness, headache, or perspiration during defecation). Detailed guidelines have been developed to ensure a common interpretation of the data sets, but their reliability remains to be evaluated. The data sets are intended for international use and,

accordingly, reliability should be tested in an international setting. For this reason, in 2011, three European spinal cord injury centers in Bologna, Italy; Buckinghamshire, UK; Viborg and Aarhus, Denmark worked to assess the inter-rater reliability of the International Spinal Cord Injury Bowel Function Basic and Extended Data Sets and to translate the original English data sets in Italian and Danish [63]. Table 29 summarizes the papers' authors and languages and Table 30 shows the quality of the studies.

3.21 Spinal Nutrition Screening Tool (SNST)

A disease-specific nutrition screening tool (NST), the spinal nutrition screening tool (SNST), was developed by dietitians working in SCI centers (SCIC). The SNST assesses eight criteria. The majority are recognized predictors or symptoms of undernutrition: the history of recent weight loss, BMI, age, level of SCI, presence of co-morbidity, skin condition, appetite, and ability to eat. Each step of screening has a score of up to 5, and the total score reflects the patient's degree of risk. A score of 0–10 indicates a low risk of undernutrition, 11–15 indicates moderate risk of undernutrition, and <15 indicates high risk of undernutrition [3]. Table 29 summarizes the papers' authors and languages and Table 30 shows the quality of the studies.

3.22 Numerical Rating Scales (NRS)

Numerical rating scales have a great deal of evidence supporting their reliability and validity as pain intensity measures. They are recommended over other existing pain intensity scales due to their relative strengths and relative lack of weaknesses. Participants are asked to rate four pain intensity domains—current and 24-hour recall of worst, least, and average pain—using 0–10 numerical rating scales, with 0 = "no pain sensation" and 10 = "most intense pain sensation imaginable." It was validated in 2015 in English language [64]. Table 29 summarizes the papers' authors and languages and Table 30 shows the quality of the studies.

3.23 Graded Chronic Pain (GCP) Disability Scale

The 7-item GCP was originally developed for primary care patients with back pain, headache, and temporomandibular disorder pain to assess pain intensity, disability, persistence, and recency of onset. In 2006, Raichle et al. validated GCP in persons with SCI in Washington, USA. They focused on the 3-item Disability scale of the GCP, composed of pain-related interference items. The first item asked participants to rate the extent to which their pain has interfered with daily activities during the prior week on a scale from 0 = "no interference" to 10 = "unable to carry out activities." The remaining two items asked respondents to rate the extent to which pain has changed their ability, within the past week, to take part in (1) recreational, social, and family activities and (2) ability to work (including housework) on a scale from 0 = "no change" to 10 = "extreme change." GCP is reliable and valid measure of pain-related interference in persons with SCI [37]. Table 29 summarizes the papers' authors and languages and Table 30 shows the quality of the studies.

3.24 Pain Medication Questionnaire (PMQ)

In 2017, BN Hand et al. worked to determine how well the PMQ measures the risk of pain medication misuse and its precision in separating individuals with SCI into meaningful classification categories, in Charleston, SC, USA. PMQ is utilized for identifying individuals at risk for pain medication misuse (PMM) in persons with SCI. The PMQ consists of 26 items rated on a five-point Likert-type scale with total scores ranging from 0 to 104. Higher scores indicate higher risk of PMM [65]. Table 29 summarizes

the authors and languages of the papers and Table 30 shows the quality of the studies.

3.25 International Spinal Cord Injury Pain (ISCIP)

In 2012, the ISCIP classification was validated in the United States, Denmark, Israel, Sweden, and Germany. ISCIP classification is designed to be comprehensive and include pain directly related to the SCI, and pain that is common after SCI but not necessarily pathologic and only casually related to the injury itself. ISCIP classification organizes pain types into a three-tiered structure. Tier 1 includes the types of nociceptive, neuropathic, other, and unknown pain. For the neuropathic and nociceptive categories, Tier 2 includes subtypes of pains identified in previous SCI pain classifications. In contract, Tier 3 is used to specify the primary pain source at the organ level and the pathology, if either is known [41]. Table 29 summarizes the papers' authors and languages and Table 30 shows the quality of the studies.

3.26 Pregnancy and Motherhood Evaluation Questionnaire (PMEQ)

The PMEQ is a tool for evaluating and measuring the impact of physical disability on pregnancy and motherhood management. It was developed in Italy in 2020 [9]. The PMEQ is a self-administered questionnaire consisting of an initial section and three subscales. It contains 31 retrospective and self-rated questions using a 5-point Likert-type scale from 1 ("not at all") to 5 ("completely"). Three subscales were concerned with practice management issues, psychological aspects, and the use of services and assistance. The questions on the practical management of pregnancy and maternity (13 items) were used to investigate the participant's degree of independence and the possible need for assistance in carrying out activities of daily living before and during pregnancy, as well as baby care and management, especially in the areas of feeding (breastfeeding, artificial feeding, and/or weaning), hygiene (bathing, diapering, dressing, and undressing), lifting, moving and carrying, and prompt night assistance. Questions on psychological aspects (3 items) dealt with fears or doubts regarding the possibility of carrying a pregnancy and giving birth to and taking care of the baby, according to one's condition or disability. The questions on the use of services and assistance (15 items) highlighted aspects related to the healthcare services received and healthcare professionals' training to investigate the women's level of satisfaction with managing her pregnancy and the postpartum period. Table 29 summarizes the papers' authors and languages and Table 30 shows the quality of the studies.

3.27 Patient Participation in Rehabilitation Questionnaire (PPRQ)

The PPRQ was developed and validated in patients with SCI by Lindberg et al. in 2013 (Switzerland) [66]. The PPRQ consisted of five scales: Respect and integrity (6 items); the staff respects patients' wishes, personality, and personal matters. The staff treats each patient as a unique individual and allows them to be alone when they so desire. Planning and decision-making (4 items); the staff acknowledges and is responsive to the patients' suggestions and opinions. The staff enquires about the patients' expectations, capabilities, and preferences. Information and knowledge (4 items); the staff explains each phase of care and rehabilitation and ensures that they receive adequate information. The information is provided so that the patient can understand and at the "right" time. Motivation and encouragement (5 items); the staff encourages, gives hope, and motivates the patient. Involvement of family (4 items); the staff allows relatives or significant others the opportunity to participate in care and rehabilitation planning if the patient so wishes. Table 29 summarizes the papers' authors and languages and Table 30 shows the quality of the studies.

3.28 Self-Care Assessment Tool (SCAT)

The Self-Care Assessment Tool (SCAT) assesses cognitive and functional skills in eight self-care areas: bathing/grooming, nutritional management, medications, mobility/transfers/safety, skin management, bladder management, bowel management, and dressing. It was validated in French (Canada) [67]. Table 29 summarizes the papers' authors and languages and Table 30 shows the quality of the studies.

3.29 Needs and Provision Complexity Scale (NPCS)

The NPCS is a 15-item measure with five subscales. It has two parts: Part A (NPCS-Needs) is completed by the treating clinician(s) to evaluate each patient's needs for health and social care in any given period. Part B (NPCS-Gets) is subsequently self-completed by the patient (or carer on their behalf) to evaluate those provision level needs over the same period. Total scores range from 0 to 50 and cover "low" to "high" levels of needs [68]. It was validated in 2014 in the English language. Table 29 summarizes the papers' authors and languages and Table 30 shows the quality of the studies.

3.30 Patient Categorization Tool (PCAT)

The PCAT was designed as a structured tool to present a more standardized evaluation of rehabilitation needs for the purpose of comparison. It comprises 18 items, each rated on a score of 1–3. In general, patients requiring rehabilitation (especially following acquired brain injury) separate into physically dependent individuals from those who are already mobile with cognitive/behavioral needs—but some, of course, will have both types of need. It was validated in English (UK) in 2019 [69]. Table 29 summarizes the papers' authors and languages and Table 30 shows the quality of the studies.

3.31 Neuropathic Pain Symptom Inventory (NPSI)

The Neuropathic Pain Symptom Inventory (NPSI) is one of the most widely used tools for characterizing neuropathic pain symptom severity, and it has been validated in over 50 different languages. The NPSI is comprised of five subscales, each representing different dimensions of neuropathic pain: burning spontaneous pain (burning), pressing spontaneous pain (pressing), paroxysmal pain (paroxysmal), evoked pain (evoked), and paresthesia/dysesthesia [70]. Table 29 summarizes the papers' authors and languages and Table 30 shows the quality of the studies.

3.32 Performing Pressure-Relief for Pressure Ulcer (PrU)

The PrU 26-item questionnaire measures a concordance attitude toward performing "pressure-relieving" activities for PrU prevention in individuals with SCI. It was created and validated in English in 2020 [71]. Table 29 summarizes the papers' authors and languages and Table 30 shows the quality of the studies.

3.33 Spinal Cord Injury Patient-Reported Outcome Measure of Bowel Function and Evacuation (SCI-PROBE)

The SCI-PROBE is comprised of 35 items and provides representative coverage of the five ICF domains—(1) activity, (2) body function and structures, (3) environmental factors, (4) participation, and (5) personal factors as well as previously identified challenges related to living with NBD following SCI. The SCI-PROBE items employ a five-point Likert-type scale (0–4), with higher ratings representing higher impact. Two "satisfaction" questions are scored inversely due to the higher ratings representing lower impacts. Five items related to intimate relationships, vocation, and caregiver assistance incorporate a "not

applicable" option; scored 0 (no impact). The SCI-PROBE has a minimum score of 0 and a maximum score of 140. Subscales for each ICF domain were also calculated [72]. Table 29 summarizes the papers' authors and languages and Table 30 shows the quality of the studies.

4 Conclusions

This chapter reports all assessment tools described in the literature to assess nursing and clinical aspects in the care of people with SCI. Among the 40 tools included in this chapter resulted in evaluating fatigue, skin management, bowel dysfunction, and pain. The most common assessment tools are the 15-item risk assessment Spinal Cord Injury Pressure Ulcers Scale (SCIPUS) created specifically to evaluate the risk of pressure ulcer development, the Neurogenic Bowel Dysfunction (NBD) score which is a symptom-based score on the severity of colorectal dysfunction clinically, and the Brief Pain Inventory (BPI) which measures both pain intensity and pain interference with different domains of the life.

References

1. King RB, Champion VL, Chen D, et al. Development of a measure of skin care belief scales for persons with spinal cord injury. Arch Phys Med Rehabil. 2012. https://doi.org/10.1016/j.apmr.2012.03.030.
2. Erdem D, Hava D, Keskinoğlu P, et al. Reliability, validity and sensitivity to change of neurogenic bowel dysfunction score in patients with spinal cord injury. Spinal Cord. 2017. https://doi.org/10.1038/sc.2017.82.
3. Wong S, Derry F, Jamous A, Hirani SP, Grimble G, Forbes A. Validation of the spinal nutrition screening tool (SNST) in patients with spinal cord injuries (SCI): result from a multicentre study. Eur J Clin Nutr. 2012. https://doi.org/10.1038/ejcn.2011.209.
4. Anton HA, Miller WC, Townson AF. Measuring fatigue in persons with spinal cord injury. Arch Phys Med Rehabil. 2008. https://doi.org/10.1016/j.apmr.2007.11.009.
5. Castelnuovo G, Giusti EM, Manzoni GM, et al. What is the role of the placebo effect for pain relief in neurorehabilitation? Clinical implications from the Italian consensus conference on pain in neurorehabilitation.

Front Neurol. 2018. https://doi.org/10.3389/fneur.2018.00310.

6. Marquez MA, De Santis R, Ammendola V, et al. Cross-cultural adaptation and validation of the "spinal cord injury-falls concern scale" in the Italian population. Spinal Cord. 2018;56(7):712–8. https://doi.org/10.1038/s41393-018-0070-6.

7. Berardi A, De Santis R, Tofani M, et al. The Wheelchair Use Confidence Scale: Italian translation, adaptation, and validation of the short form. Disabil Rehabil Assist Technol. 2018;13(4):i. https://doi.org/10.1080/17483107.2017.1357053.

8. Anna B, Giovanni G, Marco T, et al. The validity of rasterstereography as a technological tool for the objectification of postural assessment in the clinical and educational fields: pilot study. In: Advances in intelligent systems and computing. 2020. https://doi.org/10.1007/978-3-030-23884-1_8

9. Panuccio F, Berardi A, Marquez MA, et al. Development of the pregnancy and motherhood evaluation questionnaire (PMEQ) for evaluating and measuring the impact of physical disability on pregnancy and the management of motherhood: a pilot study. Disabil Rehabil. August 2020:1–7. https://doi.org/10.1080/09638288.2020.1802520.

10. Amedoro A, Berardi A, Conte A, et al. The effect of aquatic physical therapy on patients with multiple sclerosis: a systematic review and meta-analysis. In: Mult Scler Relat Disord; 2020. https://doi.org/10.1016/j.msard.2020.102022.

11. Dattoli S, Colucci M, Soave MG, et al. Evaluation of pelvis postural systems in spinal cord injury patients: outcome research. J Spinal Cord Med. 2018;43:185–92.

12. Berardi A, Galeoto G, Guarino D, et al. Construct validity, test-retest reliability, and the ability to detect change of the Canadian occupational performance measure in a spinal cord injury population. Spinal Cord Ser Cases. 2019. https://doi.org/10.1038/s41394-019-0196-6.

13. Ponti A, Berardi A, Galeoto G, Marchegiani L, Spandonaro C, Marquez MA. Quality of life, concern of falling and satisfaction of the sit-ski aid in sit-skiers with spinal cord injury: observational study. Spinal Cord Ser Cases. 2020. https://doi.org/10.1038/s41394-020-0257-x.

14. Panuccio F, Galeoto G, Marquez MA, et al. General sleep disturbance scale (GSDS-IT) in people with spinal cord injury: a psychometric study. Spinal Cord. 2020. https://doi.org/10.1038/s41393-020-0500-0.

15. Monti M, Marquez MA, Berardi A, Tofani M, Valente D, Galeoto G. The multiple sclerosis intimacy and sexuality questionnaire (MSISQ-15): validation of the Italian version for individuals with spinal cord injury. Spinal Cord. 2020. https://doi.org/10.1038/s41393-020-0469-8.

16. Galeoto G, Colucci M, Guarino D, et al. Exploring validity, reliability, and factor analysis of the Quebec user evaluation of satisfaction with assistive technology in an Italian population: a cross-sectional study.

Occup Ther Heal Care. 2018. https://doi.org/10.1080/07380577.2018.1522682.

17. Colucci M, Tofani M, Trioschi D, Guarino D, Berardi A, Galeoto G. Reliability and validity of the Italian version of Quebec user evaluation of satisfaction with assistive technology 2.0 (QUEST-IT 2.0) with users of mobility assistive device. Disabil Rehabil Assist Technol. 2019. https://doi.org/10.1080/17483107.2019.1668975.

18. Berardi A, Galeoto G, Lucibello L, Panuccio F, Valente D, Tofani M. Athletes with disability' satisfaction with sport wheelchairs: an Italian cross sectional study. Disabil Rehabil Assist Technol. 2020. https://doi.org/10.1080/17483107.2020.1800114.

19. Moher D, Shamseer L, Clarke M, et al. Preferred reporting items for systematic review and meta-analysis protocols (PRISMA-P) 2015 statement. Rev Esp Nutr Human Diet. 2016. https://doi.org/10.1186/2046-4053-4-1.

20. Mokkink LB, Terwee CB, Patrick DL, et al. The COSMIN study reached international consensus on taxonomy, terminology, and definitions of measurement properties for health-related patient-reported outcomes. J Clin Epidemiol. 2010. https://doi.org/10.1016/j.jclinepi.2010.02.006.

21. Terwee CB, Prinsen CAC, Chiarotto A, et al. COSMIN methodology for evaluating the content validity of patient-reported outcome measures: a Delphi study. Qual Life Res. 2018. https://doi.org/10.1007/s11136-018-1829-0.

22. Mokkink LB, de Vet HCW, Prinsen CAC, et al. COSMIN risk of bias checklist for systematic reviews of patient-reported outcome measures. Qual Life Res. 2018. https://doi.org/10.1007/s11136-017-1765-4.

23. Berry C, Kennedy P, Hindson LM. Internal consistency and responsiveness of the skin management needs assessment checklist post-spinal cord injury. J Spinal Cord Med. 2004. https://doi.org/10.1080/10790268.2004.11753732.

24. Gélis A, Daures JP, Benaim C, et al. Evaluating self-reported pressure ulcer prevention measures in persons with spinal cord injury using the revised skin management needs assessment checklist: reliability study. Spinal Cord. 2011. https://doi.org/10.1038/sc.2010.177.

25. Gélis A, Dupeyron A, Daures JP, et al. Validity and internal consistency of the French version of the revised skin management needs assessment checklist in people with spinal cord injury. Spinal Cord. 2018. https://doi.org/10.1038/s41393-018-0156-1.

26. Thomason SS, Luther SL, Powell-Cope GM, Harrow JJ, Palacios P. Validity and reliability of a pressure ulcer monitoring tool for persons with spinal cord impairment. J Spinal Cord Med. 2014. https://doi.org/10.1179/2045772313Y.0000000163.

27. Thomason SS, Powell-Cope G, Peterson MJ, et al. A multisite quality improvement project to standardize the assessment of pressure ulcer healing in veterans with spinal cord injuries/disorders. Adv

Ski Wound Care. 2016. https://doi.org/10.1097/01.
ASW.0000482283.85306.8f.

28. Delparte JJ, Scovil CY, Flett HM, Higgins J, Laramée MT, Burns AS. Psychometric properties of the spinal cord injury pressure ulcer scale (SCIPUS) for pressure ulcer risk assessment during inpatient rehabilitation. Arch Phys Med Rehabil. 2015. https://doi.org/10.1016/j.apmr.2015.06.020.

29. Krishnan S, Brick RS, Karg PE, et al. Predictive validity of the spinal cord injury pressure ulcer scale (SCIPUS) in acute care and inpatient rehabilitation in individuals with traumatic spinal cord injury. NeuroRehabilitation. 2016. https://doi.org/10.3233/NRE-161331.

30. Higgins J, Laramée MT, Harrison KR, et al. The spinal cord injury pressure ulcer scale (SCIPUS): an assessment of validity using Rasch analysis. Spinal Cord. 2019. https://doi.org/10.1038/s41393-019-0287-z.

31. Krogh K, Christensen P, Sabroe S, Laurberg S. Neurogenic bowel dysfunction score. Spinal Cord. 2006. https://doi.org/10.1038/sj.sc.3101887.

32. Mallek A, Elleuch MH, Ghroubi S. Neurogenic bowel dysfunction (NBD) translation and linguistic validation to classical Arabic. Prog Urol. 2016. https://doi.org/10.1016/j.purol.2016.06.008.

33. Kalpakjian CZ, Scelza WM, Forchheimer MB, Toussaint LL. Preliminary reliability and validity of a spinal cord injury secondary conditions scale. J Spinal Cord Med. 2007. https://doi.org/10.1080/10790268.2007.11753924.

34. Arora M, Harvey LA, Lavrencic L, et al. A telephone-based version of the spinal cord injury-secondary conditions scale: a reliability and validity study. Spinal Cord. 2016. https://doi.org/10.1038/sc.2015.119.

35. Conti A, Clari M, Arese S, et al. Validation and psychometric evaluation of the Italian version of the spinal cord injury secondary conditions scale. Spinal Cord. 2020. https://doi.org/10.1038/s41393-019-0384-z.

36. Hand BN, Velozo CA, Krause JS. Measuring the interference of pain on daily life in persons with spinal cord injury: a Rasch-validated subset of items from the brief pain inventory interference scale. Aust Occup Ther J. 2018. https://doi.org/10.1111/1440-1630.12493.

37. Raichle KA, Osborne TL, Jensen MP, Cardenas D. The reliability and validity of pain interference measures in persons with spinal cord injury. J Pain. 2006. https://doi.org/10.1016/j.jpain.2005.10.007.

38. Majedi H, Dehghani SS, Soleyman-Jahi S, et al. Validation of the Persian version of the brief pain inventory (BPI-P) in chronic pain patients. J Pain Symptom Manag. 2017. https://doi.org/10.1016/j.jpainsymman.2017.02.017.

39. Nielson WR, Jensen MP, Kerns RD. Initial development and validation of a multidimensional pain readiness to change questionnaire. J Pain. 2003. https://doi.org/10.1054/jpai.2003.436.

40. Nielson WR, Jensen MP, Ehde DM, Kerns RD, Molton IR. Further development of the multidimensional pain readiness to change questionnaire: the

MPRCQ2. J Pain. 2008. https://doi.org/10.1016/j.jpain.2008.01.327.

41. Bryce TN, Richards JS, Bombardier CH, et al. Screening for neuropathic pain after spinal cord injury with the spinal cord injury pain instrument (SCIPI): a preliminary validation study. Spinal Cord. 2014. https://doi.org/10.1038/sc.2014.21.

42. Franz S, Schuld C, Wilder-Smith EP, et al. Spinal cord injury pain instrument and painDETECT questionnaire: convergent construct validity in individuals with spinal cord injury. Eur J Pain (United Kingdom). 2017. https://doi.org/10.1002/ejp.1069.

43. Packham TL, Cappelleri JC, Sadosky A, MacDermid JC, Brunner F. Measurement properties of painDETECT: Rasch analysis of responses from community-dwelling adults with neuropathic pain. BMC Neurol. 2017. https://doi.org/10.1186/s12883-017-0825-2.

44. Widerström-Noga E, Biering-Sørensen F, Bryce T, et al. The international spinal cord injury pain basic data set. Spinal Cord. 2008 https://doi.org/10.1038/sc.2008.64.

45. Stampacchia G, Massone A, Gerini A, Battini E, Mazzoleni S. Reliability of the Italian version of the international spinal cord injury pain basic data set. Spinal Cord. 2019. https://doi.org/10.1038/s41393-018-0171-2.

46. Jensen MP, Widerström-Noga E, Richards JS, Finnerup NB, Biering-Sørensen F, Cardenas DD. Reliability and validity of the international spinal cord injury basic pain data set items as self-report measures. Spinal Cord. 2010. https://doi.org/10.1038/sc.2009.112.

47. Kim HR, Kim HB, Lee BS, Ko HY, Shin HI. Interrater reliability of the Korean version of the international spinal cord injury basic pain data set. Spinal Cord. 2014. https://doi.org/10.1038/sc.2014.105.

48. Widerström-Noga E, Biering-Sørensen F, Bryce TN, et al. The international spinal cord injury pain basic data set (version 2.0). Spinal Cord. 2014. https://doi.org/10.1038/sc.2014.4.

49. Widerström-Noga E, Biering-Sørensen F, Bryce TN, et al. The international spinal cord injury pain extended data set (version 1.0). Spinal Cord. 2016. https://doi.org/10.1038/sc.2016.51.

50. Berry C, Kennedy P. A psychometric analysis of the needs assessment checklist (NAC). Spinal Cord. 2003. https://doi.org/10.1038/sj.sc.3101460.

51. Kennedy P, Smithson EF, Blakey LC. Planning and structuring spinal cord injury rehabilitation: the needs assessment checklist. Top Spinal Cord Inj Rehabil. 2012;18(2):135–37. https://doi.org/10.1310/sci1802-135.

52. Kennedy P, Scott-Wilson U, Sandhu N. The psychometric analysis of a brief and sensitive measure of perceived manageability. Psychol Heal Med. 2009. https://doi.org/10.1080/13548500903012848.

53. O'Connor RJ, Cano SJ, Thompson AJ, Hobart JC. Exploring rating scale responsiveness: does the total score reflect the sum of its parts? Neurology. 2004. https://doi.org/10.1212/01.WNL.0000116136.22922.D6.

54. Post MW, van Asbeck FW, van Dijk AJ, Schrijvers AJ. Dutch interview version of the Barthel index evaluated in patients with spinal cord injuries. Ned Tijdschr Geneeskd. 1995;139:1376–80.

55. Küçükdeveci AA, Yavuzer G, Tennant A, Süldür N, Sonel B, Arasil T. Adaptation of the modified BARTHEL index for use in physical medicine and rehabilitation in Turkey. Scand J Rehab Med. 2000. https://doi.org/10.1080/003655000750045604.

56. Plantinga E, Tiesinga LJ, Van Der Schans CP, Middel B. The criterion-related validity of the Northwick Park dependency score as a generic nursing dependency instrument for different rehabilitation patient groups. Clin Rehabil. 2006. https://doi.org/10.1177/0269215506072187.

57. Alexandrescu R, Siegert RJ, Turner-Stokes L. The Northwick Park therapy dependency assessment scale: a psychometric analysis from a large multicentre neurorehabilitation dataset. Disabil Rehabil. 2015. https://doi.org/10.3109/09638288.2014.998779.

58. Soler MD, Cruz-Almeida Y, Saurí J, Widerström-Noga EG. Psychometric evaluation of the Spanish version of the MPI-SCI. Spinal Cord. 2013. https://doi.org/10.1038/sc.2013.21.

59. Widerström-Noga EG, Cruz-Almeida Y, Martinez-Arizala A, Turk DC. Internal consistency, stability, and validity of the spinal cord injury version of the multidimensional pain inventory. Arch Phys Med Rehabil. 2006. https://doi.org/10.1016/j.apmr.2005.12.036.

60. Imam B, Anton HA, Miller WC. Measurement properties of a telephone version of the modified fatigue impact scale among individuals with a traumatic spinal cord injury. Spinal Cord. 2012. https://doi.org/10.1038/sc.2012.79.

61. Palimaru AI, Cunningham WE, Dillistone M, Vargas-Bustamante A, Liu H, Hays RD. Development and psychometric evaluation of a fatigability index for full-time wheelchair users with spinal cord injury. Arch Phys Med Rehabil. 2018. https://doi.org/10.1016/j.apmr.2018.04.003.

62. Liu N, Xing H, Zhou MW, Biering-Sørensen F. Development and validation of a bowel-routine-based self-report questionnaire for sacral sparing after spinal cord injury. Spinal Cord. 2017. https://doi.org/10.1038/sc.2017.77.

63. Juul T, Bazzocchi G, Coggrave M, et al. Reliability of the international spinal cord injury bowel function basic and extended data sets. Spinal Cord. 2011. https://doi.org/10.1038/sc.2011.23.

64. Jensen MP, Tomé-Pires C, Solé E, et al. Assessment of pain intensity in clinical trials: individual ratings vs composite scores. Pain Med (United States). 2015. https://doi.org/10.1111/pme.12588.

65. Hand BN, Velozo CA, Krause JS. Rasch measurement properties of the pain medication questionnaire in persons with spinal cord injury. Spinal Cord. 2017. https://doi.org/10.1038/sc.2017.89.

66. Lindberg J, Kreuter M, Person LO, Taft C. Patient participation in rehabilitation questionnaire (PPRQ) – development and psychometric evaluation. Spinal Cord. 2013. https://doi.org/10.1038/sc.2013.98.

67. Boss BJ, Barlow D, McFarland SM, Sasser L. A self-care assessment tool (SCAT) for persons with a spinal cord injury: an expanded abstract. Axone. 1996;17:66–7.

68. Siegert RJ, Jackson DM, Turner-Stokes L. The needs and provision complexity scale: a first psychometric analysis using multicentre data. Clin Rehabil. 2014. https://doi.org/10.1177/0269215513513601.

69. Turner-Stokes L, Krägeloh CU, Siegert RJ. The patient categorisation tool: psychometric evaluation of a tool to measure complexity of needs for rehabilitation in a large multicentre dataset from the United Kingdom. Disabil Rehabil. 2019. https://doi.org/10.1080/09638288.2017.1422033.

70. Wong ML, Fleming L, Robayo LE, Widerström-Noga E. Utility of the neuropathic pain symptom inventory in people with spinal cord injury. Spinal Cord. 2020. https://doi.org/10.1038/s41393-019-0338-5.

71. Liu LQ, Chapman S, Deegan R, et al. Development and preliminary validation of a tool measuring concordance and belief about performing pressure-relieving activities for pressure ulcer prevention in spinal cord injury. J Tissue Viability. 2020. https://doi.org/10.1016/j.jtv.2020.05.002.

72. Burns AS, Delparte JJ, Hitzig SL, Shephard J, Craven BC. Development of a novel neurogenic bowel patient reported outcome measure: the spinal cord injury patient reported outcome measure of Bowel Function & Evacuation (SCI-PROBE). Spinal Cord. 2020. https://doi.org/10.1038/s41393-020-0467-x.

Research Perspectives and Considerations in Assessing Spinal Cord Injury Population

Giovanni Galeoto, Maria Auxiliadora Marquez, Marco Tofani, and Anna Berardi

1   Introduction

Measuring people's health status is of crucial importance for health professionals. Health is affected by several factors: the physical environment in which people live; the social environment—the level of social and emotional support people receive from friends and/or family; behavior and lifestyle; family genetics and individual biology [1].

Living with SCI requires strategies to face a wide range of health-related problems. Apart from the paralysis, these problems may concern various body functions, such as the bladder, bowel and sexual function, autonomic function, and pain. Functional problems can lead to limitations in activities and participation restrictions typically related to mobility, self-care activities, difficulties in regaining work, maintaining social relationships, participating in leisure activities, and being active members of the community [2, 3]. The par-

ticipation restrictions are highly dependent on environmental factors, such as mobility equipment, and transportation [4]

Thus, to identify the best treatment methods and routines to help patients return to their previous lives. The first step is to identify the correct assessment tool to robustly assess the efficacy of interventions, both at the level of the clinical treatments and in the context of clinical trials. The classic clinical trial is designed to test the efficacy of a particular intervention compared to another intervention or a control group. Facilitating comparison between groups requires a standard measure of outcome that is relevant and suited to the clinical question, valid for the population studied, and meaningful to the research team [5].

Therefore, it was decided to carry out this systematic review because clinicians and researchers need to know the most reliable, valid, and universally accepted measures currently available for evaluating people with SCI and to allow comparisons between different treatments.

Thus, this study aimed to provide clinicians and researchers information regarding the existing outcome measures to assess people with SCI based on reviewing, analyzing, comparing, and critically appraising the available outcome measures and their distribution in the international literature.

The present chapter describes different outcome measures found with the systematic review.

G. Galeoto · A. Berardi
Department of Human Neurosciences, Sapienza
University of Rome, Rome, Italy

M. Auxiliadora Marquez
Universidad Fernando Pessoa-Canarias,
Las Palmas, Spain

M. Tofani (✉)
Department of Neurorehabilitation and Robotics,
Bambino Gesù Paediatric Hospital,
Rome, Italy
e-mail: marco.tofani@uniroma1.it

Critical appraisal of findings and further perspectives was discussed

2 Materials and Methods

This study was conducted by a research group composed of medical doctors and health professionals from the "Sapienza" University of Rome and "Rehabilitation & Outcome Measure Assessment" (R.O.M.A.) association. In the last few years, the R.O.M.A. association has worked with several studies and validations of outcome measures in Italy for the spinal cord injury population [6–19]. For further details about a methodological approach, please see previous chapters. In particular see Chapter 3: Methodological Approach to Identifying Outcome Measures in Spinal Cord Injury.

3 Results

A total of 6256 records were identified and screened through the initial search strategy. After removing duplicates, 3333 papers were screened. Of these, 476 were included in this systematic review. Results show 298 assessment tools that evaluate people with SCI. All articles were categorized according to different domains.

Nineteen tools resulted for neurological status; most scales evaluate the aspect of spasticity and spasms. The most used tools are Modified Ashworth Scale (MAS) and the Spinal Cord Injury Spasticity Evaluation Tool (SCI-SET).

Forty-six tools resulted for the psychological evaluation; most scales assess the aspect of anxiety and depression, self-efficacy, and coping strategies. The most common assessment tools are the Patient Health Questionnaire-9 (PHQ-9), the Spinal Cord Lesion Related Coping Strategies Questionnaire (SCL-CSQ), and the Spinal Cord Injury—Falls Concern Scale (SCI-FCS).

Twenty-nine tools resulted for quality of life evaluation; most scales evaluate health-related QoL, community integration, and sensorimotor and prehension functions. The most common assessment tools are the World Health Organization Quality Of Life (WHOQOLBREF) and the Community Integration Questionnaire (CIQ), which addresses three central factors of integration: home competency, social integration, and productive activity.

Forty-eight tools resulted for the activity of daily living evaluation; most scales evaluate the aspect of independence, participation, and environmental factors. The most common assessment tools are the Functional Independence Measure (FIM) and the Spinal Cord Independence Measure III (SCIM-III).

Seventeen tools resulted for upper limb evaluation; most scales evaluate the arm–hand skilled performance and sensorimotor and prehension functions. The most common assessment tools are the Van Lieshout Test (VLT) and the Graded Redefined Assessment Of Strength, Sensibility And Prehension (GRASSP).

Twenty resulted for urological evaluation; most scales the aspect Intermittent Self-Catheterization, Neurogenic Bladder, and sexuality. The most common assessment tools are the Qualiveen, the Intermittent Self-Catheterization Questionnaire (ISC-Q), the Neurogenic Bladder Symptom Score (NBSS), and the Multiple Sclerosis Intimacy And Sexuality questionnaire (MSISQ).

Twenty-two tools resulted for assistive devices management evaluation; most scales evaluate the aspect of self-efficacy, mobility, and skill and they are mainly performance tests. The most common assessment tools are the Wheelchair Circuit, the Wheelchair Skills Test (WST), and the Wheelchair use Confidence Scale (WheelCon).

Thirty-eight resulted for walking and balance evaluation; most scales evaluate the aspect of amount of assistance and distance and they are mainly performance tests. The most common assessment tools are the Walking Index for Spinal Cord Injury (WISCI), the 6-minute Walking Test (6MWT), the Neuromuscular Recovery Scale (NRS), and the Berg Balance Scale (BBS).

Fifteen tools resulted for pediatric evaluation; most scales evaluate activities of daily living. The most common assessment tools are the Walking Index for Spinal Cord Injury (WISCI II), the Spinal Cord Independence Measure (SCIM) III Self-Report, and the Pediatric Neuromuscular Recovery Scale (NRS).

Four assessment tools resulted for caregiver evaluation; most scales evaluate caregiver burden and family needs, they are the Caregiver Burden Scale (CBS), the Caregiver Burden Index (CBI), the Zarit Caregiver Burden Interview Short Form (ZBI), and the Family Needs Questionnaire (FNQ).

Forty tools resulted for nursing and clinical evaluation; most scales evaluate fatigue, skin management, bowel dysfunction, and pain. The most common assessment tools are the Spinal Cord Injury Pressure Ulcers Scale (SCIPUS), the Neurogenic Bowel Dysfunction (NBD) score, and the Brief Pain Inventory (BPI).

Authors have described the flavor of the marked heterogeneity in using assessment tools and have deliberately avoided suggestions that one scale is better than another. They have focused on the most commonly used scales.

4 Conclusions

Outcome measures are frequently used to determine if patients have made meaningful changes in their recovery process and may influence care intensity and duration. Researchers use outcome measures during the investigation of the efficacy and effectiveness of a given treatment intervention. Therefore, this study aimed to provide clinicians and researchers with evidence-based recommendations regarding what outcome measures should be used to assess people with spinal cord injury (SCI).

Research in the field of outcome measures for people with SCI has increased dramatically in recent years. Many scientists have developed different systems to collect the available evidence. An example is the Rehab Measures Database (www.sralab.org/rehabilitation-measures), where outcome measures are systematized by pathology and where translation languages and psychomet-

ric properties are reported. Another concrete example is those promoted by Spinal Cord Injury Research Evidence (SCIRE), where there is a specific section for outcome measures addressed to the population with spinal cord injury. In addition, the working group has also written OUTCOME MEASURES TOOLKIT: Implementation Steps, a Guide to Implementing Evidence-Based Outcome Measures into Clinical Practice. The international community is, therefore, working to create systems for the dissemination and monitoring of outcome measures.

This systematic review has highlighted a strong heterogeneity of validated tools among the various national contexts that can be seen. This heterogeneity can be assumed to have a positive meaning if one thinks about the multiple needs of the clinical context, but certainly leads to the need to make the tools more suitable for various cultural contexts. These findings suggest that clinicians have conflicting or incomplete information available to use when making decisions in patient care; furthermore, the lack of consistency and the deficiency of standardization in outcome assessment has hindered comparative research. Further investigation of outcome measures would benefit patients, researchers, and clinicians. Universals validated outcome measures are needed to allow comparisons across practice; therefore, we recommend that future researchers use a standard outcome assessment set.

Building an international consensus in this area will improve the quality of care, rehabilitation, and efficiency of health care systems.

Therefore, the work presented in this volume aims to contribute to the construction of evidence to measure different aspects of people with spinal cord injury. We hope that researchers and academics will find in this volume a valuable tool for comparison and aggression. We also hope that students and health professionals will benefit from the topics covered in this volume, finding and selecting the most appropriate outcome measures for their work. The ultimate goal is inevitably to improve people's health and quality of life with spinal cord injury.

References

1. World Health Organization (WHO). Community health needs assessment. An introductory guide for the family health nurse in Europe. Geneva: WHO; 2001.
2. Gerhart KA, Bergstrom E, Charlifue SW, Menter RR, Whiteneck GG. Long-term spinal cord injury: functional changes over time. Arch Phys Med Rehabil. 1993. https://doi.org/10.1016/0003-9993(93)90057-H.
3. Lidal IB, Huynh TK, Biering-Sørensen F. Return to work following spinal cord injury: a review. Disabil Rehabil. 2007. https://doi.org/10.1080/09638280701320839.
4. Whiteneck G, Meade MA, Dijkers M, Tate DG, Bushnik T, Forchheimer MB. Environmental factors and their role in participation and life satisfaction after spinal cord injury. Arch Phys Med Rehabil. 2004. https://doi.org/10.1016/j.apmr.2004.04.024.
5. Harrison JK, McArthur KS, Quinn TJ. Assessment scales in stroke: Clinimetric and clinical considerations. Clin Interv Aging. 2013. https://doi.org/10.2147/CIA.S32405.
6. Castelnuovo G, Giusti EM, Manzoni GM, et al. What is the role of the placebo effect for pain relief in neurorehabilitation? Clinical implications from the Italian consensus conference on pain in neurorehabilitation. Front Neurol. 2018. https://doi.org/10.3389/fneur.2018.00310.
7. Marquez MA, De Santis R, Ammendola V, et al. Cross-cultural adaptation and validation of the "spinal cord injury-falls concern scale" in the Italian population. Spinal Cord. 2018;56(7):712–8. https://doi.org/10.1038/s41393-018-0070-6.
8. Dattoli S, Colucci M, Soave MG, et al. Evaluation of pelvis postural systems in spinal cord injury patients: outcome research. J Spinal Cord Med. 2018;43:185–92.
9. Berardi A, Galeoto G, Guarino D, et al. Construct validity, test-retest reliability, and the ability to detect change of the Canadian occupational performance measure in a spinal cord injury population. Spinal Cord Ser Cases. 2019. https://doi.org/10.1038/s41394-019-0196-6.
10. Ponti A, Berardi A, Galeoto G, Marchegiani L, Spandonaro C, Marquez MA. Quality of life, concern of falling and satisfaction of the sit-ski aid in sit-skiers with spinal cord injury: observational study. Spinal Cord Ser Cases. 2020. https://doi.org/10.1038/s41394-020-0257-x.
11. Panuccio F, Galeoto G, Marquez MA, et al. General sleep disturbance scale (GSDS-IT) in people with spinal cord injury: a psychometric study. Spinal Cord. 2020. https://doi.org/10.1038/s41393-020-0500-0.
12. Monti M, Marquez MA, Berardi A, Tofani M, Valente D, Galeoto G. The multiple sclerosis intimacy and sexuality questionnaire (MSISQ-15): validation of the Italian version for individuals with spinal cord injury. Spinal Cord. 2020. https://doi.org/10.1038/s41393-020-0469-8.
13. Galeoto G, Colucci M, Guarino D, et al. Exploring validity, reliability, and factor analysis of the Quebec user evaluation of satisfaction with assistive Technology in an Italian Population: a cross-sectional study. Occup Ther Heal Care. 2018. https://doi.org/10.1080/07380577.2018.1522682.
14. Colucci M, Tofani M, Trioschi D, Guarino D, Berardi A, Galeoto G. Reliability and validity of the Italian version of Quebec user evaluation of satisfaction with assistive technology 2.0 (QUEST-IT 2.0) with users of mobility assistive device. Disabil Rehabil Assist Technol. 2019. https://doi.org/10.1080/17483107.2019.1668975.
15. Berardi A, Galeoto G, Lucibello L, Panuccio F, Valente D, Tofani M. Athletes with disability' satisfaction with sport wheelchairs: an Italian cross sectional study. Disabil Rehabil Assist Technol. 2020. https://doi.org/10.1080/17483107.2020.1800114.
16. Berardi A, De Santis R, Tofani M, et al. The Wheelchair Use Confidence Scale: Italian translation, adaptation, and validation of the short form. Disabil Rehabil Assist Technol. 2018;13(4):i. https://doi.org/10.1080/17483107.2017.1357053.
17. Anna B, Giovanni G, Marco T, et al. The validity of rasterstereography as a technological tool for the objectification of postural assessment in the clinical and educational fields: pilot study. In: Advances in intelligent systems and computing; 2020. https://doi.org/10.1007/978-3-030-23884-1_8.
18. Panuccio F, Berardi A, Marquez MA, et al. Development of the pregnancy and motherhood evaluation questionnaire (PMEQ) for evaluating and measuring the impact of physical disability on pregnancy and the management of motherhood: a pilot study. Disabil Rehabil. 2020:1–7. https://doi.org/10.1080/09638288.2020.1802520.
19. Amedoro A, Berardi A, Conte A, et al. The effect of aquatic physical therapy on patients with multiple sclerosis: a systematic review and meta-analysis. Mult Scler Relat Disord. 2020. https://doi.org/10.1016/j.msard.2020.102022.

Printed in the United States
by Baker & Taylor Publisher Services